ANNALS OF THE NEW YORK ACADEMY OF SCIENCES
Volume 951

WEST NILE VIRUS

DETECTION, SURVEILLANCE, AND CONTROL

Edited by Dennis J. White and Dale L. Morse

D1519583

The New York Academy of Sciences
New York, New York
2001

Library of Congress Cataloging-in-Publication Data

West Nile virus : detection, surveillance, and control / editors, Dennis J. White, Dale L. Morse.
    p. cm. — (Annals of the New York Academy of Sciences ; v. 951)
    Includes bibliographical references and indexes.
    ISBN 1-57331-374-2 (cloth : alk. paper) . — ISBN 1-57331-375-0 (pbk. : alk. paper)
    1. West Nile fever—Congresses. 2. West Nile fever—United States—Congresses. I. White, Dennis J. II. Morse, Dale L. III. Series.

Q11 .N5 vol. 951
[RA644.W47]
508 s—dc21
[616.9'25]   2001051398

GYAT/PCP
Printed in the United States of America
ISBN 1-57331-374-2 (cloth)
ISBN 1-57331-375-0 (paper)
ISSN 0077-8923

ANNALS OF THE NEW YORK ACADEMY OF SCIENCES

Volume 951
December 2001

WEST NILE VIRUS

DETECTION, SURVEILLANCE, AND CONTROL

Editors
DENNIS J. WHITE AND DALE L. MORSE

This volume is the result of a conference entitled **International Conference on the West Nile Virus** held on April 5–7, 2001 in White Plains, New York, sponsored by the New York Academy of Sciences and cosponsored by the New York State Department of Health, the New York City Department of Health, and the Centers for Disease Control and Prevention.

CONTENTS

Part VII. Antiviral and Vaccine Interventions

Part VIII. Late Breaker Papers

Part IX. Poster Papers

Financial assistance was received from:

Cosponsors
- NEW YORK STATE DEPARTMENT OF HEALTH
- NEW YORK CITY DEPARTMENT OF HEALTH
- CENTERS FOR DISEASE CONROL AND PREVENTION

Major Funder
- MUSHETT FAMILY FOUNDATION INC.

Supporter
- JOSIAH MACY, JR. FOUNDATION

Contributors
- ACAMBIS INC.
- AMERICAN MOSQUITO CONTROL ASSOCIATION
- ICN PHARMACEUTICALS INC.
- IGOR N. SOUZDALTSEV

Preface

DENNIS J. WHITE

New York State Department of Health, Corning Tower,
Empire State Plaza, Albany, New York 12237

Human infection with West Nile (WN) virus was first discovered in 1937 in a Ugandan woman who survived the infection. In August and September of 1999, a cluster of human encephalitis and fatal infection in birds was detected in the metropolitan area of New York City. This cluster, first thought to be due to St. Louis encephalitis virus, was later identified and confirmed as the first introduction of WN virus in the Western Hemisphere. The introduction of this potentially fatal, mosquito-borne flavivirus into a completely naive vertebrate population resulted in large-scale epidemiologic, entomologic, ecologic, and veterinary investigations and disease control efforts. This volume of the *Annals of the New York Academy of Sciences* includes articles from many of those individuals who were most involved with the ensuing investigations of disease, ecology, natural life cycles, and management of this foreign mosquito-borne flavivirus.

Although conceived only a month after WN virus detection in this hemisphere, this first WN virus international conference was held roughly twenty months after North American investigations on WN virus commenced. Clearly, the contributions of those investigators in parts of the world where human WN virus infection was more common needed to be heard here in the United States. Despite the virus's presence in completely different zoogeographic regions of the world, relationships among the pathogen, its vectors, its pathology, epidemiology, and management observed in Europe and Africa could help explain important and useful similarities and differences here in the Western Hemisphere. Scientists from around the world were invited to discuss their experience with WN and related arboviruses, both from the Old World and from the newly affected New World perspectives.

Serious questions remain. We may never know how this virus arrived on our shores. Despite genetic determination of relationships to Old World "strains" of this virus, the actual mechanism of Western Hemisphere invasion may never be elucidated, whether the introduction was intentional or accidental. The virus may have arrived in an unsuspecting asymptomatic host, via infected mosquitoes, through an imported avian host, or by any variety of permutations of these potential routes of introduction. During the intervening months since the conference was held, as I write these comments, the virus has now been detected in avian hosts west of the Mississippi River and north into Canada. Similarly, the virus appears to have established a strong foothold in the Gulf Coast area, as well as in Florida, Georgia, and some Caribbean islands, yet seems to have virtually bypassed the Middle Atlantic states. Are certain ecologic circumstances or certain mosquito species' vector capacities supporting the establishment of WN virus in certain regions of North America? What will happen as the virus proceeds into the western United States where other aggressive mosquito species exist, especially *Culex tarsalis*? What is the role of other mosquito species, or other blood-feeding arthropods (e.g., blackflies, mites, lice, and ticks) in the natural cycle of this virus in avian hosts? What vertebrates or invertebrates may be acting as reservoir hosts? As science begins to answer these and other epidemiological questions, we will begin to understand the complex role of this virus in the natural environment of our newly affected areas. Is this another emerging infectious disease? Certainly, it seems to meet that definition here in North America. Can this virus, and our collective response to it, serve as a model for other emerging arboviral or other invading arthropod-borne infectious diseases? I believe it can.

This conference and others like it have served the medical, public health, vector control, and general communities well by providing timely and comprehensive information. We are gaining new relevant knowledge continuously. To what extent this virus serves as a model for other infectious disease processes will only be answered through time. However, through the valuable contributions of investigators from around the world, this international event will continue to build upon current knowledge.

There are numerous individuals and institutions without whom this conference could not have taken place. When the initial concept of hosting this conference was presented in October 1999 to the New York State Department of Health and the New York Academy of Sciences, I received immediate and full support from NYSDOH Commissioner Antonia Novello, M.D., M.P.H., Dr.P.H., and Deputy Commissioner Dennis Whalen as well as from Rashid Shaikh, Ph.D., Sheila Kane, and Sherryl Usmani from the Academy. Their collective strong support carried me through this personal undertaking. I am extremely appreciative of the conceptual program development that occurred through coeditor and colleague Dale Morse, M.D., and the other members of the organizing committee, including Roger Nasci, Ph.D., Marci Layton, M.D., Tracey McNamara, D.V.M., Millicent Eidson, D.V.M., Leo Grady, Ph.D., and Barbara Wallace, M.D. In addition to financial contributions from the Centers for Disease Control and Prevention, the New York State Department of Health, and the New York City Department of Health, we are grateful to the Josiah Macy, Jr. Foundation, Acambis, Inc., the American Mosquito Control Association, ICN Pharmaceuticals, Inc., and Igor N. Souzdaltsev for their valuable support. I fully appreciate the role of Commissioner Joshua Lipsman, M.D., and the Westchester County Health Department as well as the staff of the Crowne Plaza Hotel in White Plains for hosting this event. Barbara Goldman, Jennifer Tang, and Steven E. Bohall of the New York Academy of Sciences developed the information provided during this conference for publication. Most importantly, I want to thank members of my Arthropod-Borne Disease Program and my immediate supervisors, who had to put up with my day-to-day program issues while I focused on the development and completion of this conference. I am indebted to all of you. Finally, I want to thank all the conference participants for bringing their valuable knowledge to this conference and sharing it with those of us who need to learn more.

Welcoming Remarks

ANTONIA C. NOVELLO

New York State Commissioner of Health, Department of Health, Albany, New York 12237, USA

Welcome to New York—a place in which 167 languages are represented and 33 percent of the population is not native. New York City has been the epicenter of this epidemic since the West Nile virus was found here in 1999, although now the disease has appeared along the Eastern seaboard and in the District of Columbia. In the last two years, since the West Nile virus first appeared in North America, it has dispersed from the original "hot zone" in Queens through the Middle Atlantic states and is found as far north as New Hampshire and as far south as South Carolina. Last year, scientists at our Division of Epidemiology analyzed reports of more than 17,000 dead crows and nearly 54,000 dead birds from other species. In addition, scientists at New York's Wadsworth Center laboratories tested specimens from more than 3600 dead birds, approximately 1800 asymptomatic birds, and 149 mammals for West Nile virus. By the end of last year, a total of 1263 dead birds representing 55 wild species and 8 domestic or captive species had tested positive for the West Nile virus. The virus was also identified in 364 mosquito pools of more than 9900 pools submitted for testing. Scientists have also been able to confirm the infection in at least two *Culex* species and in six other mosquito species. Scientists at the Wadsworth Center investigated suspect human cases of West Nile virus by testing blood and cerebrospinal fluid from 589 New Yorkers. So the West Nile virus is here to stay and as Yogi Berra said, "The future isn't what it used to be."

One thing we have learned from the West Nile virus is that it can be anywhere, and so we must be prepared for *anything*. This is especially important in the global economy, and we must remember that New York State is a port of entry for the world. Knowledge of this potential threat may help us to prepare a strategy for countering other public health threats that may occur. The health of people in every corner of the world is tied to the health of all of the peoples in any other country of the world. Jeffrey Koplan, director of the CDC, has said "Our national public health infrastructure is the first and in many cases the only... defense because many environmental and health threats know no boundaries. We can afford no weaknesses in our line of defense. Either we are all protected or we are all at risk."

That quote brings us to what I believe is going to be crucial in this meeting: Two years ago, we received the first notice of the virus, and if we had not made sure that the departments of health in both New York City and New York State worked together with all the other agenices, but especially with the CDC and the Department of Agriculture and Markets, we would not have been able to accomplish what we have done so far. We saw at first hand that in union there is strength. Thanks to the coor-

Address for correspondence: Antonia C. Novello, M.D., M.P.H., Dr.P.H., New York State Commissioner of Health, Department of Health, Corning Tower, 14th Floor, Albany, NY 12237. Voice: 518-473-0458; fax: 518-474-5450.

dination and cooperation of these agencies we have tremendous synergy. Because infections know no boundaries, the efforts to control them should know no boundaries as well.

This meeting is being held just 30 miles from where the first case of West Nile virus was detected—a place we were petrified to be near two summers ago. Now we're here to study what we're going to do in the future. We do not know how the virus got here, but we know that it is here to stay. You know the numbers: 62 cases in 1999 and 14 in the year 2000. We have learned that it spreads rapidly and that countermeasures are critical for reducing the risk, although they will not eliminate it. We also know that the risk for humans is not distributed equally and that monitoring dead birds is going to be a critical component of surveillance. The dead crow density, the weekly number of dead crows per square mile, will help us to determine whether there is a low or a high risk of an outbreak of West Nile virus among humans. The comprehensive strategy will be crucial: we have to resist and to prevent. We have to check the human and the wild life, undertake mosquito surveillance, control the vector, and reduce the incidence of disease.

For this we obviously need money. Two and a half million dollars were given to upgrade the Wadsworth Laboratory and 30 million dollars were given last year for expenses incurred in combatting the virus. FEMA provided 3 million dollars, 3.9 million came from the CDC, and the governor of New York State has committed 22 million dollars just for the West Nile virus alone to aid local governments in monitoring risk and responding appropriately.

Above all we will continue to educate the public so that the public will in turn help us to control the mosquito. The work at the Wadsworth Laboratory is concerned with how the virus grows, replicates, and reproduces, why it prefers certain vectors, and why there are differences in the patterns of the virus in the United States and in other countries. We must have strong surveillance, and we must have strong public education. And we must have the funds to be able to accomplish this.

Even more important is having the international scientific community trying to discover how it came about, how we can control it, how we can cooperate in combatting not only the West Nile virus but any other epidemic that might visit us.

This meeting and its record in the *Annals* will address just such questions. I want to leave you with the words of Yehuda Bauer, the great historian of the Holocaust: Remember, he says, that there are three commandments that you have to follow. The first one is thou shalt not be a victim. The second one is that thou shalt not be a perpetrator. And the third one is that thou shalt not be a bystander. So, for the lives of all those people that we care for, I beg of you, when you leave this place, don't let it be said that when you came to New York, you stood as a bystander.

Welcoming Remarks

NEAL L. COHEN

Commissioner, New York City Department of Health, New York, New York 10013, USA

This feels like the kickoff for the new West Nile season, but for many of us in the room, it never ended—the season has been nonstop since September 1999. I'm struck by the fact that outside the room before we came in, I heard voices of many colleagues known only to me by their voices from the weekly conference calls with the CDC. It was around Labor Day of 1999 when we first discovered what we were dealing with, and last season we had no historical data for the Western Hemisphere, certainly for this area, for West Nile virus. There was no easy roadmap to follow for surveillance activity and for control activity. There was little experience in New York City with addressing mosquitoes as other than a nuisance and certainly not as a public health threat. For the last year and a half we've been able to reverse what had been many years of neglect with regard to the potential threat of arboviruses and put into place what is increasingly becoming a state-of-the-art mosquito surveillance and control program in New York City, the surrounding counties, and in the Northeast as well. So we've learned a lot, and we have begun to feel that the investment of time and energy in dealing with the West Nile virus will serve as a public health opportunity for us with regard to public education. We hope that our effort to inform the public on how to reduce their risk of exposures will carry over to other public health priorities, such as influenza vaccine for seniors or people at higher risk. We hope to leverage the lessons learned from the West Nile virus to encourage risk reduction by a more engaged and participatory public in a wider range of public health issues. So I'm still hopeful that our work with West Nile virus will lead to gaining advantages in other important areas as well. We are going into this season feeling that we don't have to put in place a reflexive approach to the appearance of West Nile virus. We now have data that link human risk to the appearance of infected birds and mosquitoes, and we are able to categorize the level of risk to take appropriate control measures. We are putting meaningful emphasis on the notion that prevention is the way to go. Certainly, as public health authorities who are trying to protect the health of the public, we know we are accountable to elected public officials and to our communities. We have always been under scrutiny, but nothing can compare to the recent scrutiny that we have found ourselves under in this past year and a half: the number of requests under the Freedom of Information Act is voluminous, and the feeding frenzy of the media is remarkable. My colleague at the New York City Department of Health, Dr. James Miller, described recently his own personal experience with West Nile virus this way: "A year ago, I didn't know PowerPoint. I didn't have a cell phone. I never testified in court, and I never celebrated the first frost." Dr. Miller has put his experience to good use. Expect the unexpected and realize that we need to be

Address for correspondence: Neal L. Cohen, M.D., New York State Department of Health, 125 Worth Street, New York NY 10013. Voice: 212-295-5347; fax: 212-295-5426 or 212-964-0472. ncohen@health.nyc.gov

able to anticipate changes and understand the climatic conditions and environmental factors that could make this year's experience with the virus differerent from last year's. We shouldn't expect that what we learned last year will hold us in good stead this year. Nevertheless, we're gaining confidence that we're better prepared today to detect new threats and to contain them than we were previously.

Welcoming Remarks

STEPHEN M. OSTROFF

Associate Director for Epidemiologic Science,
Centers for Disease Control and Prevention, Atlanta, Georgia 30333, USA

Let me first thank both Dr. Novello and Dr. Cohen and their colleagues at the New York State Health Department and the New York City Health Department for agreeing to cosponsor this meeting and also for their strong leadership and commitment to addressing the threats, the issues, and the complexities associated with the introduction of the West Nile virus into this hemisphere in 1999. It would also be inappropriate not to acknowledge, whether we like it or not, the role of the media and the assistance of the public as we went about our work. In my limited experience, I have not seen any other outbreak play out with the intense press scrutiny associated with the West Nile virus and the ongoing interest of the public and advocacy groups, whether in favor or against our public health efforts to minimize the health threat to the public. The key to prevention and control of the West Nile virus is to establish as strong a scientific base as possible to guide our recommendations and interventions. To the degree to which this meeting helps to build that scientific base, it will help us now and it will help us in the future. In 1999 our knowledge base was extremely limited, but it was all we had available at the time. Fortunately, the 2000 transmission season gave us the opportunity to collect and analyze high-quality data, which will permit us to refine our public health control measures. In part, this information became available because of the availability of funding, both from Congress and from the budgets of the affected states. Unfortunately, the availability of the resources to address West Nile virus is the exception rather than the rule when dealing with public health issues. Much of the information collected during 2000 will be presented over the course of this meeting and in the resulting volume of the *Annals*. It will be up to you to assess its quality and its reliability and to determine where there are knowledge gaps and how best to fill them. Although there are many questions, one thing is abundantly clear: year 2000 activities to minimize the human health impact worked. In 2000, we observed more infected birds over a wider geographic area, more infected mosquitoes, more infected horses, and other species of infected mammals, but fewer human illnesses. And, believe me, we were all looking pretty hard for human illnesses. Serosurveys conducted last fall confirmed that even in the 2000 hot zone in Staten Island there were far fewer cases than had occurred in the 1999 hot zone in northern Queens. This confirms that even when gaps in knowledge exist, we *can* act to reduce the public health risk. The outstanding question is whether we can continue to minimize the public health risk while at the same time reducing our interventions and their associated costs. We think that it is possible and hope that the

Address for correspondence: Stephen M. Ostroff, M.D., Associate Director for Epidemiologic Science, Centers for Disease Control and Prevention, 1600 Clifton Rd., N.E., Mail Stop C-12, Atlanta, Georgia 30333. Voice: 404-639-3311; fax: 404-639-4197.
smo1@cdc.gov

data presented here will convince you as well. Let me thank all of you for taking the time to participate in this free and open exchange of ideas in the best traditions of science. As the great New Yorker, Yogi Berra, also once said, "It's hard to make predictions, especially about the future." But one thing is for sure: West Nile virus isn't the first emerging disease we've seen in the United States and it surely won't be the last. Our best defense against emerging infections is to have a good offense. That means that we need a robust scientific enterprise and a healthy, capable, and responsive public health infrastructure. Our experience is that both these things are necessary and that you really can't have one without the other. In closing, let me end with a quote from Dennis Waitley: "Anticipate the best, plan for the worst, and prepare to be surprised." The coming season will continue to hold surprises for us, but we at the CDC look forward to working with all of you.

Prospects for Development of a Vaccine against the West Nile Virus

THOMAS P. MONATH

Research and Medical Affairs, Acambis Incorporated,
Cambridge Massachusetts 02139, USA

ABSTRACT: Vaccination provides the ultimate measure for personal protection against West Nile disease. The development of a West Nile vaccine for humans is justified by the uncertainty surrounding the size and frequency of future epidemics. At least two companies (Acambis Inc. and Baxter/Immuno) have initiated research and development on human vaccines. West Nile encephalitis has also emerged as a significant problem for the equine industry. One major veterinary vaccine manufacturer (Ft. Dodge) is developing formalin-inactivated and naked DNA vaccines. The advantages and disadvantages of formalin-inactivated whole virion vaccines, Japanese encephalitis vaccine for cross-protection, naked DNA, and live attenuated vaccines are described. A novel technology platform for live, attenuated recombinant vaccines (ChimeriVax™) represents a promising approach for rapid development of a West Nile vaccine. This technology uses yellow fever 17D as a live vector for envelope genes of the West Nile virus. Infectious clone technology is used to replace the genes encoding the prM and E structural proteins of yellow fever 17D vaccine virus with the corresponding genes of West Nile virus. The resulting virion has the protein coat of West Nile, containing all antigenic determinants for neutralization and one or more epitopes for cytotoxic T lymphocytes. The genes encoding the nucleocapsid protein, nonstructural proteins, and untranslated terminal regions responsible for replication remain those of the original yellow fever 17D virus. The chimeric virus replicates in the host like yellow fever 17D but immunizes specifically against West Nile virus.

KEYWORDS: West Nile virus; vaccine; Jennerian vaccine; ChimeriVax™ platform

RATIONALE FOR A WEST NILE VACCINE

Human Vaccine

The rationale for development of a vaccine is summarized in TABLE 1. The question most often asked is whether the medical impact of West Nile disease in the United States and Europe is sufficient to warrant development of a vaccine for humans. From a public health standpoint, it would appear irresponsible not to support vaccine development as long as the size and frequency of future epidemics is uncertain. The

Address for correspondence: Thomas P. Monath, M.D., Vice President, Research and Medical Affairs, Acambis Inc., 38 Sidney Street, Cambridge, MA 02139. Voice: 617-494-1339; fax: 617-494-1741.
tom.monath@acambis.com

TABLE 1. Rationale for development of a West Nile vaccin

Increased incidence of epidemics associated with severe disease.

In US, new, exotic disease; potentially lethal or disabling.

No treatment or prophylactic antiviral drug.

General intolerance to infectious diseases.

Target population subset at high risk (persons >60 years).

Urban populations affected in areas with affluent, educated populations, well-organized public health infrastructure; high media coverage.

Enzootic cycle not silent.

Promotes fear; avoidance of mosquito bite difficult.

Uncertain future medical impact; potential for larger epidemics.

Expanding geographic range.

Vector control unreliable, objectionable.

Human and veterinary indications (equids, birds).

---

marked increase in West Nile epidemic activity in the 1990s compared to earlier periods (FIG. 1), the increased severity of disease expression, the urbanization of the disease, and the likelihood of further geographic spread all suggest that, for West Nile disease, past is not prologue. At least two companies (Acambis Inc. and Baxter/Immuno) have initiated research and development on human vaccines, providing de facto evidence for a potential commercial market.

The population of the United States and other industrialized nations is generally intolerant to infectious diseases, and most people have come to expect preventative and therapeutic solutions based on modern medicine. West Nile disease strikes urban, relatively affluent areas with strong public health infrastructures and active media, and residents who demand action and solutions. There is no available treatment,

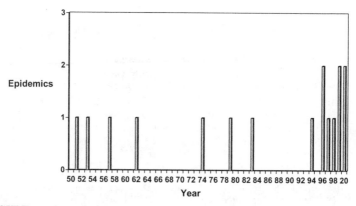

FIGURE 1. Number of reported outbreaks of West Nile virus disease by year, showing increased incidence in the 1990s.

and the clinical disease (encephalitis) is severe and potentially fatal. The West Nile virus enzootic cycle is not silent, and the occurrence of deaths in birds promotes considerable alarm in many areas. The use of pesticides for vector control has raised public concern, with fear of pesticide toxicity being nearly as prevalent as fear of acquiring the disease. There is a low likelihood that prophylactic antiviral drugs against this disease will be developed, for a variety of reasons beyond the scope of this review. Vaccination provides the ultimate measure for personal protection against West Nile disease. Those with risk factors—the elderly or infirm and residents of areas with evidence of high virus transmission—would be candidates for vaccination.

Problems for the commercialization of a human vaccine include the low disease incidence, uncertainties about the future medical impact, high cost-to-benefit ratio for immunization, and the high cost of completing vaccine development. The ideal vaccine for use in humans would be one that could be used in an impending epidemic to provide rapid immunization, preferably within a few days after a single dose.

Licensure of a human vaccine would require successful clinical trials demonstrating safety and efficacy. It is unlikely that field trials showing prevention of disease would be feasible, and licensure would thus be based on strong preclinical data in relevant animal models, the elucidation of antibody levels required for protection, and the demonstration in humans that these immunological surrogates for protection are met after vaccination.

Veterinary Vaccine

West Nile encephalitis has emerged as a significant problem for the equine industry in the United States. The direct contribution of horses engaged in recreational activities, equestrian events, and racing to the gross domestic product has been estimated at $25 billion, and direct and indirect value is over $125 billion.[1] West Nile encephalitis has caused disease in valuable animals and lost revenue due to cancelled equestrian events and restrictions in movement of horses engaged in showing and racing. Although the United States Department of Agriculture initially dismissed the need for a vaccine, there has been strong support for an initiative from the equine industry. One major veterinary vaccine manufacturer (Ft. Dodge) is developing a formalin-inactivated vaccine and is investigating a naked DNA vaccine.

A vaccine for young domestic geese, which are adversely affected by West Nile epornitics, has been investigated in Israel and is described elsewhere in this volume.[2] Other indications for vaccines include protection of zoo animals. A wide variety of exotic avian and some mammalian species are susceptible to West Nile disease.[3] Occurrence of West Nile disease has generated fear and avoidance of affected zoos by the public, causing significant loss of revenues.

A vaccine for horses will have to be safe, immunogenic, and shown to protect against West Nile virus challenge. There must be no issues for use in animals that might be used for human consumption. The antibody response to vaccination should not present problems for export controls on horses engaged in international racing and equestrian events. A marker distinguishing artificial from natural immunity would be useful. A successful West Nile vaccine might ultimately be combined with other equine vaccines, for example, those against eastern and western equine encephalitides, tetanus, or equine influenza.

APPROACHES TO VACCINE DEVELOPMENT

Inactivated and Subunit Vaccines

Formalin-inactivated whole virion vaccines produced in mouse brain tissue or cell culture have been successfully developed for other flaviviruses, including Japanese encephalitis, tick-borne encephalitis, louping ill, and Kyasanur Forest disease. Such vaccines are relatively simple to develop and manufacture, have a good safety record, and may be used in both humans and domestic livestock. For preparation of a vaccine, the virus must replicate to high titer, providing sufficient antigenic mass, and critical epitopes must not be degraded by formalin or betapropriolactone treatment. West Nile virus replicates to very high titers, often 10^{10} infectious particles/mL, in several cell substrates suitable for vaccine manufacture. In addition to the traditional killed whole virion approach, recombinant subunit or subviral particle vaccines could theoretically be developed against West Nile. However, there are no examples of commercial flavivirus products made using these approaches.

The principal disadvantage of inactivated and subunit vaccines is that they require multiple doses to elicit and sustain an effective immune response, making them less suitable for use in an impending outbreak. These vaccines also generally do not elicit strong cellular immune responses. The difficulty in patenting a classical inactivated vaccine may also reduce commercial interest in investing in product development.

Jennerian Vaccine

The use of vaccine against a related virus, Japanese encephalitis (JE), to protect against West Nile virus has received recent attention. This approach is attractive because a vaccine against JE is licensed and available in the United States and Europe (JE-VAX®, Aventis Pasteur). There is both epidemiological[4] and experimental[5] evidence that JE immunity cross-protects against West Nile. Recent, unpublished studies in birds have supported the older data demonstrating cross-protection. However, the effectiveness of cross-protection is relatively low compared to that induced by homologous immunization. More importantly, the safety of immunizing against JE in advance of sustaining a West Nile infection has not been rigorously studied. In flavivirus encephalitis, neuroinvasion and rapid accumulation of viral antigen in the critical target tissues occurs late in the course of infection and may potentially elicit inflammatory responses that enhance lesions and accelerate death. This might be the outcome in an individual who had heterologous cross-reactive immunity against West Nile below the level required to protect against brain infection. Passive transfer of JE antibodies to mice caused enhanced mortality after heterologous challenge with Murray Valley encephalitis virus.[6] This effect may be due to complement-mediated cytolysis of infected cells. Given these considerations, use of JE vaccine to prevent West Nile disease will require that a substantial body of data demonstrate safety in humans. Since it would be exceedingly difficult to obtain such data in clinical trials, further studies in animal models are indicated.

DNA Vaccine

The potential advantages include relative simplicity of development and manufacture, and the stimulation of both humoral and cellular immune responses. A recent report[7] showed that horses could be protected against West Nile challenge after a single dose of plasmid DNA that presumably expressed subviral particles *in vivo.* Disadvantages of DNA vaccines include a complex intellectual property landscape, persisting regulatory concerns, and the absence of preceding licensed products; the inefficiency of traditional vaccine delivery and requirement for special devices (gene gun, electroporation); slow onset of immunity and requirement for multiple doses; and the overall poor immunogenicity, particularly in species higher than mice, without priming and boosting with different formulations.

Live, Attenuated Vaccines

Live viral vaccines replicate in the host and elicit an immune response similar to that mounted after natural infection. The antigenic mass of the virus expands and the antigens presented mimic those of the wild-type virus. A cytokine environment is created similar to that induced by the pathogen itself. Intracellular replication elicits strong cytotoxic T cell responses and long-term memory cells. The overall result is the stimulation of durable humoral and cellular immunity. Typically, a single dose results in a strong immune response. For these reasons, we have favored a live attenuated vaccine approach for development of a West Nile vaccine for humans and horses.

CHIMERIVAX™ PLATFORM

The ChimeriVax™ technology platform uses yellow fever 17D as a live vector for envelope genes of West Nile and other flaviviruses. Chimeric vaccine candidates have been produced against West Nile, Japanese encephalitis, and dengue. Research is also underway to create a vaccine against hepatitis C.

The vector or "backbone" of ChimeriVax™ constructs, yellow fever 17D virus, is a licensed human vaccine that has been used for over 60 years in at least 400 million persons, with an excellent track record of safety and efficacy. The vaccine stimulates neutralizing antibodies (the mediator of protective immunity) in >99% of individuals within 10 days after a single dose. Immunity is very durable and probably lifelong. The vaccine may be administered to children as young as nine months of age.

To construct chimeric vaccine candidates, infectious clone technology was used to replace the genes encoding the prM and E structural proteins of yellow fever 17D vaccine virus with the corresponding genes of West Nile virus. The resulting virion has the protein coat of West Nile, containing all antigenic determinants for neutralization, and many epitopes for cytotoxic T lymphocytes. The genes encoding the nucleocapsid (C) protein, nonstructural proteins, and untranslated terminal regions (UTR) responsible for replication remain those of the original yellow fever 17D virus. The chimeric virus replicates in the host like yellow fever 17D but immunizes specifically against West Nile virus.

The construction of ChimeriVax™ West Nile virus is described diagrammatically in FIGURE 2. The donor prM-E genes from the vaccine target virus are inserted into the yellow fever infectious clone. The linearized full-length cDNA is transcribed to message sense RNA, and the RNA is then transfected into Vero cells to generate

ChimeriVax™

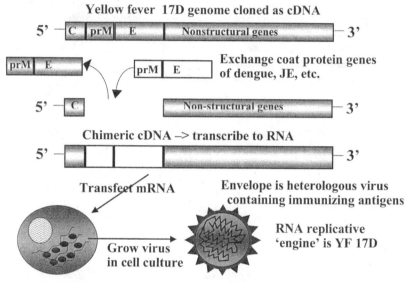

FIGURE 2. Diagrammatic representation of the construction of ChimerivaxT" vaccines using an infectious clone of yellow fever 17D virus.

progeny virus. Vero cells are used to manufacture ChimeriVax™ vaccine. Virus yields in supernatant cell culture fluids after infection at low multiplicities exceed 7 $\log_{10}$ plaque-forming units (PFU). Cellular DNA and proteins are further reduced to acceptable levels by DNase digestion and ultrafiltration. The vaccine is stabilized using conventional excipients.

Japanese Encephalitis Vaccine as a Model for West Nile

Japanese encephalitis (JE) is an important human pathogen that is very similar antigenically, clinically, and epidemiologically to West Nile. The disease occurs in Asia and Australia. A ChimeriVax™-JE vaccine has been successfully developed and is in early stage clinical trials. Because of the similarity of the technical issues, the JE vaccine provides a basis for predicting the successful development of a West Nile vaccine.

For construction of ChimeriVax™-JE, the donor genes were derived from a live attenuated vaccine strain (designated SA14-14-2) licensed in China and used in approximately 30 million children annually. Thus the JE vaccine candidate was constructed from two live attenuated vaccines. This approach was deliberately taken because yellow fever 17D has residual neurotropic properties, and it was hypothesized that insertion of the prM and E genes (which encode determinants for cell attachment) would enhance the neurotropism of the chimeric virus. Interestingly, the yellow fever/JE (SA14-14-2) chimera was less neurovirulent in mice inoculated intracerebrally than yellow fever 17D virus itself (YF-VAX® commercial vaccine)[8,9]

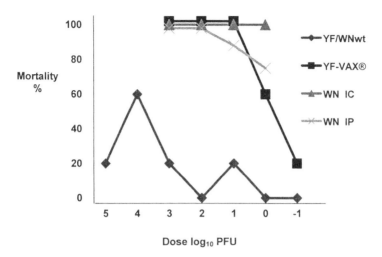

FIGURE 4. Mortality ratios, 3- to 4-week-old mice inoculated with chimeric yellow fever virus containing wild-type West Nile prM-E genes, commercial yellow fever vaccine, or wild-type West Nile virus. The chimeric vaccine is significantly less neurovirulent than either parent.

didate with wild-type prM-E sequence proves to be unsuitable after safety tests in nonhuman primates, a mutated vaccine will replace the original construct.

Timelines for ChimeriVax™–West Nile development are being foreshortened as much as possible, in order to meet unexpected needs arising from the spread of the virus in North America. It is anticipated that production of vaccine at clinical grade will be initiated in early 2002 and that clinical testing will begin at the end of that year.

ACKNOWLEDGMENTS

This work is supported by grants 1R01 AI48297-01 and 1 UC1 AI49517-01 from the National Institute of Allergy and Infectious Diseases, National Institutes of Health. Tom Chambers, St. Louis University, St. Louis MO, developed the initial JE chimera and has collaborated on many aspects of the project. The author gratefully acknowledges Juan Arroyo, the West Nile vaccine project manager at Acambis; and Farshad Guirakhoo, Chuck Miller, John Catalan, Z-X. Zhang, Michael Knauber, Simeon Ocran, Konstantin Pugachev, Richard Nichols, Ron Marchesani, Michele Areias, Karen McCarthy, and Philip Bedford at Acambis who do much of the hard work on ChimeriVax™. John Cruz, Alan Rothman, and Francis A. Ennis, University of Massachusetts Medical School, Worcester MA, kindly provide BL3 facilities enabling the work on West Nile virus. Ken Soike and Marian Ratterree at Tulane Regional Primate Center, Covington LA, Ken Draper at Sierra BioMedical, Sparks NV, and Inessa Levenbook perform studies in rhesus monkeys. John Roehrig and Duane Gubler at CDC, Ft. Collins CO, provided the West Nile virus and facilities for initial cloning of the prM-E genes of West Nile virus.

REFERENCES

1. AMERICAN HORSE COUNCIL. 1996. The Economic Impact of the Horse Industry in the United States. Barents Group. London. Vol. 1, 43 pp.
2. MALKINSON, M. 2001. Vaccination of geese against West Nile fever. Ann. N.Y. Acad. Sci. **951**. This volume.
3. MCNAMARA, T. 2001. Zoo birds. Ann. N.Y. Acad. Sci. **951**. This volume.
4. WORK, T.H. 1971. On the Japanese B-West Nile virus complex or an arbovirus problem of six continents. Am. J. Trop. Med. Hyg. **20:** 169–175.
5. GOVERNDHAN, M.K., A.B. KULKARNI, A.K. GUPTA, et al. 1992. Two-way cross-protection between West Nile and Japanese encephalitis viruses in bonnet macaques. Acta Virol. **36:** 277–283.
6. BROOM, A.K., M.J. WALLACE, J.S. MACKENZIE, et al. 2000. Immunisation with gamma globulin to Murray Valley encephalitis virus and with an inactivated Japanese encephalitis virus vaccine as prophylaxis against Australian encephalitis: evaluation in a mouse model. J. Med. Virol. **61:** 259–65.
7. DAVIS, B.S., G-J. CHANG, B. CROPP, et al. 2001. A candidate DNA vaccine expressing West Nile virus premembrane and envelope proteins protects mouse and horse from virus challenge. J. Virol. **75:** 4041–4047.
8. CHAMBERS, T.J., A. NESTOROWICZ, P.W. MASON & C.M. RICE. 1999. Yellow fever/Japanese encephalitis chimeric viruses: construction and biological properties. J. Virol. **73:** 3095–3101.
9. GUIRAKHOO, F., Z. ZHANG, T.J. CHAMBERS, et al. 1999. Immunogenicity, genetic stability and protective efficacy of a recombinant, chimeric yellow fever-Japanese encephalitis virus (ChimeriVax™-JE) as a live, attenuated vaccine candidate against Japanese encephalitis. Virology **257:** 363–372.
10. MONATH, T.P., K. SOIKE, I. LEVENBOOK, et al. 1999. Recombinant, chimaeric live, attenuated vaccine (ChimeriVax™) incorporating the envelope genes of Japanese encephalitis (SA14-14-2) virus and the capsid and nonstructural genes of yellow fever (17D) virus is safe, immunogenic and protective in non-human primates. Vaccine **17:** 1869–1882.
11. MONATH, T.P., I. LEVENBOOK, K. SOIKE, et al. 2000. Chimeric yellow fever virus 17D-Japanese encephalitis virus vaccine: dose-response effectiveness and extended safety testing in rhesus monkeys. J. Virol. **74:** 1742–1751.
12. ARROYO, J., F. GUIRAKHOO, S. FENNER, et al. 2001. Molecular basis for attenuation of neurovirulence of a yellow fever/Japanese encephalitis (ChimeriVax-JE) viral vaccine. J. Virol. **75:** 934–942.
13. CHAMBERS, T.J., M. HALEVY, A. NESTOROWICZ, et al. 1998. West Nile envelope proteins: Nucleotide sequence analysis of strains differing in mouse neuroinvasiveness. J. Gen. Virol. **79:** 2375–2380.
14. LUSTIG, S., U. OLSHEVSKY, D. BEN-NATHAN, et al. 2000. A live, attenuated West Nile virus strain as a potential veterinary vaccine. Viral Immunol. **13:** 401–410.
15. MONATH, T.P. et al. 2001. Current Drugs.

Human Arbovirus Infections Worldwide

DUANE J. GUBLER

*Division of Vector-Borne Infectious Diseases, National Center for Infectious Diseases,
Centers for Disease Control and Prevention, Public Health Service,
U.S. Department of Health and Human Services, Fort Collins, Colorado 80522, USA*

ABSTRACT: Viral diseases transmitted by blood-feeding arthropods (arboviral diseases) are among the most important of the emerging infectious disease public health problems facing the world at the beginning of the third millennium. There are over 534 viruses listed in the arbovirus catalogue, approximately 134 of which have been shown to cause disease in humans. These are transmitted principally by mosquitoes and ticks. In the last two decades of the twentieth century, a few new arboviral diseases have been recognized. More important, however, is the dramatic resurgence and geographic spread of a number of old diseases that were once effectively controlled. Global demographic and societal changes, and modern transportation have provided the mechanisms for the viruses to break out of their natural ecology and become established in new geographic locations where susceptible arthropod vectors and hosts provide permissive conditions for them to cause major epidemics. West Nile virus is just the the latest example of this type of invasion by exotic viruses. This paper will provide an overview of the medically important arboviruses and discuss several in more detail as case studies to illustrate our tenuous position as we begin the twenty-first century.

KEYWORDS: West Nile virus; arbovirus; Dengue fever; yellow fever; *Aedes aegypti* mosquito

INTRODUCTION AND OVERVIEW

The term *arbovirus* is a contraction for the phrase *arthropod-borne virus*. It has no taxonomic significance but rather is an ecologic term used to define viruses that require a hematophagous (blood-sucking) arthropod for transmission between hosts.[1] There are currently 534 viruses registered in the International Catalogue of Arboviruses; 214 (40%) are known or probable arboviruses (FIG. 1). Another 287 (54%) are listed as possible arboviruses, and 33 (6%) are listed as definitely or probably not arboviruses.[2] Most of the viruses listed in this catalogue are zoonoses or viruses that have vertebrate animals other than humans as their principal reservoir host. Of the 534 viruses, 134 (25%) have caused documented illness in humans.[2]

The arboviruses are a taxonomically diverse group; including possible arboviruses, they represent eight families and 14 genera (TABLE 1).[2,3] In addition, there are a

Address for correspondence: Duane J. Gubler, Division of Vector-Borne Infectious Diseases, National Center for Infectious Diseases, Centers for Disease Control and Prevention, Public Health Service, U.S. Department of Health and Human Services, P.O. Box 2087, Fort Collins, CO 80522. Voice: 970-221-6428: fax: 970-221-6476.
DGubler@cdc.gov

13

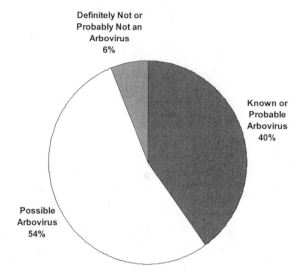

FIGURE 1. Arboviral status of viruses registered in the arbovirus catalogue.

TABLE 1. Taxonomic status of known, probable or possible arboviruses[1]

Family	Number of genera	Number of viruses
Bunyaviridae	5	248
Flaviviridae	1	61
Reoviridae	2	77
Rhabdoviridae	2	68
Togaviridae	1	28
Orthomyxoviridae	1	3
Arenaviridae	1	1
Poxiviridae	1	1
Unclassified	Unknown	13
Eight Families	14 Genera	500 Viruses

number of viruses that remain unclassified. Most of these viruses (248), however, belong to the family Bunyaviridae. Viruses of this family, along with those of the families Flaviviridae and Togaviridae, are the most important human pathogens from a public health perspective.

The arboviruses have a worldwide distribution (TABLE 2). Most known arboviruses were first isolated in Africa and South America, both tropical regions with diverse flora and fauna, where extensive studies have been conducted. Smaller numbers of viruses had been first isolated in Asia, where ecologic diversity is as great as in Af-

TABLE 2. Regions of the world where viruses registered in the arbovirus catalogue were initially isolated

Africa	135	25%
Asia	78	15%
Australasia	60	11%
Europe	35	7%
North America	91	17%
South America	135	25%

rica and tropical America, likely because fewer studies had been conducted there. The geographic distribution of each arbovirus is restricted by the ecologic parameters governing its transmission cycle. Important limiting factors include temperature, precipitation, and vegetation patterns, all of which influence the distribution of the arthropod vector and the vertebrate reservoir host required for virus maintenance.

By definition, arboviruses have at least two hosts; most arboviruses are maintained in complex cycles involving a nonhuman primary vertebrate host and a primary arthropod vector. These cycles are usually silent and undetected in nature until some environmental change allows the virus to escape the primary cycle via a secondary vector or vertebrate host, or when humans invade or encroach on the nidus of infection. Epidemics/epizootics in humans and domestic animals usually occur only after the virus is introduced into the periodomestic environment by a bridge vector, where it is transmitted by a secondary vector to secondary reservoir hosts. Humans and domestic animals, which frequently develop clinical illness, are generally incidental or dead-end hosts because they do not develop viremia high enough to infect the arthropod and contribute to the transmission cycle. Many arboviruses may have more than one vertebrate host or arthropod vector. A few arboviruses, such as dengue fever, yellow fever, and chikungunya (see TABLE 3), cause high viremia levels in humans and may be transmitted from person to person by an arthropod vector, usually a mosquito, which often, but not always, signals epidemic transmission.

Arbovirus infection, in general, causes three basic clinical syndromes in humans– systemic febrile illness, hemorrhagic fever, and meningoencephalitis (TABLE 3).[2–4] The majority of arboviruses cause a nonspecific febrile illness with sudden onset of fever accompanied or followed by headache, myalgia, malaise, and occasionally prostration. Infection may also lead to a more severe illness, presenting as hemorrhagic fever or meningoencephalitis, which may cause death or permanent neurologic sequelae. The same virus may produce different syndromes in different individuals. The illness often follows a biphasic course with a mild, nonspecific febrile phase often going unrecognized, followed by the more severe illness, which is often difficult to diagnose virologically.

TABLE 3 lists the more important arboviruses that affect humans and provides information (when known) on the vector, primary reservoir host, basic ecology, clinical presentation, and geographic distribution. Mosquitoes are by far the most important primary vectors of arboviruses, and birds and rodents are the most important vertebrate reservoir hosts.

TABLE 3. The more important arboviruses causing human disease

Family/Virus	Vector	Vertebrate Host	Ecology[b]	Disease in Humans[c]	Geographic Distribution	Epidemics
Togaviridae						
Chikungunya[a]	mosquitoes	humans, primates	U,S,R	SFI	Africa, Asia	yes
Ross River[a]	mosquitoes	humans, marsupials	R,S,U	SFI	Australia, So. Pacific	yes
Mayaro[a]	mosquitoes	birds	R,S,U	SFI	South America	yes
O'nyong-nyong[a]	mosquitoes	?	R	SFI	Africa	yes
Sinbis	mosquitoes	birds	R	SFI	Asia, Africa, Australia, Europe, Americas	yes
Barmah Forest[a]	mosquitoes	?	R	SFI	Australia	yes
Eastern equine encephalitis	mosquitoes	birds	R	SFI, ME	Americas	yes
Western equine encephalitis	mosquitoes	birds, rabbits	R	SFI, ME	Americas	yes
Venezuelan equine encephalitis[a]	mosquitoes	rodents	R	SFI, ME	Americas	yes
Flaviviridae						
Dengue 1-4[a]	mosquitoes	humans, primates	U,S,R	SFI, HF	worldwide in tropics	yes
Yellow Fever[a]	mosquitoes	humans, primates	R,S,U	SFI, HF	Africa, South America	yes
Japanese encephalitis	mosquitoes	birds, pigs	R,S	SFI, ME	Asia, Pacific	yes
Murray Valley encephalitis	mosquitoes	birds	R	SFI, ME	Australia	yes
Rocio	mosquitoes	birds	R	SFI, ME	South America	yes
St. Louis encephalitis	mosquitoes	birds	R,S,U	SFI, ME	Americas	yes
West Nile[a?]	mosquitoes	birds	R,S,U	SFI, ME	Africa, Asia, Europe, North America	yes
Kyasanar Forest disease[a]	ticks	primates, rodents, camels	R	SFI, HF, ME	India, Saudi Arabia	yes
Omsk hemorrhagic fever	ticks	rodents	R	SFI, HF	Asia	no
Tick-borne encephalitis	ticks	birds, rodents	R,S	SFI, ME	Europe, Asia, North America	no
Bunyaviridae						
Sandfly fever[a]	sandflies	?	R	SFI	Europe, Africa, Asia	yes
Rift Valley fever[a]	mosquitoes	?	R	SFI,HF,ME	Africa, Middle East	yes
La Crosse encephalitis	mosquitoes	rodents	R,S	SFI, ME	North America	no
California encephalitis	mosquitoes	rodents	R	SFI, ME	North America, Europe, Asia	yes
Crimean-Congo hemorrhagic fever[a]	ticks	rodents	R	SFI HF	Europe, Asia, Africa	yes
Oropouche[a]	midges	?	R,S,U	SFI	Central and South America	yes

[a] Arboviruses that produce significant human viremia. [b] U = urban; S = suburban; R = rural; underline designates the most important ecology. [c] SFI = systemic febrile illness; MF = meningoencephalitis; HF = hemorrhagic fever

TABLE 4. Important resurgent/emergent vector-borne viral diseases of humans at the beginning of the twenty-first century

Flaviviridae
Dengue hemorrhagic fever
Yellow fever
Japanese encephalitis
West Nile virus
Kyasanur Forest disease virus
Togaviridae
Venezuelan equine encephalitis
Epidemic polyarthritis
Barmah Forest
Mayaro
Bunyaviridae
Rift Valley fever
Oropouche
California encephalitis
Crimean-Congo hemorrhagic fever

EMERGENCE/RESURGENCE OF ARBOVIRAL DISEASE

In the waning years of the twentieth century, there was a dramatic global emergence/resurgence of arboviral diseases (TABLE 4). Although some arboviruses that cause human disease have been newly recognized, for example, Barmah Forest in Australia, the greatest problem by far has been the resurgence of diseases that were once thought to be controlled, for example, dengue/dengue hemorrhagic fever, yellow fever, Japanese encephalitis, and West Nile virus infection. In the last two decades, the geographic distribution of both vectors and viruses has expanded globally, accompanied by more frequent and intense epidemics. FIGURE 2 shows the more important arboviral epidemic activity in just the last decade of the twentieth century. It will be noted that some viruses, such as dengue, have a wide geographic distribution, being found in the tropics worldwide. Others have a more focal distribution, for example, Japanese encephalitis, yellow fever, and Venezuelan equine encephalitis. Others have been expanding their geographic distribution, for example, dengue, West Nile, and Japanese encephalitis.

The reasons for this dramatic resurgence of arboviral diseases are complex and not well understood. However, it is clear that certain demographic and societal changes in the past 30 years have had a major impact on the ecology of arboviral diseases (TABLE 5). Population growth, primarily in tropical developing countries, has been a major driving force for many of these changes, for example, uncontrolled urbanization, changing agriculture practices, new irrigation systems, and an increased rate of deforestation, which have contributed to the emergence/resurgence of these diseases. Also, modern transportation ensures faster and increased movement of humans, animals, and commodities, and with them pathogens, between regions and population centers of the world. The high rates of transmission associated with epi-

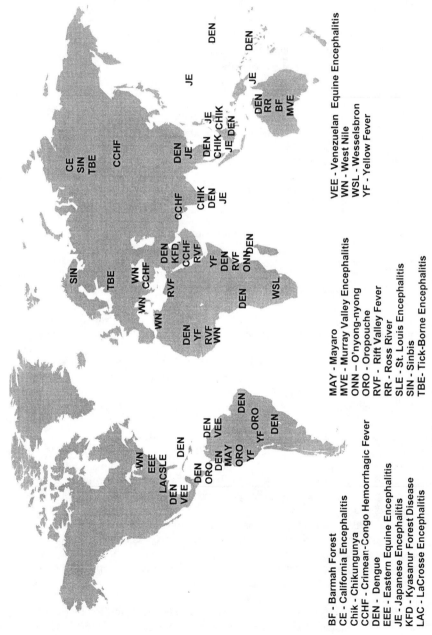

FIGURE 2. Epidemic arboviral diseases, 1990-2000.

BF - Barmah Forest
CE - California Encephalitis
Chik - Chikungunya
CCHF - Crimean-Congo Hemorrhagic Fever
DEN - Dengue
EEE - Eastern Equine Encephalitis
JE - Japanese Encephalitis
KFD - Kyasanur Forest Disease
LAC - LaCrosse Encephalitis

MAY - Mayaro
MVE - Murray Valley Encephalitis
ONN – O'nyong-nyong
ORO - Oropouche
RVF - Rift Valley Fever
RR - Ross River
SLE - St. Louis Encephalitis
SIN - Sinbis
TBE- Tick-Borne Encephalitis

VEE - Venezuelan Equine Encephalitis
WN - West Nile
WSL - Wesselsbron
YF - Yellow Fever

TABLE 5. Factors responsible for the emergence/resurgence of arbovirus diseases

Demographic changes
    Global population growth
    Movement of people within and among regions
    Unplanned and uncontrolled urbanization
Societal changes
    Human encroachment on natural disease foci
    Modern transportation of humans, animals, and commodities within and among regions
    Containerized shipping
Agricultural changes
    Land use
    Irrigation systems
    Deforestation
Changes in pathogens
    Increased movement in humans and animals
    Genetic change leading to increased epidemic potential
Changes in public health
    Lack of effective mosquito control
    Deterioration of public health infrastructure to deal with vector-borne diseases
    Disease surveillance
    Prevention programs
Climate change?
    Temperature
    Precipitation patterns
    Extreme events

demic activity and transmission by different vectors and to different vertebrae hosts in new geographic areas can result in selective pressures that lead to genetic changes in the pathogen. These new strains of virus may have greater epidemic potential and virulence. Finally, the lack of effective vector control and a deterioration in the ability of the public health infrastructure to deal with vector-borne diseases have contributed to the widespread and increased epidemic activity. Whether climate change also contributes is not known because, as yet, there are no good scientific data that confirm that changes in climate/weather have been responsible for the recent resurgence of any arboviral disease.

CASE STUDIES

Two diseases, dengue and yellow fever, will be used as case studies: dengue illustrates what has already happened, and yellow fever what the potential for the future may hold. (West Nile virus will not be discussed further since it is the subject of the other papers in this volume.)

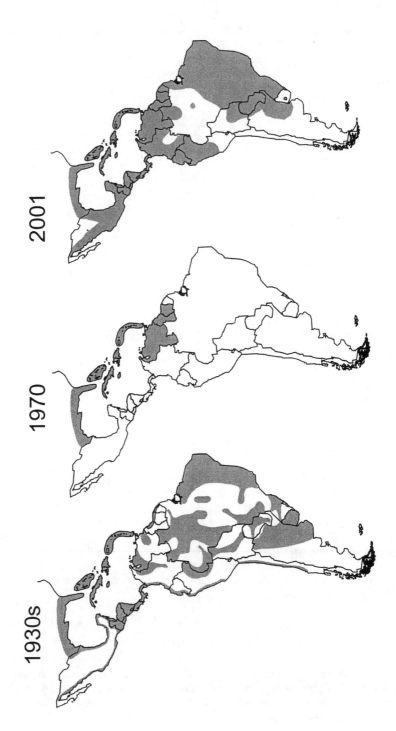

FIGURE 3. Distribution of *Aedes aegypti* in the Americas, 1930s, 1970, and 2001.

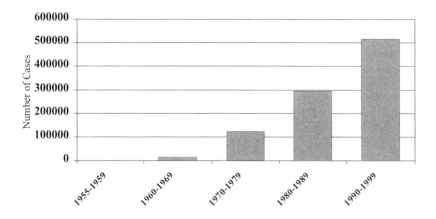

FIGURE 4. Global reports of dengue/dengue hemorrhagic fever, by decade, 1955-2000.

Dengue/Dengue Hemorrhagic Fever

Dengue fever is an old disease that has been distributed in the tropics worldwide for over 200 years and caused major epidemics from the seventeenth century through the first half of the twentieth century.[5] It is caused by infection with four closely related viruses (DEN-1, DEN-2, DEN-3, and DEN-4) that have the same epidemiology and clinical presentation. The viruses are maintained in a primary cycle involving the highly domesticated *Aedes aegypti* mosquito and humans in the large urban centers of the tropics.[6] Primitive forest cycles involving canopy-dwelling *Aedes* species mosquitoes and lower primates have been documented in Asia and Africa, but these do not appear to be important from a public health perspective.[7]

Epidemic dengue was effectively controlled in the American region when the principal mosquito vector, *Ae. aegypti,* was controlled in the 1950s and 1960s. Unfortunately, the program was disbanded in the early 1970s, and the mosquito reinfested most countries of the region over the next 30 years (FIG. 3). In Asia, epidemic dengue was never controlled. During and after World War II, a global pandemic of dengue/dengue hemmorhagic fever (DEN/DHF) began in Southeast Asia.[5,6,8] Transmission of tropical urban vector-borne diseases, such as dengue, was greatly enhanced by demographic and societal changes, and the pandemic intensified during the 1980s and 1990s.[5,6,8] Epidemic DEN/DHF expanded its distribution in Asia and moved into the Pacific and the American tropics. The result was a dramatic increase in epidemic DEN/DHF caused by multiple virus serotypes (hyperendemicity) (FIG. 4). Thus, in 20 years, both the American tropics and the Pacific Islands changed from not having a dengue problem to the point in 2001 where this disease is among the most important of public health problems in those regions. Each year, depending on epidemic activity in the world, there are an estimated 50 to 100 million cases of dengue fever and several hundred thousand cases of the severe form of the disease, DHF. The average case-fatality rate of DHF is five percent.[9]

No vaccine exists for DEN/DHF, so the only way to reverse the trend of resurgent epidemic disease is to control the mosquito vector, *Ae. aegypti*. The emphasis for mosquito control must be focused in the large urban centers of the tropics where the viruses are maintained and where the large epidemics begin and occur. A detailed discussion of mosquito control is beyond the scope of this paper, but effective control of *Ae. aegypti* has been achieved in the past, and, while it may be more difficult in the twenty-first century, it can still be achieved.[10–12] An added benefit to effective control of *Ae. aegypti* would be prevention of urban yellow fever epidemics.

Yellow Fever

Yellow fever (YF) is also an old disease caused by the yellow fever virus, which was introduced into the Western Hemisphere from Africa in the 1600s, causing major epidemics from the seventeenth to the twentieth centuries.[13] Like DEN/DHF, these epidemics were primarily urban in which the virus was transmitted by *Ae. aegypti*. The elimination of this mosquito from most countries of Central and South America in the 1950s and 1960s effectively controlled urban epidemics of YF as well as DEN in the region (FIG. 3).[10] The disease was controlled in Africa at the same time by immunization with a highly effective, safe, and economical vaccine.

YF virus is maintained in the rainforests of sub-Saharan Africa in a cycle involving monkeys and canopy-dwelling *Aedes* mosquitoes; it is periodically introduced into urban areas where it causes epidemics transmitted by *Ae. aegypti*. A similar forest cycle became established in the American tropics, involving monkeys and species of *Haemagogus* mosquitoes.

In the past 15 years, there has been a resurgence of YF in Africa; major epidemics have occurred in West Africa, and epizootic YF has occurred in Kenya for the first time in history.[14,15] The last urban YF epidemic in the Americas occurred in 1942.[13] In the intervening 60 years, however, the urban centers of tropical America have grown dramatically, and most have been reinfested with the principal urban mosquito vector, *Ae. aegypti* (FIG. 3), including large cities located in those countries of the Amazon Basin where YF is maintained in an enzootic forest cycle (FIG. 5). Thus, an estimated 150 to 300 million people, most of whom are susceptible to YF, are living in crowded urban centers of the American tropics in intimate association with equally large populations of *Ae. aegypti*. This puts the American tropics at the highest risk for urban YF epidemics in over 50 years.[16] A small outbreak was documented in Santa Cruz, Bolivia in 1998.[17] The threat is that the American tropics will once again experience major urban epidemics of YF. If that occurs in today's world in which increasing numbers of people rapidly move via modern transportation, YF virus, like dengue viruses, will likely move quickly across the Pacific to Asian and Pacific countries, most of which are also infested with *Ae. aegypti*. This scenario would result in a major global public health emergency. Because of the similarities in the clinical expression between YF and other common diseases such as DEN/DHF, leptospirosis, and rickettsial infections, and because the surveillance systems needed to detect YF are very limited in most Asian and Pacific countries, widespread epidemic transmission could occur before the disease is detected. Emergency methods for controlling adult *Ae. aegypti* mosquitoes are very ineffective,[18–20] and YF vaccine is not available in the quantities that would be required in Asia and the Pacific. Thus, major epidemics of YF could occur in these regions unless natural barriers

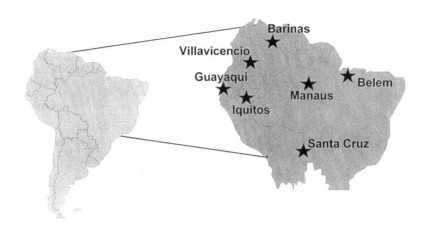

FIGURE 5. Urban centers in the Amazon basin at increased risk for epidemic yellow fever.

such as the high rate of heterotypic flavivirus antibody that occurs in those populations prevented epidemic transmission. Unfortunately, the natural barrier hypothesis
cannot be tested until it is too late.

Reversing the trend of resurgent epidemic arbovirus diseases is a major challenge
to public health officials at the beginning of the twenty-first century. Success will require a rethinking of public health priorities and of public health strategies. It will
require placing the emphasis on developing and implementing effective prevention
strategies instead of waiting until epidemics occur and then trying to stop transmission by implementing emergency response measures, which are nearly always too
little and too late.[21] It will require more resources, both human and economic, to
conduct research and develop and implement more effective prevention strategies.

REFERENCES

1. WHO. 1985. Arthropod-borne and Rodent-borne Viral Diseases. World Health Organization Technical Report Series No. 719, WHO. Geneva.
2. KARABATSOS, N. 1985. International Catalogue of Arboviruses, including certain other
   viruses of vertebrates. American Society of Tropical Medicine and Hygiene. San
   Antonio, TX. 2001 update.
3. GUBLER, D.J. & J.T. ROEHRIG. 1998. Arboviruses (Togaviridae and Flaviviridae). *In*
   Topley and Wilson's Microbiology and Microbial Infections, Vol 1. Virology. B.W.J.
   Mahy & L. Collier, Eds.: **29:** 579–600. Oxford University Press. New York.
4. MONATH, T.P. & F.X. HEINZ. 1996. Flaviviruses. *In* Fields Virology, Third Edition.
   B.N. Fields, D.M. Knipe, P.M. Howley, *et al.*, Eds.: 961–1034. Lippincott-Raven
   Publishers. Philadelphia, PA.
5. GUBLER, D.J. 1997. Dengue and dengue hemorrhagic fever: its history and resurgence
   as a global public health problem. *In* Dengue and Dengue Hemorrhagic Fever. D.J.
   Gubler & G. Kuno, Eds.: 1–22. CAB International. London, UK.
6. GUBLER, D.J. 1998. Dengue and dengue hemorrhagic fever. Clin. Microbiol. Rev.
   11(3): 480–496.

 7. RICO-HESSE, R. 1990. Molecular evolution and distribution of dengue viruses type 1 and 2 in nature. Virology **174:** 479–493.
 8. HALSTEAD, S.B. 1992. The XXth century dengue pandemic: need for surveillance and research. World Health Stat Q. **45:** 292–298.
 9. WHO. 1999. Prevention and control of dengue and dengue haemorrhagic fever. Comprehensive Guidelines. WHO Regional Publication, SEARO No. 29.
10. SCHLIESSMAN, D.J. & L.B. CALHEIROS. 1974. A review of the status of yellow fever and *Aedes aegypti* eradication programs in the Americas. Mosquito News **34:** 1–9.
11. CHAN, K.L. 1985. Singapore's dengue haemorrhagic fever control programme: a case study on the successful control of *Aedes aegypti* and *Aedes albopictus* using mainly environmental measures as part of integrated vector control. SEAMIC. Tokyo. pp. 1–114.
12. KOURI, G.P., M.G. GUZMAN, J.R. BRAVO & C. TRIANA. 1989. Dengue haemorrhagic fever/dengue shock syndrome: lessons from the Cuban epidemic, 1981. Bull. W.H.O. **67:** 375–380.
13. MONATH, T.P. 1988. Yellow fever. *In* The Arboviruses: Epidemiology and Ecology. Vol. V. T.P. Monath, Ed.: 139–231. CRC Press. Boca Raton, FL.
14. NASIDI, A., T.P. MONATH, K. DECOCK, *et al.* 1989. Urban yellow fever epidemic in western Nigeria, 1987. Trans. R. Soc. Trop. Med. Hyg. **83:** 401.
15. SANDERS, E.J. & P.M. TUKEI. 1996. Yellow fever: an emerging threat for Kenya and other east African countries. East Afr. Med. J. **73**(1): 10–12.
16. GUBLER, D.J. 1998. Resurgent vector-borne diseases as a global health problem. Emerg. Infect. Dis. **4:** 442–450.
17. VAN DER STUYFT, P., A. GIANELLA, M. PIRARD, *et al.* 1999. Urbanization of yellow fever in Santa Cruz, Bolivia. Lancet **353:** 1558–1562.
18. GUBLER, D.J. 1989. *Aedes aegypti* and *Aedes aegypti*-borne disease control in the 1990s: top down or bottom up. Am. J. Trop. Med. Hyg. **40:** 571–578.
19. NEWTON, E.A.C. & P. REITER. 1992. A model of the transmission of the dengue fever with an evolution of the impact of ultra-low volume (ULV) insecticide application on dengue epidemics. Am. J. Trop. Med. Hyg. **47:** 709–720.
20. REITER, P. & D.J. GUBLER. 1997. Surveillance and control of urban dengue vectors. *In* Dengue and Dengue Hemorrhagic Fever. D.J. Gubler & G. Kuno, Eds.: 425–462. CAB International. London, UK.
21. GUBLER, D.J. 2001. Prevention and control of tropical diseases in the 21st century: back to the field. Presidential address delivered at the 49th annual meeting of the American Society of Tropical Medicine and Hygiene, Houston TX, 31 October 2000. Am. J. Trop. Med. Hyg. **65**(1): v–vi.

West Nile Virus: Uganda, 1937, to New York City, 1999

Infectious Diseases Directorate, Naval Medical Research Center,
Silver Spring, Maryland 20910-7500

ABSTRACT: West Nile virus, first isolated in 1937, is among the earliest arthropod-borne viruses discovered by humans. Its broad geographical distribution,
not uncommon infection of humans, transmission by mosquitoes, and association with wild birds as enzootic hosts were well documented by the mid-1960s.
However, West Nile virus was not considered to be a significant human pathogen because most infections appeared to result in asymptomatic or only mild
febrile disease. Several epidemics had been documented prior to 1996, some involving hundreds to thousands of cases in mostly rural populations, but only a
few cases of severe neurological disease had been reported. The occurrence between 1996 and 1999 of three major epidemics, in southern Romania, the Volga
delta in southern Russia, and the northeastern United States, involving hundreds of cases of severe neurological disease and fatal infections was totally unexpected. These were the first epidemics reported in large urban populations.
A significant factor that appeared in common to all three outbreaks was the apparent involvement of the common house mosquito, *Culex pipiens*, as a vector.
This species had not previously been implicated as important in the transmission of West Nile virus. In addition the epidemic in the northeastern United
States was unusual in the association of West Nile virus infection with fatal disease of birds, suggesting a change in the virulence of the virus toward this host.
Understanding the risk factors that contributed to these three urban epidemics
is important for minimizing the potential for future occurrences. This review
will attempt to compare observations on the biology of West Nile virus made
over about 60 years prior to the recent epidemics to observations made in association with these urban epidemics.

KEYWORDS: West Nile virus; review; epidemic; vectors; hosts; disease;
epidemiology

West Nile (WN) virus has recently emerged as a major public health concern in Europe and the United States with the occurrence of epidemics involving hundreds of cases of meningoencephalitis and encephalitis in three large urban areas since 1996. More human cases of severe neurological disease and more deaths have been reported in these three recent epidemics than in all known past outbreaks of West Nile disease. These are also the first reported epidemics to occur in large urban areas and the first to have the common house mosquito, *Culex pipiens*, implicated as a major vector.

Address for correspondence: Curtis G. Hayes, Infectious Diseases Directorate, Naval Medical
Research Center, Silver Spring, Maryland 20910-7500. Voice: 301-319-7455; fax: 301-319-7460.
hayesc@nmrc.navy.mil

THE VIRUS

Previous Observations

West Nile virus was originally isolated in 1937 from the blood of an adult female in Uganda.[1] The next isolates of WN virus were not obtained until 13 years later in Egypt from the blood of three apparently healthy children.[2] However, after that slow beginning, hundreds of additional isolates of WN virus have been obtained, particularly from humans, birds, and mosquitoes, over a wide geographic area ranging from Africa, through the Middle East and Europe, to Asia.[3–5]

Shortly after the original isolation of WN virus was made, researchers were able to show that this virus was antigenically related to two other arboviruses that were known to cause encephalitis, St. Louis encephalitis (SLE) virus and Japanese encephalitis (JE) virus.[6] Later, cross-neutralization studies expanded the relationship of WN virus with other flaviviruses, placing it in an antigenic group with SLE, JE, Murray Valley encephalitis, Kunjin, Usutu, Kokobera, Stratford, and Alfuy viruses.[7]

Antigenic variation among selected isolates of WN viruses was shown to exist in 1965 when 21 isolates from 6 different countries were compared in a kinetic hemagglutination-inhibition assay.[8,9] The isolates were divided into two major groups, the African–Middle-Eastern and Indian antigenic groups, with the exception of one of three isolates tested from South Africa, which was not placed in either group. Several studies have suggested that virulence differences also existed among isolates of WN virus, but interpretation of these studies is complicated by the fact that the isolates compared had undergone different passage histories, usually by intracerebral inoculation of mice, in the laboratory.

With the availability of the improved nucleic acid sequencing technology, an envelope protein gene fragment was compared from 20 WN virus isolates from nine African countries and one isolate from France made between 1951 and 1990.[10] This study classified the WN isolates into two lineages (I and II). West Nile viruses belonging to both lineages were found to circulate widely in Africa and overlapped in some areas. This study also classified the closely related Australian flavivirus, Kunjin, as a WN subtype in lineage I.

Current Observations

Improved nucleic acid sequencing capability also has allowed researchers to rapidly determine the genetic relationship of the WN virus isolates made during the course of the three urban epidemics that occurred between 1996 and 1999. Only two WN isolates, one from a mosquito and one from a human, were obtained during the 1996 epidemic in Romania.[11] Both isolates, although slightly different from each other, were shown to belong to lineage I of WN viruses. These two isolates were most closely related to several earlier isolates from countries in sub-Saharan Africa, suggesting that they could have been introduced into Romania from migrating birds from that region.

An analysis of gene fragments from WN virus isolates obtained during the 1999 epidemic/epizootic in New York, Connecticut, and New Jersey also showed that they belonged to lineage I.[12] All of these isolates had a very high degree of homology (>99.8%) over the 1278 nucleotide regions sequenced, even though they were obtained from humans, birds, and mosquitoes. Unexpectedly, these isolates shared the same high degree of homology with an isolate obtained from a dead goose in Israel in 1998, suggesting that the origin of the WN virus circulating in the northeastern United States was the Mediterranean region.

Nucleic acid sequences of WN virus gene fragments amplified from the brain tissues of seven fatal cases during the Volgograd epidemic were identical to each other and also were placed in lineage I.[13] The 165 nucleotide base sequence of the envelope gene used for this analysis was 100% homologous to the same region from the 1996 mosquito isolate made during the Romania epidemic, and showed >98% homology with two isolates obtained in 1999 from a bird and a human in New York City.

THE VECTOR

Previous Observations

Because WN virus was known to be antigenically related to other viruses transmitted by mosquitoes,[6] experimental vector studies were undertaken shortly after its discovery. These studies demonstrated that several species of mosquitoes could be experimentally infected and successfully transmit WN virus in the laboratory.[14,15]

The first field studies that implicated mosquitoes as important vectors of WN virus were conducted in Egypt from 1952 to 1954.[16,17] Over the three years of this study, 17 isolates of WN virus were made from pools of mosquitoes, 5 from *Culex antennatus,* 9 from *Culex univittatus,* and 3 from mixed pools of *Culex pipiens* and *Culex univittatus.* These isolates were made during the same time of the year that WN virus infections were documented in children in the study area. During this same study a number of pools of other arthropods, including ticks, also were tested for WN virus isolation but were negative. Subsequent field studies in South Africa from 1961 to 1964 and Israel from 1964 to 1966 further supported the role of mosquitoes belonging to the *Culex unvittatus* complex as major vectors of WN virus.[18,19]

Other species of mosquitoes, such as *Culex modestus* during an outbreak of WN in the early 1960s in France[20] and *Culex vishnui* complex mosquitoes in India and Pakistan, also have been implicated as important vectors of WN virus in different geographical areas.[21,22] WN virus has been isolated from many other species of mosquitoes, but their role as vectors has often remained poorly defined.

West Nile virus also has been isolated occasionally from ticks, but their role in the ecology of the virus remains unknown.[3–5] Conceivably they could play a role in the dissemination of virus via migrating birds or in the overwintering of WN virus in temperate areas.

Current Observations

In all three major WN epidemics that occurred between 1996 and 2000, *Culex pipiens pipiens* was thought to play a major role as a vector for the first time. During the Romanian epidemic, *Culex pipiens pipiens* was the most abundant mosquito species collected, and the single WN virus isolate obtained from mosquitoes was from this species.[11] The minimum WN virus infection rate for *Culex pipiens pipiens* per 1000 adult female mosquitoes tested was only 0.19, but all of these females were collected in October at the end of the epidemic. In the epidemic/epizootic that occurred in the northeastern United States in 1999–2000, multiple isolates of WN virus were made from pools of *Culex pipiens pipiens* females collected during the time that transmission to humans and birds also was occurring.[23,24] Limited vector competence studies have been conducted with four different species of mosquitoes collected in the New York City metropolitan area in 1999 using an isolate of WN virus recovered from the brain of a dead crow found in New York City during 1999.[25] This study supported the field virus isolation data that *Culex pipiens* is a competent vector of WN virus. No entomological observations have been reported from the 1999 epidemic in the Volgograd region of Russia.

Earlier experimental infection studies had demonstrated that *Culex pipiens pipiens* could become infected and transmit WN virus after ingesting a high-titered blood meal.[26–28] However, only a few isolates of WN virus had been reported previously from this species, and it was generally not considered an important vector because of its low field virus isolation rate compared to the isolation rates from other sympatric mosquito species.[17–19]

Two other interesting observations were made on mosquito vectors during the 1999–2000 WN epidemic in the northeastern United States. West Nile virus was isolated from overwintering *Culex pipiens pipiens* females collected in New York City,[29] and WN virus was isolated or WN virus nucleotide sequences were detected in 12 different species of mosquitoes.[30] The role of *Culex pipiens pipiens* as an overwintering vector for WN virus had previously been suggested by investigators in Egypt when they obtained a single isolate of WN virus from this species during January.[17] However, they speculated that *Culex pipiens pipiens* continued to transmit WN virus at a low level throughout the winter (instead of hibernating), since some females of this species remained active at the ambient winter temperatures in this part of Egypt, and a few children were documented to develop antibodies against WN virus during the winter months. The number of mosquito species from which WN virus has been isolated in the northeastern United States far exceeds the number reported from any other area of the world in association with epidemic or epizootic activity, although WN virus isolates have been reported from a large number of different mosquito species in some tropical countries where endemic/enzootic activity has been monitored.[5]

THE HOST

Previous Observations

Humans were the first vertebrate hosts recognized to become infected with WN virus by virus isolations obtained from blood as well as the presence of WN neutralizing antibody in blood.[1,2,31] Subsequent studies in Israel, however, suggested that humans naturally infected with WN virus usually do not circulate high enough titers of virus in their blood to efficiently infect mosquito vectors.[32] By contrast, experimental infection studies conducted on advanced cancer patients in New York City showed that titers of WN virus in the blood high enough to theoretically infect mosquitoes could occur.[33] Interestingly, this study also found that the clinical severity of a patient's WN virus infection correlated with the length of their viremia. Many other studies have confirmed that humans become infected with WN virus in different areas throughout the range of this virus, but their role in the transmission of WN virus remains undefined.[3–5]

The detailed village-based study on the ecology of WN virus conducted in the Sindbis sanitary district, Egypt from 1952–1954 showed for the first time that wild birds were important hosts in the transmission cycle of WN virus.[34] In this highly endemic site for WN virus, neutralizing antibody rates in blood samples collected from six of the area's most abundant bird species were found to range from 48% to 100%. They also found that the antibody rate in the hooded crow population increased from 40% during the late spring to 87% in the summer and winter and suggested the lower rate in late spring reflected the yearly introduction of susceptible juveniles into the population. This also was the first study that isolated WN virus from wild birds and the first to show that experimentally infected wild birds developed titers of WN virus in their blood high enough to infect mosquitoes.

A number of field studies conducted in different geographical areas corroborated the importance of birds in the transmission cycle of WN virus based on the presence of high rates of antibody.[35–39] In particular, a study conducted in South Africa immediately following a large outbreak of WN in the human population found very high antibody rates among wild birds, suggesting that an avian epizootic had occurred concurrently with the human infections.[40] Studies in South Africa on the experimental infection of wild birds also showed that nearly all birds were highly susceptible to WN virus and developed high levels of virus in their blood.[41]

Antibody surveys have shown that many species of wild and domestic mammals, other than humans, become infected with WN virus, and a few WN virus isolates also have been made from naturally infected mammals other than humans.[3–5] Experimental infection studies have been conducted with a few domestic mammals as well as wild rodents.[17,42–46] The WN viremia levels have generally been undetectable or low, but only a very limited number of subjects have been included in these studies. On the basis of these early studies most researchers have concluded that the role of mammals, including humans, in the transmission cycle of WN virus is probably not critical to the long-term survival of the virus.

Current Observations

High WN antibody rates (41%) were found in domestic birds immediately following the 1996 epidemic in Romania.[11] These birds were mostly tested from locations where human cases had occurred. A very limited sampling of wild birds was done, and only one out of twelve birds tested was positive for WN virus antibody. These limited results suggested birds played a role in this epidemic. Other than humans, testing of mammals for WN virus antibody was not reported. On the basis of serosurvey results, thousands of human infections occurred during this epidemic.[47]

A large epizootic in birds clearly occurred in the northeastern United States during the 1999–2000 epidemic. For the first time, thousands of bird deaths attributable to natural WN virus infection were reported during this outbreak.[30] The largest number of deaths were reported in the common crow, but dozens of other species of birds also were involved. Interestingly, WN virus was recovered from the brain of a dead red-tailed hawk collected during the middle of the winter in New York, suggesting a prolonged infection or a route of transmission other than mosquitoes.[48] Birds also have clearly played a major role in spreading WN virus during this epizootic from the four states originally involved in 1999 to twelve states in 2000.[30] Earlier studies had suggested that wild birds were involved in the geographic dispersal of WN virus during their migratory flights, but definitive data were lacking. A number of humans and horses and a few other mammals have been reported infected with WN virus during this epidemic/epizootic. Until better serosurvey data becomes available to determine more accurate infection rates in different species, comparisons are difficult to make, but the preliminary data strongly suggest that birds have been the important vertebrate hosts for WN virus transmission during the epidemic/epizootic in the northeastern United States.

THE DISEASE

Previous Observations

The earliest isolates of WN virus from humans were associated with a mild febrile disease or asymptomatic infections.[1,2] Several studies were conducted during the early to mid-1950s that provided more detailed information on the clinical presentation of WN virus infection in humans. In Egypt, village-based studies conducted from 1952–1954 on children presenting to a medical clinic found that most WN virus infections in this age group presented as mild acute febrile episodes.[17] These investigators found no evidence of central nervous system involvement in WN virus infections. From these studies it was clear that many asymptomatic infections or infections too mild for the patient to seek medical care also occurred.

Around the same time period, a series of WN epidemics were described in Israel.[49] The first virologically proven epidemic occurred in 1951 among the inhabitants of an agricultural community.[50] Out of 303 inhabitants, 123 (41%) clinical cases were described. Both children and adults presented with acute self-limited febrile disease, but recovery was noted to be more rapid in children compared to adults. Most adults in this study were under the age of 30 years. No fatal cases occurred, and no cases of frank meningitis or encephalitis were diagnosed, although 10 of the children did present with a positive Brudzinski's sign. A detailed clinical description of 50 additional hospitalized cases of WN confirmed by serology or virus isolation was made during a 1952 epidemic.[51] Most of the patients were young adult soldiers and presented with a typical acute febrile disease course. Only one case of mild aseptic meningitis was reported among these 50 cases.

In 1957 another large epidemic of WN occurred in Israel, and clinical data were described from three distinct patient groups, soldiers living in army camps, children and adults living in and around the town of Hadera, and elderly persons living in two nursing homes.[52] Most patients in the first two groups presented with typical clinical episodes of WN fever similar to what had been described earlier in Israel, although three cases were complicated by meningoencephalitis. From the third group of 45 elderly patients, 12 had a severe course of meningoencephalitis, but all recovered. The other 33 elderly patients presented with only fever. Interestingly, none of these 45 patients presented with lymphadenopathy or rash that had been commonly associated with WN virus infections in the past in Israel. In addition to these 45 serologically confirmed WN infections, four more elderly patients died from diffuse encephalitis during this epidemic, but serological confirmation of these cases was lacking. These four fatal cases almost certainly represent the first human deaths ever attributed to naturally acquired WN virus infection. This epidemic also provided the first evidence that WN infection may be more severe in elderly persons.

The 1957 epidemic in Israel was the only epidemic of WN prior to the 1996 Romania epidemic in which severe neurological disease, particularly associated with fatalities, was a prominent clinical presentation. However, other sporadic severe cases of WN virus infection have been reported, including fatal cases of encephalitis in children in India[53] and fatal cases of hepatitis in the Central African Republic.[54]

In addition to disease associated with natural WN virus infections, disease occurring following the experimental infection of advanced cancer patients also has been described.[33] Of 78 patients experimentally infected with one of the earliest human isolates of WN virus from Egypt, 89% developed fever as their only clinical evidence of disease. However, 11% did develop signs of diffuse encephalitis, but no fatalities were attributed to the WN virus infections.

Other than humans the only animals that had been reported to develop illness following natural WN virus infection prior to the 1999 New York City epidemic/epizootic were horses and a single bird. An isolate of WN virus was recovered from the brain of a 12-year-old horse that died of encephalitis in Egypt in 1959,[42] and another isolate was obtained from the lumbar spinal column of a 6-month-old horse with encephalitis in France in 1965.[44] During the 1952–1954 field study in Egypt, WN virus was recovered from the brain, spleen, and blood of a sick pigeon.[17]

In addition to natural infections, several animal species have been experimentally infected with WN virus; however, these studies should be interpreted with caution, since the dose and route of infection usually do not mimic natural exposure. Both horses and wild birds have been reported to develop disease following inoculation of WN virus. In Egypt, two mules, six donkeys, three horses, two sheep, and a water buffalo were infected with WN virus by subcutaneous and/or intravenous inoculation or were exposed to the bites of WN virus–infected mosquitoes, but only two of the donkeys developed low grade fever.[42] Apparently some foals inoculated subcutaneously with WN virus in France developed a severe encephalomyelitis, but adult horses did not develop severe disease.[44]

In Egypt, 13/13 hooded crows and 10/16 house sparrows died after being fed on by WN virus–infected mosquitoes.[34] Most deaths occurred between four and seven days postexposure. No deaths were recorded in kestrels, buff-backed herons, and palm doves, which were also infected during these same experiments. In experiments in South Africa, 13 species of wild birds were inoculated intramuscularly with WN virus.[41] Although almost all of the birds became infected and some of the birds died during the viremic period, the authors attributed the mortality to handling, not to the infection. Neither house sparrows nor crows were included in these experiments.

Current Observations

Within a period of less than five years, epidemics of WN occurred in and around three large urban areas, producing hundreds of more cases of severe disease in infected humans than had been identified since the discovery of this virus in 1937.[13,23,47] Based on serosurvey data collected after the epidemics in southeastern Romania and the northeastern United States, many asymptomatic or mild infections also occurred for each case presenting with neurological disease (less than 1% of infections presented with severe neurological disease).[47,55] The most severe and particularly fatal infections mostly occurred in elderly patients, similar to the situation reported during the 1957 epidemic in Israel. The case fatality ratio in the southeastern Romania epidemic was 4.3%, and for the northeastern U.S. epidemic for 1999 the case fatality rate was approximately 11%. On the basis of the limited data presented, the case fatality rate in the Volgograd epidemic was similar. A clinical presentation of severe muscle weakness resembling Guillain-Barré syndrome was prominent during the northeastern U.S. epidemic,[56,57] and apparently a few similar cases were reported during the 1996 Romania epidemic.[58] Prior to these recent cases, only one other WN infection had been described with a similar clinical presentation in a young adult from Israel.[59] Unfortunately, reliable population-based data on the clinical/subclinical infection ratio and age-specific case fatality rates are not available from earlier epidemics of WN virus infection to compare with these recent epidemics.

Of the three major urban epidemics of WN that have occurred since 1996, only in the northeastern United States has disease been reported in animals other than humans. The most striking feature of the epidemic/epzootic that occurred in New York and surrounding states during 1999–2000 was the thousands of dead and moribund birds that were found infected with WN virus.[30] This is the first time that significant bird mortality has been attributed to natural infection with this virus. The common crow has been the species most frequently reported to be killed by WN virus, but 75 other species have also been found infected with WN virus. Pathological studies of birds have shown that not only the brain but many extraneural tissues, as well, had lesions caused by WN virus infection.[60] The reason why WN virus has been so deadly for birds during this epizootic is not known, but possible reasons are that birds in the Western Hemisphere have not been evolutionarily selected for resistance in the absence of WN virus circulation in this part of the world or that the particular strain of WN virus causing this epizootic has enhanced virulence for birds. The latter possibility is supported by the fact that a WN virus strain recently associated with bird deaths in Israel has been shown by nucleotide sequence comparison to be almost identical to the strain circulating in the northeastern United States.[12]

Clinical cases of WN infection in horses also were reported during the 1999–2000 epidemic/epizootic in the northeastern United States. During this period over 80 clinical cases were confirmed, exceeding the number of cases reported in any past epizootic.[61,62] Apparently all except one of the horses developing neurological disease have been adults, and their mean age was several years higher than horses that were infected but that did not develop neurological signs.

Interestingly, for the first time during the northeastern U.S. epidemic/epizootic, fatal WN virus infections were identified in mammals other than humans and horses. Fatal infections have apparently been diagnosed in a cat, skunk, squirrel, chipmunk, rabbit, and bats.[62]

THE EPIDEMIOLOGY

Previous Observations

Epidemiological investigations on West Nile virus were conducted in the Nile delta of Egypt from 1952–1954.[17] Villages located in the southern part of the delta were found to be highly endemic for WN virus infection. Transmission was found to be most intense during the summer months from June through September, with the peak occurring during July. Serosurveys showed that 50% of the four year olds had neutralizing antibody to WN virus that increased to over 90% in twenty year olds, and seroconversion rates exceeding 20% were documented over a three-month period. By contrast, in villages along the northern rim of the Nile delta close to the Mediterranean coast, WN virus activity was found to be much lower. Several factors were found to differ between these two regions that might account for the differences in transmission intensity. Compared to the northern delta villages, the southern villages had a greater human population density (600 versus 200 per square kilometer), a greater amount of land under irrigated cultivation, and a much higher density of the main mosquito vector, *Culex univittatus*.

Around this same time the first epidemics of WN were described in Israel at two major areas located north and south of Tel Aviv along the Mediterranean coastal plain.[49] The seasonal occurrence of these epidemics followed the same summertime pattern as the endemic transmission cycle observed in Egypt. The reason that these epidemics were geographically circumscribed to these two main sites was not determined. Apparently both sites were located in regions previously covered by swamps. Many of the swamps had been converted to fish ponds that still retained some of the earlier ecological characteristics of the swamp habitat.[63]

The isolation of WN virus from sick humans and a horse in the Rhone delta of France and from sick humans in the Volga delta of Russia in the 1960s considerably extended the known epidemic range of WN virus. It is not clear from these early studies if such outbreaks represented a periodic introduction of WN virus into these regions, possibly via migrating birds, or a flare-up of low-level enzootic activity.[3-5]

Prior to the 1996 epidemic in southern Romania, the largest known epidemic occurred in the Cape province of South Africa in 1974.[40] This epidemic occurred following unusually heavy rains in this normally arid part of the country. Factors contributing to this epidemic were thought to be the unusually heavy rainfall, an increased density of the main mosquito vector, *Culex univittatus*, and the high summer temperatures that prevail in the area where the epidemic occurred.

Prior to the 1974 epidemic, sporadic WN virus infections of humans had been recognized in South Africa, but usually in the moister high inland plateau region. Ecological studies conducted in this region during the 1960s had already provided insight into how manmade modifications of the environment, weather conditions, and mosquito behavior can all impact on the transmission cycle of WN virus.[18,64]

Studies conducted in other countries from the late 1950s through the early 1990s revealed the widespread geographical distribution of WN virus throughout Africa and its presence in southern Europe and South Asia.[3-5] However, only a few cases of human disease attributable to WN virus infection, usually among residents of rural areas, were reported during this period.

Current Observations

Since 1996 large epidemics caused by WN virus have occurred in southern Romania (1996),[47] in the Volgograd region of Russia (1999),[13] and in the northeastern United States (1999).[23,30] All of these epidemics involved densely populated urban areas as well as surrounding suburban/rural areas and have been characterized by a large number of cases of severe neurological disease. All three sites were located adjacent to large rivers, presumably providing a favorable wetland habitat for attracting both resident and migratory species of wild birds.[65] As mentioned earlier, wild or domestic birds have been implicated as important hosts in both the southern Romania and northeastern U.S. epidemics.

These are the first epidemics reported from large cities and the first epidemics in which *Culex pipiens* has been implicated as a major vector. Apparently all three urban areas had lower than normal rainfall the summers of the epidemics. Such dry conditions presumably could have increased the number of favorable breeding sites available to *Culex pipiens,* which readily lay eggs in stagnant and polluted water sources.

Detailed risk factor data have only been reported from the southern Romania epidemic.[66] A case-control study comparing asymptomatically infected and uninfected persons identified the presence of mosquitoes in the home, more mosquito bites per day, and, for apartment dwellers, having a flooded basement as risk factors for acquiring infection. Several apartment buildings in Bucharest were noted to have basements flooded with a mixture of drinking water and sewage from leaking pipes. A second case-control study comparing patients with WN meningoencephalitis to WN-infected asymptomatic cases found spending a greater amount of time outdoors as a significant risk factor for developing severe disease. Risk factor data has not been published from the epidemics in the Volgograd region or the northeastern United States; however, an initial investigation carried out by the New York City Department of Health on the first cluster of eight cases reported in that city found that all of the patients were active outdoors.[56]

CONCLUSION

Comparing knowledge acquired during the three recent urban epidemics about vectors, enzootic/epizootic hosts, virulence of viral strains, and environmental conditions to knowledge gained over the previous 60 years during studies on the ecology of West Nile virus will, we trust, lead to a greater understanding of the factors that contributed to this sudden eruption in epidemic activity. However, to successfully accomplish this, detailed epidemiological and virological studies must be continued and expanded to address the many questions that have arisen from the recent epidemics, such as (1) the role of different mosquito species in the transmission of West Nile virus to birds, humans, horses, and possibly other mammals; (2) the contribution of humans and horses to the infection of mosquitoes with West Nile virus; (3) the importance of nonmosquito transmission, such as direct bird to bird or predator to prey transmission; (4) the importance of genetic differences seen between lineages I and II West Nile viruses and between different clades of West Nile virus within the same lineage in virulence expression and other aspects of the ecology of these viruses; (5) the role of mosquitoes and birds in the overwintering of West Nile virus in temperate regions; (6) the importance of migrating birds in introducing or reintroducing West Nile virus into areas of Europe; and (7) the influence of different natural and man-made environmental conditions on the intensity of West Nile virus transmission. Clearly much research remains to be done on this important emerging human pathogen.

REFERENCES

1. SMITHBURN, K.C., T.P. HUGHES, A.W. BURKE, *et al.*, 1940. A neurotropic virus isolated from the blood of a native of Uganda. Am. J. Trop. Med. Hyg. **20**: 471–472.
2. MELNICK, J.L., J.R. PAUL, J.T. RIORDAN, *et al.* 1951. Isolation from human sera in Egypt of a virus apparently identical to West Nile virus (18884). Proc. Soc. Exp. Biol. Med. **77**: 661–665.
3. HAYES, C.G. 1988. West Nile viruses. *In* The Arboviruses: Epidemiology and Ecology. T.P. Monath, Ed.: 59–88. CRC Press, Inc. Boca Raton, FL.
4. MALIK PEIRIS, J.S. & F.P. AMERASINGHE. 1994. West Nile fever. *In* Handbook of Zoonoses: Viral: 139–148. CRC Press, Inc. Boca Raton, FL.
5. HUBALEK, Z. & J. HALOUZKA. 1999. West Nile fever—a reemerging mosquito-borne viral disease in Europe. Emerg. Infect. Dis. **5**: 643–650.
6. SMITHBURN, K.C. 1942. Differentiation of the West Nile virus from the viruses of St. Louis and Japanese B encephalitis. J. Immunol. **44**: 25–31.
7. DE MADRID, A.T. & J.S. PORTERFIELD. 1974. The flaviviruses (group B arboviruses): a cross-neutralization study. J. Gen. Virol. **23**: 91–96.
8. HAMMAM, H.M., D.H. CLARKE & W.H. PRICE. 1965. Antigenic variation of West Nile virus in relation to geography. Am. J. Epidemiol. **82**: 4–55.
9. HAMMAM, H.M. & W.H. PRICE. 1965. Further observations on geographic variation in the antigenic character of West Nile and Japanese B Viruses. Am. J. Epidemiol **83**: 113–122.
10. BERTHET, F.X., H.G. ZELLER, M.T. DROUET, *et al.* 1997. Extensive nucleotide changes and deletions within the envelope glycoprotein gene of Euro-African West Nile viruses. J. Gen. Virol. **78**: 2293–2297.
11. SAVAGE, H.M., C. CEIANU, G. NICOLESCU, *et al.* 1999. Entomologic and avian investigations of an epidemic of West Nile fever in Romania in 1996, with serologic and molecular characterization of a virus isolate from mosquitoes. Am. J. Trop. Med. Hyg. **61**: 600–611.
12. LANCIOTTI, R.S., J.T. ROEHRIG, V. DEUBEL, *et al.* 1999. Origin of the West Nile virus responsible for an outbreak of encephalitis in the northeastern United States. Science **286**: 2333–2337.
13. PLATONOV, A.E., G.A. SHIPULIN, O.Y. SHIPULINA, *et al.* 2001. Outbreak of West Nile virus infection, Volgograd Region, Russia, 1999. Emerg. Infect. Dis. **7**: 128–132.
14. PHILIP, C.B. & J.E. SMADEL. 1943. Transmission of West Nile virus by Infected *Aedes albopictus*. Proc. Soc. Exp. Biol. Med. **53**: 49–50.
15. KITAOKA, M. 1950. Experimental transmission of the West Nile virus by the mosquito. Jpn. J. Med. **3**: 77–81.
16. TAYLOR, R.M. & H.S. HURLBUT. 1953. Isolation of West Nile virus from *Culex* mosquitoes. J. R. Egyptian Med. Assoc. **36**: 199–208.
17. TAYLOR, R.M., T.H. WORK, H.S. HURLBUT, *et al.* 1956. A study of the ecology of West Nile virus in Egypt. Am. J. Trop. Med. Hyg. **5**(4): 579–620.
18. MCINTOSH, B.M., P.G. JUPP, D.B. DICKINSON, *et al.* 1967. Ecological studies on Sindbis and West Nile viruses in South Africa. I. Viral activity as revealed by infection of mosquitoes and sentinel fowls. S. Afr. J. Med. Sci. **32**: 1–14.
19. NIR, Y., R. GOLDWASSER, Y. LASOWSKI, *et al.* 1968. Isolation of West Nile virus strains from mosquitoes in Israel. Am. J. Epidemiol. **87**: 496–501.
20. HANNOUN, C., R. PANTHER, J. MOUCHET, *et al.* 1964. Isolement en France du virus West Nile a partir de malades et du vecteur *Culex modestus* Ficalbi. C.R. Acad. Sci. Paris **259**: 4170–4172.
21. DANDAWATE, C.N., P.K. RAJAGOPALAN, K.M. PAVRI, *et al.* 1969. Virus isolations from mosquitoes collected in North Arcot district, Madras state, and Chittoor district, Andhra Pradesh between November 1955 and October 1957. Indian J. Med. Res. **57**: 1420–1426.
22. HAYES, C.G. & M.I. BURNEY. 1981. Arboviruses of public health importance in Pakistan. J. Pakistan Med. Assoc. **31**: 16–26.
23. CDC. 1999. Weekly update: West Nile virus encephalitis—New York, 1999. Morb. Mortal. Wkly. Rep. **48**: 944–947.

24. CDC. 2000. Weekly update: West Nile virus activity—Northeastern United States, 2000. Morb. Mortal. Wkly. Rep. **49:** 820–822.
25. TURELL, M.J., M. O'GUINN & J. OLIVER. 2000. Potential for New York mosquitoes to transmit West Nile virus. Am. J. Trop. Med. Hyg. **62:** 413–414.
26. HURLBUT, H.S. 1956. West Nile virus infection in arthropods. Am. J. Trop. Med. Hyg. **5:** 76–85.
27. TAHORI, A.S., V.V. STERK & N. GOLDBLUM. 1955. Studies on the dynamics of experimental transmission of West Nile virus by *Culex molestus*. Am. J. Trop. Med. Hyg. **4:** 1015–1027.
28. JUPP, P.G. 1976. The susceptibility of four South African species of *Culex* to West Nile and Sindbis viruses by two different infecting methods. Mosquito News **36:** 166–173.
29. CDC. 2000. Notice to readers: update: West Nile virus isolated from mosquitoes—New York, 2000. Morb. Mortal. Wkly. Rep. **49:** 211.
30. CDC. 2000. Weekly update: West Nile virus activity—Eastern United States, 2000. Morb. Mortal. Wkly. Rep. **49:** 1044–1047.
31. SMITHBURN, K.C. & H.R. JACOBS. 1942. Neutralization-tests against neurotropic viruses with sera collected in central Africa. J. Immunol. **44:** 9–23.
32. GOLDBLUM, N., V.V. STERK & W. JASINSKA-KLINGBERG. 1957. The natural history of West Nile fever II. Virological findings and the development of homologous and heterologous antibodies in West Nile infection in man. Am. J. Hyg. **66:** 363–380.
33. SOUTHAM, C.M. & A.E. MOORE. 1954. Induced virus infections in man by the Egypt isolates of West Nile virus. Am. J. Trop. Med. Hyg. **3:** 19–50.
34. WORK, T.H., H.S. HURLBUT & R.M. TAYLOR. 1955. Indigenous wild birds of the Nile Delta as potential West Nile virus circulating reservoirs. Am. J. Trop. Med. Hyg. **4:** 872–888.
35. NIR, Y., R. GOLDWASSER, Y. LASOWSKI, *et al.* 1966. Isolation of arboviruses from wild birds in Israel. Am. J. Epidemiol. **86:** 372–378.
36. MCINTOSH, B.M., G.M. MCGILLIVRAY, D.B. DICKINSON, *et al.* 1968. Ecological studies on Sindbis and West Nile viruses in South Africa. IV. Infection in a wild avian population. S. Afr. J. Med. Sci. **33:** 105–112.
37. NIR, Y., Y. LASOWSKI, A. AVIVI, *et al.* 1969. Survey for antibodies to arboviruses in the serum of various animals in Israel during 1965–1966. Am. J. Trop. Med. Hyg. **18:** 416–422.
38. GHOSH, S.N., P.K. RAJAGOPALAN, G.K. SINGH, *et al.* 1975. Serological evidence of arbovirus activity in birds of KFD epizootic–epidemic area, Shimoga District, Karnataka, India. Indian J. Med. Res. **63:** 1327–1334.
39. HAYES, C.G., S. BAQAR, T. AHMED, *et al.* 1982. West Nile virus in Pakistan. 1. Seroepidemiological studies in Punjab province. Trans. R. Soc. Trop. Med. Hyg. **76:** 431–436.
40. MCINTOSH, B.M., P.G. JUPP, I. DOS SANTOS, *et al.* 1976. Epidemics of West Nile and Sindbis viruses in South Africa with *Culex (Culex) univittatus* Theobald as vector. S. Afr. J. Sci. **72:** 295–300.
41. MCINTOSH, B.M., D.B. DICKINSON & G.M. MCGILLIVRAY. 1969. Ecological studies on Sindbis and West Nile viruses in South Africa v. the response of birds to inoculation of virus. S. Afr. J. Med. Sci. **34:** 77–82.
42. SCHMIDT, J.R. & H.K. MANSOURY. 1963. Natural and experimental infection of Egyptian equines with West Nile virus. Ann. Trop. Med. Parasitol. **57:** 415–427.
43. MCINTOSH, B.M. 1961. Susceptibility of some African wild rodents to infection with various arthropod-borne viruses. R. Soc. Trop. Med. Hyg. **55:** 63–68.
44. HANNOUN, C., R. PANTHIER & B. CORNIOU. 1969. Epidemiology of West Nile infections in the south of France. Institute Pasteur Paris: 379–387.
45. RODHAIN, F., J.J. PETTER, R. ALBIGNAC, *et al.* 1985. Arboviruses and lemurs in Madagascar: experimental infection of *Lemur fulvus* with yellow fever and West Nile viruses. Am. J. Trop. Med. Hyg. **34:** 816–822.
46. BLACKBURN, N.K., F. REYERS, W.L. BERRY, *et al.* 1989. Susceptibility of dogs to West Nile virus: a survey and pathogenicity trial. J. Comp. Pathol. **100:** 59–66.
47. TSAI, T.F., F. POPOVICI, C. CERNESCU, *et al.* 1998. West Nile encephalitis epidemic in southeastern Romania. Lancet **352:** 767–771.

48. GARMENDIA, A.E., H.J. VAN KRUININGEN, R.A. FRENCH, *et al.* 2000. Recovery and identification of West Nile virus from a hawk in winter. J. Clin. Microbiol. **38:** 3110–3111.
49. KLINGBERG, M.A., W. JASINSKA-KLINGBERG & N. GOLDBLUM. 1959. Certain aspects of the epidemiology and distribution of immunity of West Nile virus in Israel. Proc. 6th Int. Cong. Trop. Med. Malaria **5:** 132–140.
50. BERNKOPF, H., S. LEVINE & R. NERSON. 1953. Isolation of West Nile virus in Israel. J. Infect. Dis. **93:** 207–218.
51. MARBERG, K., N. GOLDBLUM, V.V. STERK, *et al.* 1956. The natural history of West Nile fever. I. Clinical observations during an epidemic in Israel. Am. J. Hygiene **64:** 259–269.
52. SPIGLAND, W., W. JASINSKA-KLINGBERG, E. HOFSHI, *et al.* 1958. Clinical and laboratory observations in an outbreak of West Nile fever in Israel. Harefuah **54:** 275–281.
53. GEORGE, S., M. GOURIE-DEVI, J.A. RAO, *et al.* 1984. Isolation of West Nile virus from the brains of children who had died of encephalitis. Bull. W. H. O. **62:** 879–882.
54. GEORGES, A.J., J.L. LESBORDES, M.C. GEORGES-COURBOT, *et al.* 1987. Fatal hepatitis from West Nile virus. Ann. Inst. Pasteur/Virol. **138:** 237–244.
55. CDC. 2001. Weekly update: serosurveys for West Nile virus infections—New York and Connecticut counties, 2000. Morb. Mortal. Wkly. Rep. **50:** 37–39.
56. ASNIS, D.S., R. CONETTA, A.A. TEIXEIRA, *et al.* 2000. The West Nile virus outbreak of 1999 in New York: the Flushing Hospital experience. Clin. Infect. Dis. **30:** 413–418.
57. AHMED, S., R. LIBMAN, K. WESSON, *et al.* 2000. Guillain-Barré syndrome: an unusual presentation of West Nile virus infection. Neurology **55:** 144–146.
58. CEAUSU, E., S. ERSCOIU, P. CALISTRU, *et al.* 1997. Cinical manifestations in the West Nile virus outbreak. Rom. J. Virol. **48:** 3–11.
59. GADOTH, N., S. WEITZMAN & E.E. LEHMANN. 1979. Acute anterior myelitis complicating West Nile fever. Arch. Neurol. **36:** 172–173.
60. STEELE, K.E., M.J. LINN, R.J. SCHOEPP, *et al.* 2000. Pathology of fatal West Nile virus infections in native and exotic birds during the 1999 outbreak in New York City, New York. Vet. Pathol. **37:** 208–224.
61. USDA. 1999. Summary of West Nile virus in the United States—Animal and Plant Health Inspection Service Report: 1–6.
62. USDA. 2001. Update on the current status of West Nile virus—Animal and Plant Health Inspection Service Report: 1–10.
63. NIR, Y., R. GOLDWASSER, Y. LASOWSKI, *et al.* 1967. Isolation of arboviruses from wild birds in Israel. Am. J. Epidemiol. **86:** 372–378.
64. JUPP, P.G. & B.M. MCINTOSH. 1967. Ecological studies on Sindbis and West Nile viruses in South Africa. II. Mosquito bionomics. S. Afr. J. Med. Sci. **32:** 15–33.
65. RAPPOLE, J.H., S.R. DERRICKSON & Z. HUBALEK. 2000. Migratory birds and spread of West Nile virus in the Western Hemisphere. Emerg. Infect. Dis. **6:** 319–328.
66. HAN, L.L., F. POPOVICI, J.P. ALEXANDER JR., *et al.* 1999. Risk factors for West Nile virus infection and meningoencephalitis, Romania, 1996. J. Infect. Dis. **179:** 230–233.

"Neon Needles" in a Haystack

The Advantages of Passive Surveillance for West Nile Virus

MILLICENT EIDSON

Zoonoses Program, New York State Department of Health, Albany, New York 11237, USA

ABSTRACT: Passive surveillance is usually viewed as less efficient for case ascertainment than active surveillance. However, for diseases with nonhuman animal reservoirs, active surveillance can be like looking for a needle in a haystack and may be prohibitively expensive. Fortunately for surveillance of West Nile virus (WNV) in the northeast US, the dead crows have served as "neon needles in a haystack"—indicators of viral activity that call attention to themselves. In 2000, laboratory testing of dead birds, including all species, birds found singly, with signs of trauma, or no compatible pathology, provided the first confirmation of viral activity in most areas. The surveillance factor most closely associated with the number of human cases was the dead crow density. In 2001, dead crow densities will be used as an additional index for monitoring human risk and need for prevention and control activities. If there are few crows in an area, if their case-fatality rate is reduced, or if there is public complacency about reporting dead crow sightings, this passive surveillance indicator may not be helpful in identifying areas likely to have occasional human cases or an outbreak.

KEYWORDS: West Nile virus; epidemiology; surveillance; arbovirus; rabies

West Nile virus (WNV) and rabies are both viral diseases with animal reservoirs that circulate in the environment with infrequent spillover to humans. Thus viral activity is largely hidden from public view, unless specific surveillance systems are developed to detect it. In both diseases, the occasional human clinical cases represent the tip-of-the-iceberg for infection and serve as a reminder of the diseases' continuing presence. Because these are encephalitic infections in humans, with an estimated case fatality rate of 11% for WNV (in the United States)[1,2] and nearly 100% for rabies, prediction of human risk and development of prevention measures are critically important.

New York State (NYS) leads the nation with the highest number of identified WNV and rabies infections.[1,3] Since 1990 there have been three human rabies deaths in the state,[4–6] and eight deaths from WNV in 1999 and 2000.[1,2] Without costly prevention and control programs for both diseases, these mortality rates could be much higher. Thus it is critical to identify which areas of NYS (and the US) are at the great-

Address for correspondence: Millicent Eidson, Zoonoses Program, New York State Department of Health, Albany, New York 12237. Voice: 518-474-3186; fax: 518-473-6590.
mxe04@health.state.ny.us

est risk of human cases in order to prioritize scarce public health prevention resources.

This summary reviews some "lessons learned" about surveillance for WNV since its introduction into NYS and the Western Hemisphere in 1999, in reference to the perspective gained from the state's much longer experience with another zoonotic virus, rabies.

TYPES OF SURVEILLANCE

Public health surveillance programs can be characterized as one of four types: passive, active, sentinel, and special.[7] Passive systems rely on receipt of reports by public health agencies, rather than active efforts to obtain reports or specimens for laboratory testing. Sentinel systems use a sample of providers, or in the case of arboviruses, a sample of birds, to provide an indication of the disease occurrence. Special systems involve special focused studies, for example, special surveys to gather disease data. In general, passive systems are viewed as the most feasible and economical disease surveillance systems, but at the cost of lower case ascertainment. As a general rule, it is believed that active surveillance provides a better view of disease occurrence if there are sufficient resources for its implementation.

However, these generalizations do not appear to be applicable for relatively rare zoonotic diseases like rabies and WNV. If the disease is hidden in the animal population and occurs in only a few animals or vector species such as mosquitoes (like "needles in a haystack"), active surveillance will have to be extraordinarily thorough and extensive to find the few positives. This applies also to sentinel systems, such as sentinel birds for arboviruses. Even if the sentinel bird species is a reservoir species for the virus, the number of birds and the variety of placements would have to be huge to detect a rare virus. In addition, if the active surveillance system is for laboratory-confirmed infections to meet a specific clinical case definition, disease detection will be inherently delayed during the time for specimen collection, processing, testing, and reporting of results. Thus the number of samples to be taken and the resources for determining disease status can be cost prohibitive.

WNV-POSITIVE BIRDS

Value of Testing

A major component of New York State's dead bird surveillance system for WNV was necropsy evaluation and laboratory testing. In 1999, NYS reported 142 WNV-positive birds from all five New York City (NYC) boroughs and four surrounding counties.[8] These positives and the additional 78 WNV-positive birds from New Jersey and 75 WNV-positive birds from Connecticut represented 20 different avian species, but 89% of the positive birds were American crows.[8] In 2000, NYS reported 1263 WNV-positive birds from 61 of the state's 62 counties, including all five NYC boroughs,[9] representing 63 different avian species.[10]

Dead bird surveillance provided the first laboratory confirmation of the introduction of WNV to the US in 1999[11,12] and the first genomic sequencing of the virus.[13]

Compared to other surveillance systems, dead bird surveillance provided the earliest laboratory confirmation of viral activity in most of the state. Of the 61 NYS counties with laboratory-confirmed viral activity, all but one had this confirmation first with WNV-positive dead birds (the other county had viral activity first confirmed by WNV-positive mosquitoes).

In most of the state, WNV-positive dead birds also provided the only confirmation of viral activity, because WNV-positive mosquitoes were detected only in NYC and the six counties near NYC or in the lower Hudson River valley.[14] Although final analyses are still ongoing, NYS also reported very few WNV-positive sentinel chickens and mammals. Twenty case horses were reported in 1999 and twenty-three in 2000 from NYS,[15] but these cases occurred late in the transmission season and did not provide an early indication or the only indication of WNV in any NYS county.

We cannot be certain whether the date of detection for the first WNV-positive bird indicates with any precision the date of introduction of the virus to an area. Those areas with more infected birds may be more likely to have them reported and submitted for testing, so areas with more infected birds may have viral activity detected earlier than areas with fewer infected birds, even though the virus arrived in the areas at the same time. As indicated in FIGURE 1A, in 2000 WNV-positive birds were first detected in the areas with viral activity in 1999 (townships with darker coloration on the map, in and around NYC). Based on the dates the first WNV-positive bird was found, the virus appeared to spread first north along the Hudson River valley and then west along the Mohawk River valley to the Finger Lakes in central NYS and the Great Lakes on its western border (as indicated by lighter coloration on the map for the townships with WNV-positive birds first found later in the year). Although WNV-positive birds were frequently found in townships with waterways, those are also the areas of human settlement in NYS with the highest population densities (darker colored townships in FIG. 1C). In comparing two areas with similar viral activity, the area with the higher population density may be more likely to have dead birds reported and submitted for testing.

Which Birds to Test

Laboratory testing of dead birds for WNV is a surveillance system with both passive and active components. Most of the birds collected for testing were reported via a passive reporting system of their sightings by the public to local health agencies. However, active efforts and decision making are required to determine whether to pick up the dead bird for possible testing, to submit the bird for necropsy, to conduct the necropsy, to decide whether the bird is a priority for sample submission for WNV testing, and to complete laboratory testing. In NYS, birds were prioritized for evaluation and testing, although there were no absolute indications against possible submissions. Thus, analyses of possible submission criteria could be made with the 2000 data. The ultimate choice about submission criteria will depend on whether the surveillance needs to be sensitive (for example, for early verification of viral activity in each new mosquito season in order to rapidly mobilize appropriate prevention and control activities) or specific (for example, to conserve on laboratory resources especially later in the mosquito season after viral activity has already been confirmed).

Initially, NYS and other jurisdictions were concerned about being overwhelmed with dead birds for processing and WNV testing and thus established restrictions

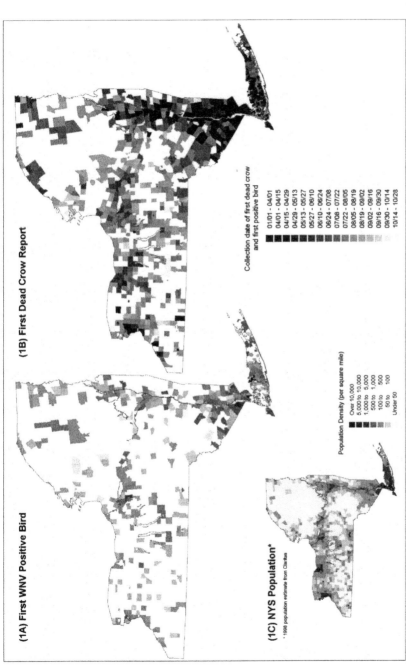

FIGURE 1. West Nile virus, New York State, 2000. (A) Date first WNV-positive bird was found, by township or zip code. (B) Date first dead crow found for those reported, by township or zip code. (C) NYS population density (per square mile). (NOTE: Information is noted by township in all counties except in New York City and Nassau and Suffolk counties, where information is noted by zip code.)

based on the number of dead birds reported from an area. Specifically, in 1999 to submit dead birds for WNV testing, NYS required two or more birds to be found within one mile of each other within 72 hours. However, none of the WNV-positive birds in 2000 were part of a reported large group die-off, and there were only 13 pairs of positive birds (two positive birds, same general location, same date). Thus, it appears that even with large numbers of birds dying and confirmed in specific areas, WNV has not yet been documented to cause mass die-offs of birds at a single time and place.

Birds were initially also excluded for submission if showing causes of death, including trauma. The purpose of this exclusion was to avoid using up necropsy and testing resources on tests of birds that died of causes other than WNV. However, in 2000, 38% of the WNV-positive birds in NYS had evidence of trauma on necropsy. In hindsight, it is understandable that birds with an encephalitic disease would fly into buildings, or walk on roads to be hit by cars, or behave erratically and come to the attention of hunters.

Also to maximize testing resources, selecting only those birds with characteristic signs on necropsy[16] could be considered a reasonable strategy. However, in an analysis of NYS dead bird submissions in 2000 prior to the onset date of the first positive human case (July 20, 2000), the sensitivity of gross pathology results for WNV-positivity was only 40%.[17] The positive predictive value (proportion of those birds with pathologic indications that tested WNV-positive) was also low (27.9%). The specificity was higher, with 90.3% of WNV-negative birds having no gross pathologic indications of WNV, and the negative predictive value for necropsy evaluation was 85.3%. In the time period after human cases began to occur, the sensitivity of the pathologic exam increased to 68%, and was 79% for American crows. The positive predictive value increased to 55.1%, and the negative predictive value decreased to 73.9%. The specificity decreased to 62.1%.[17]

A final important factor to consider in determining the birds to submit for WNV testing is species. Although two-thirds of the WNV-positive birds in NYS in 2000 were American crows, they represented the first WNV-positive bird species in only 30 of the 61 counties with WNV-positive birds. Corvids (including fish crows and blue jays) represented the first WNV-positive bird species in 39 of the 61 counties.[17] If only American crows had been tested, this would have led to a delay of days to weeks in confirmation of viral activity in those counties. Even more important, 15 of the counties never had positive American crows (nor any WNV-positive mosquitoes or mammals) and would have concluded that they were not at risk for WNV in 2000 if other species of birds had not been tested for WNV.[17] Of these counties, all but three submitted crows for testing, but they were negative for WNV, so detection occurred only in other species.

Based on these analyses on 2000 dead bird testing data, NYS in 2001 is continuing to test all species of birds, although American crows have a priority for testing resources. NYS is also not excluding birds because they were found singly, showed evidence of trauma, or were negative for compatible signs on a gross pathologic exam. These policies are particularly critical early in the transmission season when it is important to verify viral activity as soon as possible to focus prevention and control efforts. Once viral activity has been confirmed in an area, limitations in testing resources may require more specific and less sensitive triage requirements, such as a reduction in number of submissions and a greater focus on American crows and birds with pathologic indications of WNV.

DEAD CROW SIGHTINGS

Forecasting of Human Cases

Although WNV testing of dead birds was found to be the optimal method for early confirmation of viral presence in NYS in 1999 and 2000, the outbreak of human WNV cases was not distributed statewide, as the WNV-positive birds were. In addition, for the areas of NYS, New Jersey, and Connecticut with human cases, confirmation of viral activity was not universally received in time to prevent onset of the human cases, owing to the inherent time required for dead bird collection, processing, testing, and reporting results. These findings raise questions about whether there are any circumstances in which human risk is lower and there is less need for expensive surveillance, prevention, and control activities, and whether there is any component of existing dead bird surveillance systems that could help forecast human case risk.

In addition to recording reports of birds submitted for WNV testing, NYS also recorded reports of dead bird sightings in which the birds were not collected for possible WNV testing. In 1999, 17,339 dead birds were reported after surveillance was established at the end of September, with dates the birds were found ranging from May 1 to November 30. A third (5697) of the ill or dead birds sighted were crows.[8] In 2000, when the state used a real-time web-based reporting system for data entry at the local level,[18] there were 71,332 sightings of ill or dead birds reported, with one-quarter of them (17,571) being American crows.[17]

Dead birds of species other than American crows, with a much smaller proportion testing positive for WNV, were a much less specific indicator of the possible presence of the virus. Thus, for an early index of possible WNV activity, dead crow sightings were examined. Townships in NYS in 2000 reported their first dead crow sighting many weeks earlier (darker coloration in Fig. 1B) compared to viral confirmation (lighter coloration for same townships in Fig. 1A), and the dead crow sightings provide the same pattern for the spread of WNV throughout the state as the WNV-positive birds. Dead crow sightings have the same limitations as tested birds in the reliance on the public to see and report them, perhaps partially accounting for the observed relationship between the sightings (Fig. 1B) and human population density (Fig. 1C).

Various dead bird surveillance factors were assessed for their correlations with the number of human WNV cases by county (TABLE 1). The number of human cases were high in Staten Island (10), moderate (0–2) in areas of the state with viral activity both in 1999 and 2000 (the other boroughs of NYC and the four counties immediately to the east and north of NYC), and low (0) in upstate New York. For WNV-positive birds, both the number of positive birds per square mile and the proportion of birds testing positive were significantly correlated ($P < 0.01$) with the number of human cases by county. However, these factors were not consistently associated with the number of human cases. For the dead bird sightings (TABLE 1), the number of dead birds sighted and the number of dead birds sighted per 100,000 population were

TABLE 1. Associations between number of human WNV cases and dead bird surveillance factors by county/region, New York State, 2000

	Human cases	Cases/ 100,000	Number of positive birds			Number of dead birds sighted		
			All spp.	Am. crow	Corvid^c	All spp.	Am. crow	Corvid^c
Staten Island	10	2.42	60	45	51	5258	1967	2131
Brooklyn	2	0.09	38	35	37	3460	826	869
Manhattan	1	0.06	37	29	30	1577	202	238
Queens	1	0.05	29	15	20	5362	671	796
North^a	0	0	120	92	111	4601	1197	1513
East^a	0	0	149	133	146	10,170	3550	4046
Upstate^a	0	0	8	3	5	406	61	82
Correlation^b			0.13	0.13	0.12	0.28^e	0.28^e	0.26^e

	Human cases	Cases/ 100,000	Number of positive birds per square mile^d			Number of dead birds sighted per square mile^d		
			All spp.	Am. crow	Corvid^c	All spp.	Am. crow	Corvid^c
Staten Island	10	2.42	1.02	0.76	0.86	89.12	33.34	36.12
Brooklyn	2	0.09	0.54	0.49	0.52	48.73	11.63	12.24
Manhattan	1	0.06	1.32	1.04	1.07	56.32	7.21	8.50
Queens	1	0.05	0.27	0.14	0.18	49.19	6.16	7.30
North^a	0	0	0.55	0.43	0.51	21.27	5.53	6.99
East^a	0	0	0.25	0.22	0.24	16.98	5.93	6.75
Upstate^a	0	0	0.01	<0.01	0.01	0.48	0.07	0.10
Correlation^b			0.50^f	0.48^f	0.47^f	0.76^f	0.92^f	0.90^f

	Human cases	Cases/ 100,000	Number of positive birds/ 100,000 human population^d			Number of dead birds sighted/ 100,000 human population^d		
			All spp.	Am. crow	Corvid^c	All spp.	Am. crow	Corvid^c
Staten Island	10	2.42	14.52	10.89	12.34	1272.26	475.95	515.63
Brooklyn	2	0.09	1.68	1.54	1.63	152.54	36.42	38.31
Manhattan	1	0.06	2.38	1.87	1.93	101.62	13.02	15.34
Queens	1	0.05	1.45	0.75	1.00	268.01	33.54	39.79
North^a	0	0	15.06	11.62	14.01	579.06	150.69	190.38
East^a	0	0	11.08	9.89	10.86	756.44	264.01	300.90
Upstate^a	0	0	6.42	2.60	3.70	312.51	46.65	63.08
Correlation^b			0.02	0.07	0.06	0.37^f	0.48^f	0.43^f

	Human cases	Cases/ 100,000	Proportion of birds testing positive			Proportion of dead birds sighted	
			All spp.	Am. crow	Corvid^c	Am. crow	Corvid^c
Staten Island	10	2.42	0.58	0.87	0.84	0.37	0.41
Brooklyn	2	0.09	0.43	0.69	0.70	0.24	0.25
Manhattan	1	0.06	0.49	0.85	0.86	0.13	0.15
Queens	1	0.05	0.22	0.54	0.53	0.13	0.15
North^a	0	0	0.46	0.57	0.52	0.26	0.33
East^a	0	0	0.50	0.63	0.58	0.35	0.40
Upstate^a	0	0	0.20	0.19	0.20	0.15	0.20
Correlation^b			0.31^e	0.43^f	0.40^f	0.19	0.14

[a] North: average of counties without WNV human cases in and north of New York City (Bronx, Rockland, Westchester). East: average of counties east of NYC (Nassau, Suffolk). Upstate: average of upstate counties ($n = 53$).

[b] Pearson correlation with the number of human WNV cases by county ($n = 62$, except for proportion of birds testing positive for American crow ($n = 59$) and for corvid ($n = 61$)).

[c] Corvid: American crow, fish crow, and bluejay.

[d] 1990 census land area data and 1999 census population estimate.

[e] $P < 0.05$

[f] $P < 0.01$

significantly ($P<0.05$ and $P<0.01$, respectively) correlated with the number of human cases by county, but these factors also did not consistently separate the state into three areas of risk. The dead bird surveillance factor most strongly associated ($r=0.92$) with the number of human cases was the number of dead crow sightings per square mile, or dead crow density (the total number of dead crow sightings for the county divided by the square mile size of the county).[9]

Although total dead crow density for 2000 was strongly associated with the total number of human cases, to be useful for forecasting human cases, a relationship must be demonstrated between surveillance factors and the number of human cases in real time. It is critical that the surveillance factors used for forecasting the number of human cases successfully provide an indication of risk prior to the human case onset in time for prevention and control activities to be undertaken. It is also important that such surveillance factors do not falsely forecast human cases so that control expenditures are incurred without sufficient gain. Thus in addition to examining the overall relationship between various dead bird surveillance factors and the number of human cases by county, the surveillance factors with the highest correlations with human cases for the year were graphed by week to examine their relationship to the onset of the human cases. Again, the only dead bird surveillance factor that appeared to clearly distinguish between areas with different numbers of human cases was the dead crow density.[9]

Weekly dead crow densities appeared to divide NYS into three clearly distinct areas (FIG. 2). The highest weekly dead crow density level ever reached by an upstate county with viral activity only in 2000 was 0.1 for Monroe County. The highest

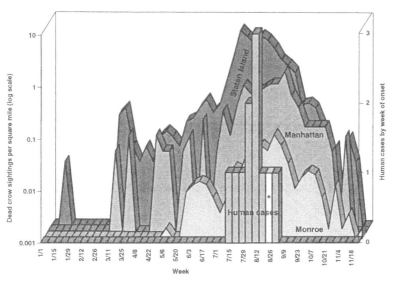

* Only human case in Manhattan, all others in this figure were in Staten Island.

FIGURE 2. Weekly number of dead crow sightings per square mile (dead crow density) [log scale] for highest representative three counties (Staten Island > 1.5; Manhattan < 1.3; and Monroe, < 0.1) and the human cases (based on onset week) for those counties.

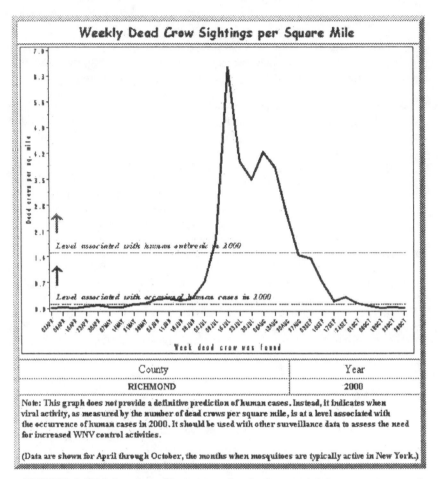

FIGURE 3. Web-based tracking system for dead crow sightings per square mile
(dead crow density), NYS, 2001. (A) Real-time automated graph of dead crow densities per
week, per county.

weekly dead crow density level ever reached by counties or NYC boroughs surrounding Staten Island was 1.25 for Manhattan. Staten Island's dead crow density
level began to rise above this level approximately two weeks before the appearance
of their first human case. The increase in dead crow densities in Staten Island preceded confirmation of viral activity with a WNV-positive bird or any special public-
ity about WNV, although the peak in dead crow densities occurred in the same week
that the first WNV-positive bird was reported and the media released information on
a false-positive human case. [9]

It remains to be determined whether increased dead crow densities will be found
prior to human case onset in other years or other geographic areas. However, in order

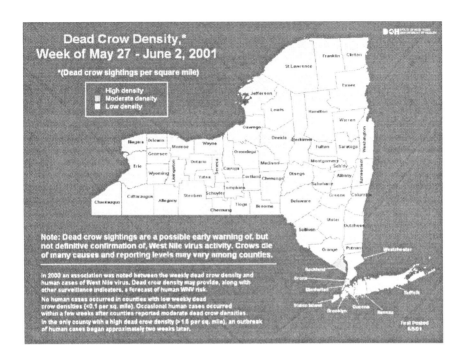

FIGURE 3. (B) Weekly updated summary map of dead crow densities for each county for public website.

to assist local health agencies in their planning and control prioritization, real-time automated graphs of weekly dead crow densities have been developed for all NYS counties to use in their decision making in 2001. An example, with Staten Island (Richmond County) data in 2000, is provided in FIGURE 3A. This graph is automatically generated for each county by the dead crow sightings that the local health agencies enter on the state's web-based information interchange for WNV reporting.[18] For the state's public WNV website (www.health.state.ny.us), in addition to a summary map used in 2000 to provide the results of WNV testing, a similar map has been developed for 2001 to summarize the prior week's dead crow densities (FIG. 3B). Both the weekly dead crow density graphs for the internal state–local web-based interchange and the dead crow density map for the public website include a warning that dead crow densities do not provide a definitive prediction of human cases, but instead provide an indication when viral activity and other risk factors are at a level associated with the occurrence of human cases in 2000. A weekly dead crow density monitoring system should be used with other WNV surveillance data to determine the need for increased WNV education, prevention, and control activities. However, the 2000 data in NYS indicate that if control activities are delayed until increasing dead crow densities are verified by viral confirmation, it may be too late to prevent onset of the initial human cases.[9]

Assessment of Control Efficacy

The bottom-line indication of whether prevention and control efforts for WNV have been beneficial is whether human cases occur. In addition to prevention and control activities directed to human behavior and self-protective measures, a number of mosquito control options are available, including cleanup of breeding sites and use of chemicals to kill mosquito larvae (larviciding) or adult mosquitoes (adulticiding). In order to help assess the balance between a need to control mosquitoes to prevent WNV in humans and domestic animals and concerns about the effects of chemicals in the environment, measures of mosquito control efficacy would be helpful. Logically, the ideal measures will include systematic assessments of mosquito counts before and after various control measures. However, in the face of a WNV outbreak, identifying and prioritizing sufficient resources for such systematic mosquito sampling may not be feasible. If dead bird surveillance information is already being collected as part of an early warning for viral activity and possible forecasting of human cases, can such information also be useful for providing insights into control efficacy? If control measures are successful in reducing the number of mosquitoes, the number of infected and dead crows should be reduced. Although it is not known when precisely we might expect to see such an effect, because the time between infection and death for WNV in American crows is believed to be relatively short, on the order of a few days to a week,[19] such reductions in dead crow sightings might be expected to be seen within a week or two after a control measure is applied, such as adulticiding.

To begin an examination of the usefulness of dead crow densities for providing insights into adulticide efficacy, spray dates and dead crow densities were graphed for two townships in Rockland County (FIG. 4A) and two areas of contiguous zip codes in Staten Island (FIG. 4B). The number of nights within the week in which temperatures reached below 50°F are also indicated, as an index for climatic conditions that may discourage mosquito activity and thus decrease crow infections. For the areas examined, upward trends of dead crow densities appear to be reversed after adulticide use. However, between adulticide applications, dead crow densities sometimes rebounded. Frequent repeated sprayings used in Staten Island appear to be associated with reductions in dead crow densities. As expected, dead crow densities decreased when colder weather developed in mid- to late-September.

A problem in interpreting cause and effect between the adulticide applications and decreases in dead crow densities is the possibility of other factors systematically influencing the dead crow densities. Ideally, these dead crow density patterns in sprayed areas would be compared with counties that did not spray. However, there are no counties with a similar level of dead crow densities that did not use adulticide at some point in 2000. Thus, these initial graphs of dead crow densities and adulticide use in 2000 provide some indication that dead crow densities may provide an economical crude index of control success, but not a definitive method for assessment compared to more costly rigorously designed mosquito studies. Although monitoring dead crow densities may not provide a precise measure of control success owing to other unidentified factors influencing the reporting of dead crows, an area that continues to see steep rises in dead crow densities, despite extensive control efforts, may need to reevaluate the effectiveness of those control efforts.

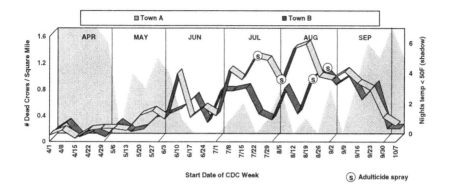

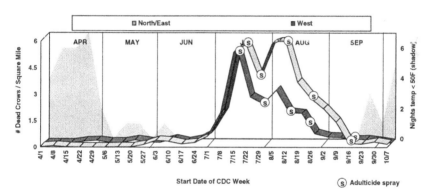

FIGURE 4. Weekly number of dead crow sightings per square mile (dead crow density) by number of nights with colder temperatures (<50°F) and adulticide use, NYS, 2000. (**A**) Two townships in Rockland County; (**B**) groups of zip codes in Staten Island.

SUMMARY

Dead bird surveillance for WNV is a surveillance system with both active and passive surveillance components. The active surveillance aspects of collecting dead birds for WNV testing has been shown extremely beneficial for early verification of viral activity. Analyses in NYS indicate that to maximize early detection of WNV, birds of all species should be tested, and birds should not be excluded from testing because they are found singly, have trauma, or do not have signs of WNV on necropsy examination. Based on evidence from 1999 and 2000, once viral activity has been definitively verified in a new area or a new mosquito season, additional testing of dead birds is not required because viral activity appears to persist until the end of the mosquito season, except if the testing is needed for special studies or to maintain public attention on prevention and control activities. At that point to save on collection and laboratory resources, a more specific collection scheme is recommended that focuses only on American crows or corvids and perhaps requires additional factors for testing such as signs of WNV on necropsy examination.

However, most active surveillance systems are more costly to implement than passive systems. Bird testing relies on the passive component of public reporting of dead bird sightings and thus has appeared to be more efficacious in early viral detection than other more active surveillance systems such as mosquito or mammal testing. The reason for the unusual advantages of this passive dead bird sighting system for WNV is the high case fatality rate in American crows. The dead crows are serving as "neon needles in the haystack," allowing more cost-effective identification and verification of viral activity. In fact, weekly dead crow densities, a more clearly passive surveillance system than dead bird testing, was the surveillance factor most highly associated in 2000 with the number of human cases. Despite standard statewide recommendations for surveillance, it is impossible for these surveillance systems to be applied in precisely the same manner in all jurisdictions. In comparison to dead bird sightings, the testing system has inherently more delays and may be subject to even greater variabilities across jurisdictions, owing to the decision making process for making choices about specimen collection, processing, and testing.

With the retrospective analyses indicating that dead crow density may be particularly useful for forecasting the occurrence of human cases and possibly for crude monitoring of control efficacy in the New York area, it is critical that such monitoring systems be tested in real time for 2001. Several graphic and map summaries of data have been developed using New York's real-time web-based infrastructure for WNV surveillance that allows for timely local data entry of dead crow reports, statewide sharing and monitoring of data, and automatically generated reports of dead crow densities.

As indicated, using the passive reporting of dead crow sightings for WNV surveillance has several advantages. Passive surveillance systems are generally cheaper and less labor-intensive than active systems. There is no need to collect, process, or test specimens. There is no need to identify areas of viral activity for sampling—the dead crows "select" themselves, so there is a higher specificity for testing than if testing samples were identified in other ways. Because successful active surveillance requires research of the factors that influence success (such as the types of sentinel birds or cage placement), passive surveillance has the advantage that such research studies are not required before its implementation. Finally, the surveillance results, such as weekly dead crow densities, can be generated much more quickly in comparison to laboratory test results, which is particularly critical for a mosquito-borne disease with a relatively short incubation period that requires rapid interventions for control.

On the other hand, there are a number of factors that may limit the value of dead crow densities for passive surveillance of WNV. If the public does not know to report dead crows, or if there is not a system set up to receive such reports, this surveillance will not be effective. In addition, if there is a time lag between receipt of the report and data entry and analysis, identification of sharp increases in dead crow densities may be delayed, and interventions may be too late to prevent the initial human cases. Another problem is the inherent difficulty in explaining a surveillance system to the public that relies on sightings of dead crows rather than on laboratory testing. Restrictions on testing, such as individuals not being allowed to get "their" dead bird tested that was found in the yard or neighborhood, may reduce public interest in providing reports of dead bird sightings. Lack of good geolocating information for the reports (such as precise addresses, zip codes, or latitude/longitude coordinates) can make it difficult to interpret dead crow densities for specific areas. For areas newly infected with WNV, if there are low infection rates, the number of infected crows may be small and there will be inherent instability and difficulty in interpreting small numbers (e.g., one additional dead crow report in a week can make a huge difference in the dead crow densities, especially in small areas of a few square miles because of the small denominator).

One potential limitation to monitoring dead crow density is not knowing how to interpret it in very small areas (such as individual zip codes) or very big areas (such as a region). A large county in terms of geographic size, or a region, will need to have a huge number of dead crows in one particular area or a moderately high number of dead crows throughout the area in order for the overall dead crow density to reach levels of concern seen in 2000. On the other hand, dead crow densities can become extremely high in one small area like a single neighborhood or zip code (as occurred in 2000) without identification of a human case from that small area. Such focal differences in dead crow densities and viral activity may not be valuable for forecasting human cases owing to movement of people and birds within larger areas. These types of analyses will be enhanced by development of statistical cluster recognition techniques that do not require comparison of rates in artifically defined geographic areas such as zip codes, townships, counties, or states.

One frequently raised concern about the use of dead crows for monitoring human risk is the dependence of the surveillance system on having sufficient human population nearby to see and report them. This would be a problem if the dead crow densities were being used to compare the underlying viral activity in two areas with different human population densities. Even if they had the same level of viral activity, the area with the larger human population density would be more likely to receive dead crow reports and would then have a higher dead crow density and forecasted number of human cases. But this is not an issue if the purpose of the surveillance system is to forecast the number of human cases rather than an underlying statistical probability of risk for an individual, because the factor that is required for the surveillance system (people to see and report dead crows) is also required for human cases to occur (people to become infected and seriously ill through mosquito bites). Given the frequency of asymptomatic infections in humans, sparsely populated areas may be unlikely to have a large outbreak of human WNV cases and may always have lower dead crow densities. Thus if the goal is to forecast the actual occurrence of human cases with current case definitions requiring serious illness, as opposed to a theoretical probability of risk based on viral activity, the dependence on humans to see and report the dead crows may actually be one of the strengths of this passive surveillance system for forecasting human case risk (within the limitations listed above of the public knowing to report and having a system to receive and process the reports).

Two factors with potentially the greatest impact on the success of a dead crow surveillance system are biologic—no crows in an area or a reduced case fatality rate over time (no more neon needles in the haystack), and behavioral—a tendency towards complacency about health risks as they become more familiar. It takes effort on the part of members of the public to determine where to report a dead bird sighting and to do it. Thus it will become even more critical as the WNV hysteria wears off that public health agencies develop mechanisms to make dead crow reporting very easy. Systems that should be considered include web-based reporting, as used by the NYC Department of Health, and a central toll-free telephone hotline, as piloted by the USDA Wildlife Services in New York for 2001.

Rabies appears to be similar to WNV, with both diseases having a relatively low incidence in the general animal or vector population at large but critical public health impacts when there is spillover to humans and domestic animals. Thus, active surveillance methods can be hit-or-miss, and yield little about patterns of risk in a cost-effective and timely fashion. Random or systematic collection of trapped animals in an area, or bats in a cave or house, for rabies testing has been demonstrated less useful for determining the impact of rabies on an area than testing animals that present themselves with signs of rabies. Similarly, surveillance focused on the neon needles in the haystack (dead crows) appears to be of more value for timely surveillance of WNV than testing of other species that do not provide a ready-made indicator of infection with mortality. Active surveillance methods for WNV, including collection and testing of mosquitoes, mammals, and healthy birds (either wild-caught or sentinel flocks), may provide critical information about the maintenance and transmission of WNV in nature. Ultimately, it is hoped that such information will provide important insights into better WNV prevention and control. However, in the interim, local and state agencies wishing to use a less costly surrogate index for forecasting human cases are advised to emphasize reporting of dead crow sightings and timely data processing of such data to monitor dead crow densities.

ACKNOWLEDGMENTS

These conclusions are based on surveillance data reported by local health agencies, including J. Miller and staff of the New York City Department of Health and M. Anand and staff of the Rockland County Department of Health; bird necropsies conducted by W. Stone and staff of the New York State Department of Environmental Conservation's Wildlife Pathology Unit; laboratory testing conducted by L. Kramer and staff of the NYSDOH Wadsworth Center Arbovirus Laboratory and B. McLean and staff of the National Wildlife Health Center; analyses and mapping by Y. Hagiwara, L. Smith, and K. Schmit of NYSDOH's Zoonoses Program; data system development by I. Gotham and staff of NYSDOH; and surveillance plan conceptualization and development by P. Smith, B. Wallace, D. White, and A. Willsey of NYSDOH's Division of Epidemiology. C. Trimarchi, Wadsworth Center Rabies Laboratory, is acknowledged for rabies data and surveillance concepts.

This publication was supported in part by Cooperative Agreement Number U50/CCU212415 from the Centers for Disease Control and Prevention (CDC). Its contents are solely the responsibility of the authors and do not necessarily represent the official views of the CDC.

REFERENCES

1. CENTERS FOR DISEASE CONTROL AND PREVENTION. 2001. Human West Nile virus surveillance—Connecticut, New Jersey, and New York, 2000. Morb. Mortal. Wkly. Rep. **50:** 265–268.
2. NASH, D., F. MOSTASHARI, A. FINE, et al. & THE 1999 WEST NILE OUTBREAK RESPONSE WORKING GROUP. 2001. The outbreak of West Nile virus infection in the New York City area in 1999. N. Engl. J. Med. **344:** 1807–1814.
3. KREBS, J.W., C.E. RUPPRECHT & J.E. CHILDS. 2000. Rabies surveillance in the United States during 1999. J. Am.Vet. Med. Assoc. **217:** 1799–1811.
4. CENTERS FOR DISEASE CONTROL AND PREVENTION. 1993. Human rabies—New York, 1993. Morb. Mortal. Wkly. Rep. **42:** 799–806.
5. CENTERS FOR DISEASE CONTROL AND PREVENTION. 1996. Human rabies—Connecticut, 1995. Morb. Mortal. Wkly. Rep. **45:** 207–209.
6. CENTERS FOR DISEASE CONTROL AND PREVENTION. 2000. Human rabies—California, Georgia, Minnesota, New York, and Wisconsin, 2000. Morb. Mortal. Wkly. Rep. **49:** 1111–1115.
7. ISTRE, G. 1992. Disease surveillance at the state and local levels. *In* Public Health Surveillance. W.H. Halperin & E.L. Baker, Eds.: 45–49. Van Nostrand Reinhold. New York.
8. EIDSON, M., N. KOMAR, F. SORHAGE, et al. & THE WEST NILE VIRUS AVIAN MORTALITY SURVEILLANCE GROUP. 2001. Crow deaths as a sentinel surveillance system for West Nile virus in the Northeastern United States, 1999. Emerg. Infect. Dis. **7:** 615–620.
9. EIDSON, M., J. MILLER, L. KRAMER, et al. & THE WEST NILE VIRUS BIRD MORTALITY ANALYSIS GROUP. 2001. Dead crow densities and human cases of West Nile virus, New York State. Emerg. Infect. Dis. **7:** 662–664.
10. BERNARD, K.A., J.G. MAFFEI, S.A. JONES, et al. & THE NY STATE WNV SURVEILLANCE TEAM. 2001. Comparison of West Nile virus infection in birds and mosquitoes, New York State, 2000. Emerg. Infect. Dis. **7:** 679–685.
11. CENTERS FOR DISEASE CONTROL AND PREVENTION. 1999. Outbreak of West Nile-like viral encephalitis—New York, 1999. Morb. Mortal. Wkly. Rep. **48:** 845–849.
12. ANDERSON, J.F., T.G. ANDREADIS, C.R. VOSSBRINCK, et al. 1999. Isolation of West Nile virus from mosquitoes, crows, and a Cooper's hawk in Connecticut. Science **286:** 2331–2333.
13. LANCIOTTI, R.S., J.T. ROEHRIG, V. DEUBEL, et al. 1999. Origin of the West Nile virus responsible for an outbreak of encephalitis in the northeastern United States. Science **286:** 2333–2337.
14. WHITE, D.J., L.D. KRAMER, P.B. BACKENSON, et al. & THE STATEWIDE WEST NILE VIRUS RESPONSE TEAMS. 2001. Mosquito surveillance and polymerase chain reaction detection of West Nile virus, New York State. Emerg. Infect. Dis. **7:** 643–649.
15. TROCK, S.C., B.J. MEADE, A.L. GLASER, et al. 2001. West Nile virus outbreak among horses in New York State, 1999 and 2000. Emerg. Infect. Dis. **7:** 745–747.
16. STEELE, K.E., M.J. LINN, R.J. SCHOEPP, et al. 2000. Pathology of fatal West Nile virus infections in native and exotic birds during the 1999 outbreak in New York City, New York. Vet. Pathol. **37:** 208–224.
17. EIDSON, M., L. KRAMER, W. STONE, et al. & THE NEW YORK STATE WEST NILE VIRUS AVIAN SURVEILLANCE TEAM. 2001. Dead bird surveillance as an early warning system for West Nile virus. Emerg. Infect. Dis. **7:** 631–635.
18. GOTHAM, I.J., M. EIDSON, D.J. WHITE, et al. 2001. West Nile virus: A case study in how NY State health information infrastructure facilitates preparation and response to disease outbreaks. J. Pub. Hlth. Mgmt. Practice **7:** 79–89.
19. WORK, T.H., H.S. HURLBUT & R.M. TAYLOR. 1955. Indigenous wild birds of the Nile delta as potential West Nile virus circulating reservoirs. Am. J. Trop. Med. Hyg. **4:** 872–888.

West Nile Virus Transmission and Ecology in Birds

ROBERT G. McLEAN,[a] SONYA R. UBICO,[a] DOUGLAS E. DOCHERTY,[a]
WALLACE R. HANSEN,[a] LOUIS SILEO,[a] AND TRACEY S. McNAMARA[b]

[a]United States Geologic Survey, National Wildlife Health Center,
Madison, Wisconsin 53711, USA

[b]Wildlife Conservation Society, The Bronx, New York 10460, USA

ABSTRACT: The ecology of the strain of West Nile virus (WNV) introduced into
the United States in 1999 has similarities to the native flavivirus, St. Louis encephalitis (SLE) virus, but has unique features not observed with SLE virus or
with WNV in the old world. The primary route of transmission for most of the
arboviruses in North America is by mosquito, and infected native birds usually
do not suffer morbidity or mortality. An exception to this pattern is eastern
equine encephalitis virus, which has an alternate direct route of transmission
among nonnative birds, and some mortality of native bird species occurs. The
strain of WNV circulating in the northeastern United States is unique in that it
causes significant mortality in exotic and native bird species, especially in the
American crow (*Corvus brachyrhynchos*). Because of the lack of information on
the susceptibility and pathogenesis of WNV for this species, experimental studies were conducted at the USGS National Wildlife Health Center. In two separate studies, crows were inoculated with a 1999 New York strain of WNV, and
all experimentally infected crows died. In one of the studies, control crows in
regular contact with experimentally inoculated crows in the same room but not
inoculated with WNV succumbed to infection. The direct transmission between
crows was most likely by the oral route. Inoculated crows were viremic before
death, and high titers of virus were isolated from a variety of tissues. The significance of the experimental direct transmission among captive crows is unknown.

KEYWORDS: West Nile virus; ecology in birds

The introduction of West Nile virus (WNV, *Flavivirus*, Flaviviridae) into the
United States in 1999 initiated a human epidemic and caused extensive bird mortal-
ity, particularly in the American crow (*Corvus brachyrhynchos*) in New York City
(NYC)[1] and brought a new perspective to the status of arboviruses in North America.
Originally, the virus responsible for the human epidemic was thought to be St. Louis
encephalitis (SLE), a virus closely related to WNV, which regularly occurs through-

Address for correspondence: Robert G. McLean, Ph.D., United States Geologic Survey,
National Wildlife Health Center, 6006 Schroeder Road, Madison, Wisconsin 53711. Voice: 608-
270-2401; fax: 608-270-2415.

bob_mclean@usgs.gov

out the United States.[2] However SLE virus does not cause mortality in birds. Historical data on WNV in birds from Africa, the Middle East, and Europe suggested that
most of the viral strains circulating in nature were not pathogenic to birds either, including hooded crows (*Corvus corone*).[3,4] The virus appeared to be a highly virulent
strain of WNV introduced possibly from Israel.[5] The crow emerged as a symbol of
WNV activity in the northeastern United States because of its high susceptibility to
infection with WNV. Enhanced surveillance for the detection of WNV expansion out
of the original focus in NYC was established subsequently using mortality in crows
as an indicator of WNV activity.[6] In addition, public health departments began using
WNV-positive crows to make public health decisions about human risk. A number
of other bird species in New York were found infected with WNV, and many may
have died from the infection, including in zoological avian collections in the affected
area.[7] Thousands of birds, a total of 19 species, died from WNV in the NYC area in
1999, and when the virus reemerged in 2000 and expanded to 12 states, tens of thousands of birds of 54 native bird species died, mostly crows.[8,9]

The apparent transmission patterns and ecology of WNV that are now occurring
within the ecosystems shared by the traditional viruses of SLE and eastern equine
encephalitis (EEE) that regularly occur in the United States[10] have become unique
to these viruses. The basic transmission cycle for some of the major arboviruses of
public health importance in the United States, WNV, SLE, EEE, and western equine
encephalitis (WEE), involves birds as the natural hosts and mosquitoes as the primary vectors (FIG. 1). Humans are incidental and dead-end hosts for these viruses; however, except for SLE, the other viruses also cause morbidity and mortality in equines
(FIG. 2). West Nile and EEE viruses also cause mortality in birds, although less for
EEE than for WNV. Little is known about WNV infections in wild birds, and there
is no information available on the effects of this virus on North American bird species or on exotic bird species in zoological collections or endangered species, like
the whooping crane. This lack of information on susceptibility and pathogenesis in
native birds will hinder efforts to predict possible persistence and reemergence of the
virus in affected areas. It will also make it difficult to predict which bird species are
at risk from infection, to know which bird species are the best sentinels for detecting
virus activity, and to establish effective surveillance networks.

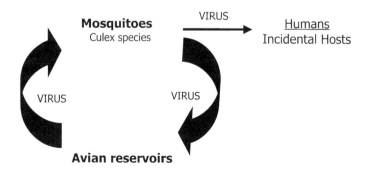

**FIGURE 1. Basic transmission cycle for some major mosquito-borne arboviruses of
birds.**

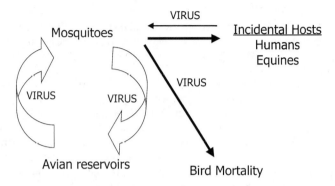

FIGURE 2. Transmission cycle for eastern equine encephalitis and western equine encephalitis and West Nile viruses.

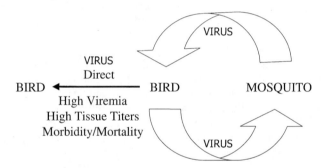

FIGURE 3. Direct transmission of West Nile and eastern equine encephalitis viruses between birds.

Experimental infection studies were conducted with American crows at the BSL-3 animal facilities at the USGS National Wildlife Health Center to determine their susceptibility and reservoir competence to WNV (R.G. McLean, personal communication). A New York 1999 strain of WNV was inoculated subcutaneously into 10 crows individually held in cages along with 4 control birds in separate cages. All inoculated crows died within seven days, and none of the control birds became infected. Viremias in infected crows were of sufficient titer to infect mosquitoes before the birds died, making them reservoir competent, and high titers of virus were isolated from a variety of tissues. In a second experiment (R.G. McLean, personal communication), nine experimental and seven control crows were housed together in a free-flying arrangement in the same room where they had regular contact with each other. The nine experimental birds were inoculated with the same WNV strain and dosage as in the first experiment, and all nine died between days 5 and 8 postinoculation (PI). Noninoculated control crows began dying at 10 days from the start of the experiment, and 5 of the 7 controls died by day 21 PI. The method of direct transmission between inoculated crows and controls was likely from WNV-laden discharge in feces or oral secretions and to other crows through oral ingestion and/or by mutual grooming of feathers. The significance of this direct transmission of WNV among crows is unknown at this time. Direct transmission of EEE virus also occurs among exotic game birds in captivity,[11] and EEE and WNV virus may share this method of transmission (FIG. 3).

REFERENCES

1. CENTERS FOR DISEASE CONTROL AND PREVENTION. 1999b. Update: West Nile–like viral encephalitis—New York, 1999. Morb. Mortal. Wkly. Rep. **48:** 890–892.
2. CENTERS FOR DISEASE CONTROL AND PREVENTION. 1999a. Outbreak of West Nile–like viral encephalitis—New York, 1999. Morb. Mortal. Wkly. Rep. **48:** 845–849.
3. TAYLOR, R.M., T.H. WORK, H.S. HURLBUT & F. RIZK. 1956. A study of the ecology of West Nile Virus in Egypt. Am. J. Trop. Med. Hyg. **5:** 579.
4. WORK, T.H., H.S. HURLBUT & R.M. TAYLOR. 1955. Indigenous wild birds of the Nile Delta as potential West Nile circulating reservoirs. Am. J. Trop. Med. Hyg. **4:** 872–878.
5. LANCIOTTI, R.S., J.T. ROEHRIG, V. DEUBEL, *et al.* 1999. Origin of the West Nile virus responsible for an outbreak of encephalitis in the northeastern United States. Science **286:** 2333–2337.
6. CENTERS FOR DISEASE CONTROL AND PREVENTION. 1999c. Update: West Nile–like viral encephalitis—New York, 1999. Morb. Mortal. Wkly. Rep. **48:** 944–946, 955.
7. STEELE, K.E., M.J. LINN, R.J. SCHOEPP, *et al.* 2000. Pathology of fatal West Nile virus infections in native and exotic birds during the 1999 outbreak in New York City, New York. Vet. Pathol. **37:** 208–224.
8. CENTERS FOR DISEASE CONTROL AND PREVENTION. 2000a. Update: West Nile virus activity— northeastern United States, January–August 7, 2000. Morb. Mortal. Wkly. Rep. **49:** 714–717.
9. CENTERS FOR DISEASE CONTROL AND PREVENTION. 2000b. Update: West Nile virus activity–northeastern United States, 2000. Morb. Mortal. Wkly. Rep. **49:** 1044–1047.
10. MOORE, C.G., R.G. MCLEAN, C.J. MITCHELL, *et al.* 1993. Guidelines for arbovirus surveillance in the United States. U.S. DHHS, Public Health Service, CDC, NCID, DVBID. Fort Collins, CO. 83 pp.
11. MCLEAN R.G. 1991. Arboviruses of wild birds and mammals. Bull. Soc. Vector Ecol. **16:** 3–16.

West Nile Virus Surveillance using Sentinel Birds

NICHOLAS KOMAR

Centers for Disease Control and Prevention, Fort Collins, Colorado 80522, USA

ABSTRACT: Captive and free-ranging birds have been used for decades as living sentinels in arbovirus surveillance programs. This review summarizes information relevant to selecting sentinel bird species for use in surveillance of West Nile (WN) virus. Although experience using avian sentinels for WN virus surveillance is limited, sentinels should be useful for both detecting and monitoring WN virus transmission; however, sentinel bird surveillance systems have yet to be adequately tested for use with the North American strain of WN virus. Captive chickens are typically used for arbovirus surveillance, but other captive species may be used as well. Serosurvey and experimental infection data suggest that both chickens and pigeons show promise as useful captive sentinels; both species were naturally exposed during the epizootics in New York City, 1999–2000, and both species develop antibodies after infection without becoming highly infectious to *Culex pipiens* vectors. Wild bird species that should be targeted for use as free-ranging sentinels include house sparrows and pigeons. The ideal wild bird should be determined locally on the basis of seroprevalence studies. Interpreting serological data generated from studies using free-ranging sentinel birds is complex, however. Sentinel bird monitoring sites should be selected in enzootic transmission foci. Several years of observation may be required for selection of effective sentinel monitoring sites.

KEYWORDS: Arbovirus; Flaviviridae; West Nile virus; birds; sentinels

INTRODUCTION

Sentinel birds have been used to monitor arthropod-borne virus transmission for decades.[1] West Nile (WN) virus is maintained in nature by birds[2] and thus lends itself to being monitored through the use of sentinel birds. WN virus infections in avian hosts (the principal reservoir hosts, FIG. 1) should occur more frequently (and therefore, earlier) than the disease events in people and horses. Controlled use of sentinels also lends itself to the quantitative evaluation of infection rates, which are used for recommending public and animal health interventions.

The ideal sentinel bird is a species that is uniformly susceptible to infection, is resistant to disease, rapidly develops a detectable immune response, is easily maintained, presents negligible health risks to handlers, does not contribute to local pathogen transmission cycles, and seroconverts to the target pathogen prior to the onset of disease outbreaks in the community. There is probably no ideal sentinel spe-

Address for correspondence: Nicholas Komar, Sc.D., P.O. Box 2087, Fort Collins, CO 80522. Voice: 970-221-6496; fax: 970-221-6476.

nkomar@cdc.gov

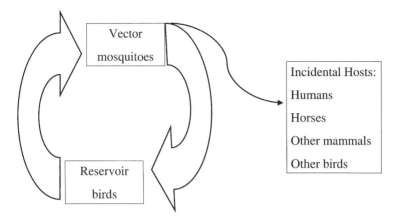

FIGURE 1. The basic transmission cycle of West Nile virus. Certain birds, mainly members of the Passeriformes order, serve as principal amplifying reservoir hosts for infection of vector mosquitoes, mainly ornithophilic *Culex* species. Important reservoir and vector hosts may vary regionally. People, horses, other mammals, and other birds are incidental hosts that do not normally participate in the transmission cycle.

cies for any zoonotic pathogen. Perhaps the greatest challenge in using sentinel birds is the lack of knowledge of the locations of enzootic transmission foci. Such knowledge would be key to successful placement of sentinel bird monitoring sites (FIG. 2).

WN virus is a reemerging public and animal health threat in Europe,[3] North Africa,[3,4] the Middle East,[5] and is now emerging in North America.[2,6] Sentinel birds should be useful for monitoring enzootic transmission and predicting epizootic and epidemic WN virus activity. Sentinel bird–based surveillance systems for WN virus may target captive birds or free-ranging birds, or even morbidity/mortality events in bird populations. Dead crows, and closely related corvid species, have been a hallmark of the North American WN virus outbreak in 1999 and 2000 and have been used effectively as sentinels for detection of local WN virus activity.[7–9] This article reviews the use of sentinel birds, alive and dead, captive and free-ranging, in detecting and monitoring WN virus transmission, with emphasis on the North American experience. Particular attention is given to the difficulties that arise when interpreting flavivirus serological results from birds.

AVIAN MORBIDITY/MORTALITY

The North American strain of WN virus was first identified in brain tissue from a dead American crow (*Corvus brachyrhynchos*) collected September 8, 1999 in Westchester County, New York.[10] Subsequently, many other isolates were made from other crows[7] and exotic birds from a zoological collection in New York City (NYC).[10,11] These carcasses were used as public health sentinels,[7] establishing locations where WN virus may be circulating. Although monitoring crow deaths, combined with rapid diagnostic testing of these specimens, has been a useful sentinel

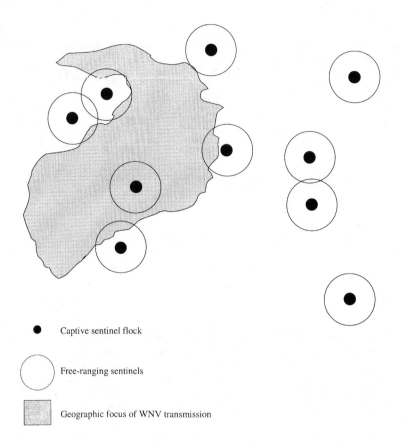

● Captive sentinel flock

◯ Free-ranging sentinels

▨ Geographic focus of WNV transmission

FIGURE 2. Placement of sentinel monitoring sites for West Nile virus. In this schematic, the knowledge of the geographic limits of a transmission focus was unknown when the sentinel monitoring sites were placed. As a result, only 1 of 10 captive sentinel flocks will be exposed to natural transmission. Free-ranging sentinels sampled at the same locations will demonstrate exposure at half of the locations.

system, it is far from ideal, in that quantification of infection rates is infeasible. Accurate quantification of infection rates would require knowing the size of the local crow population and knowing the mortality rate in crows. The variables are even more difficult to assess when carcasses of other species are included in the surveillance system.

The success of avian morbidity/mortality surveillance for WN virus depends on participation of the public in reporting carcasses to the public health system. The public will not participate equally in every region or at all times and may not participate at all at certain times or locations. Nonetheless, an analysis of the dead crow reports in 2000 found a significant association between high densities of dead crows at the county level (greater than 1 per square mile) and occurrence of human cases several weeks later.[12] In 2000, dead crows infected with WN virus appeared in April and May in New York and New Jersey,[13,14] several weeks earlier than other surveillance indicators.[14] In areas of high population density, it is clear that dead crows are effective sentinels when the public is actively engaged in reporting them. Thus, dead crows can indicate early season WN virus transmission weeks before the occurrence of human cases, which began in July in New York in 2000.[14]

However, the future success of dead bird sentinels for detecting WN virus is uncertain for several reasons: (1) the public may lose interest in reporting dead crows; (2) those birds genetically predisposed to fatal WN virus infection may be removed from the population by attrition; (3) crows in regions where closely related flaviviruses circulate (*e.g.*, St. Louis encephalitis virus in southern latitudes of North America) may already have developed cross-reactive immunity, or even innate resistance to severe flavivirus infection; and (4) new evolving strains of WN virus may be less virulent. Thus, other sentinel bird systems should be developed, ones that reliably estimate WN virus infection rates in the avian community.

CAPTIVE SENTINELS

Captive sentinel birds are typically chickens held in cages designed to permit the entry and egress of mosquitoes while affording protection from natural predators. General guidelines for use of sentinel chickens are available from the Centers for Disease Control and Prevention (CDC).[1] In North America, arbovirus surveillance programs using chickens have been described in Arizona,[15] California,[16] Florida,[17] Iowa,[18] New Jersey,[19] Utah,[20] and Canada.[21] Other programs are currently in place in Alabama, Colorado, Delaware, Louisiana, Maryland, Nebraska, Nevada, North Carolina, Tennessee, and Texas. These programs have been monitoring eastern equine encephalitis, western equine encephalitis, and/or St. Louis encephalitis virus activity. The number of chickens in a flock range from two to thirty, and numerous caging strategies are used (FIG. 3). Some programs keep individual birds in separate compartments of the cages, while others allow direct contact between the birds. Cages are typically maintained above ground on stilts to avoid attack by predators. Some programs provide pens for ground-level chickens, with sheds for shelter and sleeping. Both hens and roosters of many different breeds have been used. Blood samples are collected periodically (usually biweekly) and tested for antibodies specific to the arbovirus(es) being monitored. Numerous blood sampling schemes and diagnostic testing strategies have been described elsewhere.[22–31]

Placement of chickens is key to success of the sentinel program. Common sense indicates that chickens should be located adjacent to mosquito resting sites and near arbovirus vector breeding sites. Ideal habitats, however, are not always intuitive. In Florida, one study demonstrated that penned chickens were more likely to seroconvert to SLE virus in open, well-drained habitats than in forested, moist habitats with greater mosquito densities. This likelihood was probably a function of rainfall-associated behaviors of the vector mosquito, *Culex nigripalpis*.[32] Another study in Florida failed to identify habitat as an important factor influencing SLE virus transmission rates in sentinel chickens.[33] Most importantly, the sentinels should be located in regions where arboviruses are maintained in enzootic transmission cycles (FIG. 2). In this manner, enzootic activity may be monitored. Increasing levels of enzootic activity or levels above the historical mean, measured in units of percent se-

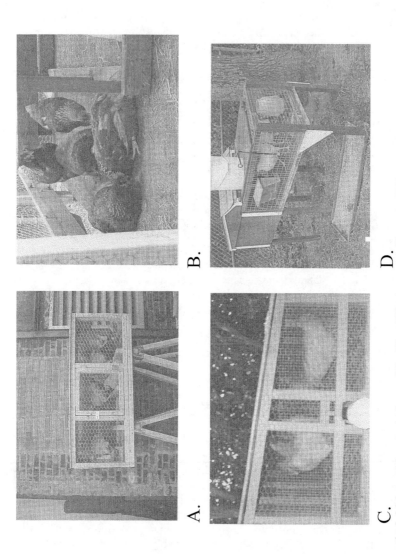

FIGURE 3. Sentinel chicken caging strategies used for West Nile virus surveillance in 2000. (A) New York City (photo courtesy of S. Trock). **(B)** Rockland County, New York (photo courtesy of E.O. Alleyne). **(C)** Bay County, Florida (photo courtesy of Florida Bureau of Epidemiology and Beach Mosquito Control District). **(D)** Cape May County, New Jersey (photo courtesy of P. Bosak).

roconversion or seroconversions per days of exposure, would serve as a red flag for potential epizootic activity. Some jurisdictions have chosen to place flocks close to population centers (away from enzootic foci), such that a single infection in the sentinel flock would indicate epizootic/epidemic risk. However, this strategy may result in late notification of the risk and may underestimate risk in nearby population centers that lack sentinel flocks. There is no established formula for determining the appropriate number of flocks in a jurisdiction. As with the specific locations of flocks, this number is determined empirically and may require several years of experience to establish an effective regimen in a jurisdiction. Preexisting privately owned flocks ("backyard flocks") may serve as sentinels if they are located in appropriate sentinel site locations.

   Other species of birds have been used as captive sentinels for arbovirus monitoring, including pheasants,[34] bobwhite,[35] Japanese quail,[36] pigeons,[37] and wild birds.[38] Captive mammals have been used as well, such as horses,[39] dogs,[40] rabbits,[38,41] hamsters,[42] and mice.[38,43] Sentinel mammals might better indicate risk of transmission to mammals, whereas sentinel birds effectively monitor transmission to birds—another justification for using sentinel birds to monitor enzootic, rather than epizootic, transmission of avian arboviruses; in theory, risk of epizootic transmission to humans would be best monitored using sentinel mammals.

   West Nile virus has been monitored using captive sentinels in several locations around the world. In South Africa, both chickens and pigeons were used briefly as sentinels.[44,45] In Australia, chickens are used as sentinels for Kunjin virus, a subtype of West Nile virus.[46,47] In Romania, sentinel chicken surveillance was established briefly in Bucharest subsequent to the outbreak recorded in 1996, with successful results.[48] Seroconversion rates in these chickens (determined by an experimental ELISA procedure) reached a maximum of 40% in late July 1997 and occurred up to six weeks prior to the appearance of human cases. In Russia, a variety of wild bird species were used experimentally as captive sentinels in order to evaluate which wild birds were involved in the local transmission cycle.[38]

   In North America, experimental infection studies demonstrated the utility of chickens as sentinels for the New York strain of WN virus.[49,50] Chickens were used to monitor WN virus transmission in the American states of New York, New Jersey, Pennsylvania, Delaware, Maryland, Virginia, North Carolina, Florida, Louisiana, and Texas and in several provinces of Canada in 2000. Seroconversions were recorded only in New York and New Jersey.[14] However, in the other states and Canada, no WN virus activity was recorded in counties where chickens were concurrently placed, except in Pennsylvania.

   The North American experience using chickens as sentinels for WN virus in 2000 was disappointing. On the basis of the results of an avian serosurvey in 1999 in the borough of Queens in NYC, in which a single flock of chickens had a prevalence of infection of 63% in the middle of September,[51] it was hoped that a relatively few number of chickens in the program would serve for early detection of WN virus activity. However, in 2000 early detection in chickens failed, with the first seroconversion on August 4 in Westchester County, NY;[52] although no human cases were recorded in Westchester County in 2000, human cases occurred nearby in adjacent NYC, where the first patient had onset of symptoms on July 20 in Staten Island (Richmond County).[14] Although seroconversion rates in sentinel chicken flocks did

TABLE 1. WNV seroconversion rates and timing in sentinel chickens used in New York and New Jersey, 2000; the counties listed in the table are all located in New York State

Location	No. birds	No. positive[a]	Percent positive	Date of earliest seroconversion	Date of earliest human case onset[14]
New Jersey[b]	129	4	2.3	September 27	August 6
New York City[53, c]	114	9	7.9	August 23	July 20
Westchester County[d]	70	1	1.4	August 4	—
Rockland County[e]	12	0	—	—	—
Suffolk County[f]	60	0	—	—	—
Onondaga County[d]	47	0	—	—	—

[a]Seropositive chickens were confirmed by neutralization testing.
[b]Chickens were placed in flocks throughout all of New Jersey's 21 counties. Data provided by C. Farello, N. J. Department of Health and Senior Services.
[c]Sentinel chickens were sampled in all five boroughs of NYC.
[d]Data provided by G. Ebel, NYS Department of Health.
[e]Data provided by M. Anand, Rockland County Health Department.
[f]Data provided by S. Campbell, Suffolk County Health Department.

eventually exceed 1% in some locations,[53] seroconversions were generally detected late in the transmission season, after the onset of human cases (TABLE 1).

The success of sentinel chickens, or other captive bird species, for monitoring WN virus transmission in North America will depend on placement of flocks within microhabitats conducive to mosquito attack and determination of enzootic WN virus transmission foci, at which flocks should be placed. It may require several years before these foci, sites that support annual low-level WN virus transmission among avian reservoir hosts, are located. Other factors that may influence success of captive sentinel systems include cage design, relative attractiveness of sentinel species to vector attack, height above ground level, and flock size.

FREE-RANGING SENTINELS

Free-ranging sentinel birds are wild birds that are captured, blood-sampled, and released. General guidelines for use of wild birds as sentinels are available from the CDC.[1] These birds are marked, usually by federally authorized aluminum leg bands, so that individuals are recognized upon recapture. In the United States, bands and authorization are provided by the U.S. Fish and Wildlife Service Bird Banding Laboratory, although permission for bird capture and banding is also required by state authorities and property owners where the work takes place. However, certain non-native species are exempt from federal statutes, including the house sparrow (*Passer domesticus*), European starling (*Sturnus vulgaris*), and rock dove or domestic pigeon (*Columba livia*). These three species were all introduced to the United States from Europe in previous centuries and have become abundant in a variety of habitats. All three are well adapted to human environments and, in many cases, should make good arbovirus sentinels.

One advantage that free-ranging sentinels have over captive sentinels is the freedom to move about, increasing the probability that they may at some point during their lives spend some time in an arbovirus transmission focus. Thus, a program that monitors free-ranging sentinels effectively monitors a larger region than that which relies solely on captive sentinels, even if the same study sites are used (FIG 2). Unfortunately, it is impossible to know the travel history of each wild bird that is sampled, but some generalizations may be made regarding bird movement. For example, nonmigratory species, such as pigeons and house sparrows, are presumed to remain resident within a small region. Migratory species, such as starlings and many others, must be regarded with caution when presuming location of exposure to arboviruses. Investigators should keep in mind that the time between exposure and capture will be at least a week, due to the delay in antibody production after infection. Frequently, an individual banded bird's local residence status may be ascertained by its recapture, although seasonal movements must be considered. For example, a starling banded in July and recaptured in August is most certainly a summer resident. However, if it is recaptured the following June, one cannot assume that it has been locally resident throughout the year, as it may have migrated hundreds of miles in the fall and returned to its breeding territory the following spring.

Recapturing wild birds affords a mechanism for detecting seroconversion (a change from negative to positive antibody status), the main objective of sentinel bird sampling programs. However, most wild birds are not recaptured, and seroconversion may not be observed. To solve this problem of free-ranging sentinel programs, it is important to consider the age of each bird being sampled. A bird in its first summer of life that circulates arbovirus antibodies either was infected in the current summer or acquired maternal antibodies. Maternal antibodies usually do not persist beyond a few weeks of life and generally have low neutralization titers.[54] Adult birds (greater than one year old) that circulate antibodies do not provide information on which year the infection took place unless these birds have been recaptured and have seroconverted. A guide for aging North American passerine and related wild birds is available,[55] but a single manual for aging all birds is not. In general, most birds can be assigned to categories of ages, such as "hatching year" and "after hatching year," which is sufficient to indicate whether circulating antibodies are due to a recent infection acquired during the current virus-transmission season or to an old infection acquired previous to the current season. In subtropical and tropical regions where transmission may occur year-round, even this basic aging scheme may be insufficient to determine useful information on the timing of transmission except where free-ranging birds may be frequently recaptured. Occasionally, older individual birds that have been repeatedly sampled show waning of antibody responses over time until the antibodies are no longer detected (seroreversion).[56] Even more occasionally, these same individuals seroconvert a second time (seroreconversion). The mechanism for seroreconversion is unknown. It has been speculated to result from reexposure to mosquito-borne infection or from relapse of a latent infection, sometimes referred to as recrudescence.[57,58]

In North America, arbovirus-monitoring programs using free-ranging sentinel birds have been described in Alabama,[59] California,[58,60] Florida,[61] Maryland,[35] Massachusetts,[56] New Jersey,[57] and Tennessee.[62] Other similar programs have been operated in Louisiana, Texas, Ohio, Michigan, Indiana, and Illinois. These programs have been monitoring eastern equine encephalitis, western equine encephalitis, and

St. Louis encephalitis virus activity. Blood samples are typically taken from the jugular vein of passerine birds (such as house sparrows). A variety of diagnostic tests have been used and have been described elsewhere.[24,29] Species-specific diagnostic tests (such as IgM-capture ELISA for chickens) are not effective for use with serum collected from multiple avian species.

West Nile virus has not been monitored consistently using free-ranging sentinels, although wild birds have been the targets of many serosurveys conducted in several continents. In 2000, NYC reported several seropositive hatching year wild birds, indicating recent infection (B. Cherry, personal communication). However, these birds were not sampled consistently in the same locations. Also in 2000, an ecologic study of WN virus transmission in northern New Jersey and southern New York used house sparrows as free-ranging sentinels. Sparrow populations were sampled three times at six-week intervals in ten locations (in six counties). WN virus activity was observed in sparrows at just two of these locations, and the seroprevalence in a location never exceeded 2%. Positive sparrows were detected in two of the six counties, while horse and human cases were each reported from three of these. Infected sentinel chickens, mosquitoes, and dead birds were detected in two, five, and five of these counties, respectively (CDC, unpublished data).

The use of free-ranging sentinel birds for WN virus may become more feasible in North America in future years. To be successful, public health authorities in the affected regions must know the locations of the WN virus enzootic transmission foci and the species that are most frequently infected at these locations. These data require investigations that may take several years to accomplish successfully. Serosurvey data during both epizootic and interepizootic periods will be useful in targeting appropriate wild bird sentinels in different regions. Lastly, knowledge of the important reservoir hosts in a surveillance region will be useful, as these species may be targeted for surveillance purposes.

USE OF SEROSURVEY DATA FOR ESTABLISHING SENTINEL PROGRAMS

In a region where little is known of WN virus transmission dynamics, and where transmission foci have not been located, avian serosurvey data will be useful in selecting both captive and free-ranging sentinel species for monitoring WN virus transmission. These data, as well as avian mortality and mosquito infection rate data, will also direct the placement of sentinel monitoring sites, which ideally will be located in WN virus transmission foci. Other data to consider for the placement of sentinel monitoring sites are (1) breeding sites of vector mosquitoes, (2) proximity of high-risk human and animal populations, and (3) feasibility. For example, it is infeasible to place chicken flocks where they are likely to be vandalized or where they could generate complaints from the public. Wild bird monitoring sites will have to be restricted to locations where wild birds can be readily captured. The experience of conducting an avian serosurvey in a region where WN virus may require monitoring will provide valuable information with regard to feasibility issues as well as determining which domestic and wild bird species have high levels of exposure in a given region.

TABLE 2. West Nile virus–neutralizing antibodies (Ab) in resident birds in Queens during September 1999, by species (adapted from Komar *et al.* 2001[51]), and their status as captive or free-ranging ("free")

Common name	Total tested	No. (Percent) Ab positive	Captive or free
Domestic goose	7	6 (86)	captive
Domestic chicken	141	89 (63)	captive
House sparrow	20	12 (60)	free
Other species[a,b]	13	5 (38)	
Canada goose	7	2 (29)	free
Rock dove[b]	49	13 (26)	
Mallard/domestic duck[b]	16	1 (6)	

[a]Comprised of American robin, brown-headed cowbird, domestic turkey, European starling, mourning dove, and red-winged blackbird.
[b]These birds had both captive and free-ranging individuals sampled

After the discovery of WN virus introduction into the United States in 1999, several avian serosurveys were undertaken to determine the geographic extent of WN virus transmission. One of these surveys targeted the center of the 1999 epizootic in northeastern Queens in mid-September.[51] Only resident bird species were sampled in order to compare the involvement of these local birds in the WN virus transmission cycle in Queens. Both captive and free-ranging birds of 12 species were evaluated (TABLE 2). From this survey, it was clear that populations of several species of birds had been heavily exposed during the course of the epizootic and would be candidates for sentinels, including captive chickens and geese, and wild house sparrows and pigeons. The survey also served to identify neighborhoods where bird exposure was particularly intense. However, one year's data is insufficient to identify permanent enzootic transmission foci. One of the locations in this study was revisited in July of 2000 and both free-ranging birds and captive birds were sampled. House sparrows were targeted and 1 of 87 yearlings circulated neutralizing antibody, indicating continued transmission at this location in 2000 (CDC, unpublished data). Such a location, hence, would be a reasonable sentinel bird monitoring site.

The 1999 September avian serosurvey in NYC also sampled birds in four locations peripheral to northeastern Queens.[51] WN virus seropositive birds were encountered in each of the locations, although seroprevalences were lower than that encountered in northeastern Queens. One of these locations, on Staten Island in NYC, was revisited in October 2000, after epizootic transmission had occurred there during the summer of 2000. Both free-ranging and captive bird species were readily sampled there. The findings at this site in 2000 demonstrated relatively high levels of exposure to a variety of bird species.[63] Thus, this site too may warrant selection as a permanent sentinel monitoring site.

The WN virus avian serosurvey in Staten Island during October 2000 identified several other bird populations that were heavily exposed (TABLE 3). This study identified captive pigeons and several wild passerine bird species (northern cardinal, gray catbird, and house finch) as candidate sentinels. Chickens and house sparrows

TABLE 3. West Nile virus–neutralizing antibodies (Ab) in resident birds in Staten Island during October 2000, by species (adapted from Komar *et al.* 2001[63]), and their status as captive or free-ranging ("free")

Common name	Total tested	No. (Percent) Ab positive	Captive or free
Northern cardinal	13	9 (69)	free
Rock dove	55	30 (54)	captive
House finch	5	2 (40)	free
Gray catbird	17	6 (35)	free
Common peafowl	10	2 (20)	captive
House sparrow	93	8 (9)	free
Mallard/domestic duck	13	1 (8)	free
Domestic chicken	55	3 (6)	captive
European starling	7	0 (0)	free

were not as heavily exposed as they had been in the previous year in Queens. These data serve to underscore the geographic variability in arbovirus transmission dynamics that must be considered when planning sentinel bird surveillance for WN virus or other arboviruses.

INTERPRETATION OF SEROLOGIC RESULTS

Serologic data require careful evaluation, as several elements serve to complicate their interpretation. First, serologic data are based on the humoral immune responses of living systems, each of which is unique. Second, serologic data are derived from available laboratory tests, none of which is perfect. Third, cross-reactivity among closely related viruses confounds flavivirus serology. Finally, knowing the age of the sentinel bird is essential to accurate interpretation of the serology, yet determining ages in some sentinel birds is challenging, and sometimes impossible. This issue is discussed above with regard to free-ranging wild birds used as sentinels.

The first complex issue is the variability of the humoral immune response among and within species. Humoral immunity may be evaluated for the serum levels of IgM, IgG, hemagglutination inhibiting (HI), and/or neutralizing (N) antibodies (Ab). Each sentinel bird species should be evaluated experimentally for its ability to develop Ab that are detectable by the available laboratory tests. IgM and HI antibodies typically increase in titer shortly after infection and are relatively short-lived compared with IgG and N Ab. Thus, a sentinel bird-monitoring program that relies on serial sampling of birds at frequent intervals may select a strategy of detecting either IgM or HI Ab. A program that samples individual sentinel birds infrequently (such as free-ranging birds) should sample for either IgG or N Ab. However, none of these Ab types are reliably detected less than seven days after infection. Some of these Ab types for flaviviruses may be ephemeral in some species.[58,64] Consequently, false negative test results are common due to the failure of birds with histories of infection to consistently circulate all types of Ab.

Recent experimental infection studies of chickens, turkeys, and domestic geese, using WNV-NY99, have confirmed that N Ab is consistently detected at 14 days postinfection.[49,50,65,66] Similar observations were made with 14 species of free-ranging North American birds (CDC, unpublished studies). However, these studies generally did not evaluate the duration of detectable N Ab and did not evaluate the detectability of other Ab types. In chickens experimentally infected with SLE virus, detectability of IgM and N Ab was roughly equivalent from 12–21 days postinfection.[23] Preliminary evaluation of IgM production in WNV-NY99-infected chickens indicates that IgM may not endure reliably beyond 19 days postinfection (CDC, unpublished data). Thus, bleeding captive sentinel chickens every two weeks could miss a WN virus infection. Weekly or 10-day interval bleeding regimens is recommended.

The second complex issue is the variable sensitivity and specificity of laboratory tests. When interpreting serologic test results it is important to remember that no diagnostic test is perfect. IgM-capture ELISA, IgG immunoassays (such as immunofluorescence tests), and HI tests for flaviviruses are generally highly sensitive but often have low specificity, even when there is no evidence of previous heterologous flavivirus infection, resulting in false positive test results. IgG-capture ELISA is generally not useful because of low sensitivity. N antibody tests have the greatest sensitivity and specificity but generally require BSL3 laboratory safety designation (for working with infectious WN virus preparations). All positive test results should be confirmed by neutralization. Neutralization test results should be replicated for confirmation.

Cross-reactivity of antibodies to more than one virus needs to be considered when planning serologic tests and also when interpreting test results. WN virus cross-reacts with a group of closely related viruses that are members of the Japanese encephalitis (JE) serocomplex.[67] In North America, WN virus appears to be sympatric with St. Louis encephalitis (SLE) virus in some regions. Cross-reactivity is common between WN and SLE viruses using ELISA-based and HI assays. In the plaque-reduction neutralization assay, about 6% of WN-positive avian serum specimens also tested positive for SLE. However, titers of WN virus N Ab were about eightfold greater than titers of SLE virus N Ab.[51] Thus, it is essential to confirm an N Ab titer to WN virus by comparing the titer to SLE virus. A fourfold difference in titer is considered sufficient to implicate one of the cross-reactive viruses as the etiologic agent. If titers to heterologous JE serocomplex viruses are observed to be less than fourfold different or equivalent, a specific etiologic agent cannot be determined, and the diagnosis should simply be "flavivirus infection." Flavivirus serology becomes even more confusing when a single host is infected by more than one flavivirus, as heterologous flavivirus antibody responses due to the previous infection may be greater than the homologous antibody response due to the current infection, a phenomenon known as "original antigenic sin."[68] This phenomenon will be most important where WN virus becomes established in regions that are enzootic for SLE virus, such as the southeastern United States.

THE FUTURE FOR SENTINEL BIRD USE IN
WEST NILE VIRUS SURVEILLANCE

The main purpose of captive sentinel bird systems for WN virus surveillance should be monitoring risk levels, rather than detection of virus activity in new regions. To achieve this purpose, sentinel monitoring sites must be placed in enzootic transmission foci; finding these foci is paramount to a successful sentinel program. Unfortunately, use of sentinel birds for WN virus surveillance can be complex and is hindered by lack of experience with this virus in North America. As the virus spreads into new regions of North America (such as Florida), where sentinels are already in use for monitoring SLE virus transmission, new experience will be gained. Ultimately, rigorous comparison of sentinel bird systems will be required to determine the best sentinel system in particular locations. Unfortunately, due to the complexity of arbovirus transmission dynamics, these systems may require variation in different regions.

REFERENCES

1. MOORE, C.G., R.G. MCLEAN, C.J. MITCHELL, et al. 1993. Guidelines For Arbovirus Surveillance in the United States. Fort Collins, CO: U.S.D.H.H.S./P.H.S./C.D.C./N.C.I.D./D.V.B.I.D.
2. KOMAR, N. 2000. West Nile viral encephalitis. Rev. Sci. Tech. 19: 166–176.
3. HUBALEK, Z. & J. HALOUZKA. 1999. West Nile fever—a reemerging mosquito-borne viral disease in Europe. Emerg. Infect. Dis. 5: 643–650.
4. LE GUENNO, B., A. BOUGERMOUH, T. AZZAM & R. BOUAKAZ. 1996. West Nile: a deadly virus? Lancet 348: 1315.
5. WEINBERGER, M., S.D. PITLIK, D. GANDACU, et al. 2001. West Nile fever outbreak, Israel, 2000: epidemiologic aspects. Emerg. Infect. Dis. 7: 686–691.
6. PETERSEN, L.R. & J.T. ROEHRIG. 2001. West Nile virus: a reemerging global pathogen. Emerg. Infect. Dis. 7: 611–614.
7. EIDSON, M., N. KOMAR, F. SORHAGE, et al. 2001. Crow deaths as a sentinel surveillance system for West Nile virus in the northeastern United States, 1999. Emerg. Infect. Dis. 7: 615–620.
8. BERNARD, K.A., J.G. MAFFEI, S.A. JONES, et al. 2001. West Nile virus infection in birds and mosquitoes, New York State, 2000. Emerg. Infect. Dis. 7: 679–685.
9. EIDSON, M., L. KRAMER, W. STONE, et al. 2001. Dead bird surveillance as an early warning system for West Nile virus. Emerg. Infect. Dis. 7: 631–635.
10. CENTERS FOR DISEASE CONTROL AND PREVENTION. 1999. Outbreak of West Nile-like viral encephalitis-New York, 1999. Morbid. Mortal. Wkly. Rep. 48: 845–849.
11. STEELE, K.E., M.J. LINN, R.J. SCHOEPP, et al. 2000. Pathology of fatal West Nile virus infections in native and exotic birds during the 1999 outbreak in New York City, New York. Vet. Pathol. 37: 208–224.
12. EIDSON, M., J. MILLER, L. KRAMER, et al. 2001. Dead crow densities and human cases of West Nile virus, New York State, 2000. Emerg. Infect. Dis. 7: 662–664.
13. CENTERS FOR DISEASE CONTROL AND PREVENTION. 2000. West Nile virus activity-New York and New Jersey, 2000. Morbid. Mortal. Wkly. Rep. 49: 640–642.
14. MARFIN, A.A., L.R. PETERSEN, M. EIDSON, et al. 2001. Widespread West Nile virus activity, Eastern United States, 2000. Emerg. Infect. Dis. 7: 730–735.
15. SMITH, H.H., R.J. JANSSEN, G.A. MAIL & S.A. WOOD. 1969. Arbovirus activity in southern Arizona. Isolations of virus and observations of sentinel chickens. Am. J. Trop. Med. Hyg. 18: 448–454.
16. REISEN, W.C. 1995. Guidelines for Surveillance and Control of Arboviral Encephalitis in California. Sacramento, CA: California Mosquito Vector Control Assoc.
17. DAY, J.F. 1989. The use of sentinel chickens for arbovirus surveillance in Florida. J. Fla. Anti-Mosq. Assoc. 60: 56–61.
18. GILLILAND, T.M., W.A. ROWLEY, N.S. SWACK, et al. 1995. Arbovirus surveillance in Iowa, USA, during the flood of 1993. J. Am. Mosq. Control. Assoc. 11: 157–161.
19. CRANS, W.J. 1982. The use of sentinel chickens for St. Louis encephalitis surveillance in New Jersey. Proc. N. J. Mosq. Control Assoc. 69: 39–41.

20. WAGSTAFF, K.H., S.L. DICKSON & A. BAILEY. 1986. Western equine encephalitis surveillance in Utah. J. Am. Mosq. Control. Assoc. **2:** 201–203.
21. WONG, F.C., L.E. LILLIE & R.A. DRYSDALE. 1976. Sentinel flock monitoring procedures for western encephalomyelitis in Manitoba-1975. Can. J. Public Health **67:** 15–20.
22. VIGLIANO, R.R. & D.B. CARLSON. 1986. An adjustable restrainer for sentinel chickens used in encephalitis surveillance. J. Am. Mosq. Control Assoc. **2:** 357–359.
23. REISEN, W.K., S.B. PRESSER, J. LIN, et al. 1994. Viremia and serological responses in adult chickens infected with western equine encephalomyelitis and St. Louis encephalitis viruses. J. Am. Mosq. Control Assoc. **10:** 549–555.
24. HOLDEN, P., D. MUTH & R.B. SHRINER. 1966. Arbovirus hemagglutinin-inhibitor in avian sera: inactivation with protamine sulfate. Am. J. Epidemiol. **84:** 67–73.
25. PAPADOPOULOS, O., R.O. ANSLOW & R.P. HANSON. 1970. Application of the immunodiffusion procedure to rapid identification of arboviruses and to detection of specific antibody in sentinel animals. Am. J. Epidemiol. **92:** 145–150.
26. CALISHER, C.H., H.N. FREMOUNT, W.L. VESELY, et al. 1986. Relevance of detection of immunoglobulin M antibody response in birds used for arbovirus surveillance. J. Clin. Microbiol. **24:** 770–774.
27. BROOM, A.K., J. CHARLICK, S.J. RICHARDS & J.S. MACKENZIE. 1987. An enzyme-linked immunosorbent assay for detection of flavivirus antibodies in chicken sera. J. Virol. Methods **15:** 1 9.
28. OPRANDY, J.J., J.G. OLSON & T.W. SCOTT. 1988. A rapid dot immunoassay for the detection of serum antibodies to eastern equine encephalomyelitis and St. Louis encephalitis viruses in sentinel chickens. Am. J. Trop. Med. Hyg. **38:** 181–186.
29. BEATY, B.J., C.H. CALISHER & R.E. SHOPE. 1989. Arboviruses. In Diagnostic Procedures for Viral, Rickettsial and Chlamydial Infections, 6th edit. N.J. Schmidt & R.W. Emmons, Eds.: 797–855. American Public Health Association. Washington.
30. OLSON, J.G., T.W. SCOTT, L.H. LORENZ & J.L. HUBBARD. 1991. Enzyme immunoassay for detection of antibodies against eastern equine encephalomyelitis virus in sentinel chickens. J. Clin. Microbiol. **29:** 1457–1461.
31. HALL, R.A., A.K. BROOM, A.C. HARTNETT, et al. 1995. Immunodominant epitopes on the NS1 protein of MVE and KUN viruses serve as targets for a blocking ELISA to detect virus-specific antibodies in sentinel animal serum. J. Virol. Methods **51:** 201–10.
32. DAY, J.F. & D.B. CARLSON. 1985. The importance of autumn rainfall and sentinel flock location to understanding the epidemiology of St. Louis encephalitis virus in Indian River County, Florida. J. Am. Mosq. Control Assoc. **1:** 305–309.
33. DAY, J.F., R. WINNER, R.E. PARSONS & J.T. ZHANG. 1985. Distribution of St. Louis encephalitis viral antibody in sentinel chickens maintained in Sarasota County, Florida: 1978-1988. J. Med. Entomol. **28:** 19–23.
34. MORRIS, C.D., W.G. BAKER, L. STARK, et al. 1994. Comparison of chickens and pheasants as sentinels for eastern equine encephalitis and St. Louis encephalitis viruses in Florida. J. Am. Mosq. Control. Assoc. **10:** 545–548.
35. WILLIAMS, J.E., O.P. YOUNG, D.M. WATTS & T.J. REED. 1971. Wild birds as eastern (EEE) and western (WEE) equine encephalitis sentinels. J. Wildl. Dis. **7:** 188–194.
36. KOMAR, N. & A. SPIELMAN. 1995. Japanese quail as EEE sentinels. Proc. N.J. Mosq. Control Assoc. **82:** 32–36.
37. REISEN, W.K., J.L. HARDY & S.B. PRESSER. 1992. Evaluation of domestic pigeons as sentinels for detecting arbovirus activity in southern California. Am. J. Trop. Med. Hyg. **46:** 69–79.
38. BEREZIN, V.V., M.P. CHUMAKOV, B.F. SEMENOV, et al. 1971. Study of the ecology of mosquito-borne arboviruses by using sentinel animals in the Volga Delta. Vopr. Virusol. **1971:** 739–745 (Russian).
39. MONATH, T.P., M.S. SABATTINI, R. PAULI, et al. 1985. Arbovirus investigations in Argentina, 1977–1980. IV. Serologic surveys and sentinel equine program. Am. J. Trop. Med. Hyg. **34:** 966–975.
40. TAKEDA, T., T. ITO, M. CHIBA, et al. 1998. Isolation of tick-borne encephalitis virus from Ixodes ovatus (Acari: Ixodidae) in Japan. J. Med. Entomol. **35:** 227–231.

41. PINGER, R.R., W.A. ROWLEY, Y.W. WONG & D.C. DORSEY. 1975. Trivittatus virus infections in wild mammals and sentinel rabbits in central Iowa. Am. J. Trop. Med. Hyg. 24: 1006–1009.
42. VENTURA, A.K. & N.J. EHRENKRANZ. 1975. Detection of Venezuelan equine encephalitis virus in rural communities of Southern Florida by exposure of sentinel hamsters. Am. J. Trop. Med. Hyg. 24: 715–717.
43. TOMORI, O., A. FAGBAMI & A. FABIYI. 1978. Isolations of West Nile virus from man in Nigeria. Trans. R. Soc. Trop. Med. Hyg. 72: 103–104.
44. MCINTOSH, B.M., P.G. JUPP, D.B. DICKINSON, et al. 1967. Ecological studies on sindbis and West Nile viruses in South Africa. I. Viral activity as revealed by infection of mosquitoes and sentinel fowls. S. Afr. J. Med. Sci. 32: 1–14.
45. MCINTOSH, B.M. & P.G. JUPP. 1979. Infections in sentinel pigeons by Sindbis and West Nile viruses in South Africa, with observations on Culex (Culex) univittatus (Diptera: Culicidae) attracted to these birds. J. Med. Entomol. 16: 234–239.
46. DOHERTY, R.L., J.G. CARLEY, B.H. KAY, et al. 1976. Murray Valley encephalitis virus infection in mosquitoes and domestic fowls in Queensland, 1974. Aust. J. Exp. Biol. Med. Sci. 54: 237–243.
47. RUSSELL, R.C. 1998. Mosquito-borne arboviruses in Australia: the current scene and implications of climate change for human health. Int. J. Parasitol. 28: 955–969.
48. CERNESCU, C., N.I. NEDELCU, G. TARDEI, et al. 2000. Continued transmission of West Nile virus to humans in southeastern Romania, 1997–1998. J. Infect. Dis. 181: 710–712.
49. SENNE, D.A., J.C. PEDERSEN, D.L. HUTTO, et al. 2000. Pathogenicity of West Nile virus in chickens. Avian Dis. 44: 642–649.
50. LANGEVIN, S.A., M. BUNNING, B. DAVIS & N. KOMAR. 2001. Experimental infection of chickens as candidate sentinels for West Nile virus. Emerg. Infect. Dis. 7: 726–729.
51. KOMAR, N., N.A. PANELLA, J.E. BURNS, et al. 2001. Serologic evidence for West Nile virus infection in birds in the New York City vicinity during an outbreak in 1999. Emerg. Infect. Dis. 7: 621–625.
52. CENTERS FOR DISEASE CONTROL AND PREVENTION. 2000. Update: West Nile Virus Activity—Northeastern United States, 2000. Morb. Mort. Wkly. Rep. 49: 820–822.
53. CHERRY, B., S.C. TROCK, A. GLASER, et al. 2001. Sentinel chickens as a surveillance tool for West Nile virus in New York City, 2000. Ann. N.Y. Acad. Sci. 951. This volume.
54. LUDWIG, G.V., R.S. COOK, R.G. MCLEAN & D.B. FRANCY. 1986. Viremic enhancement due to transovarially acquired antibodies to St. Louis encephalitis virus in birds. J. Wildl. Dis. 22: 326–334.
55. PYLE, P. 1997. Identification Guide to North American Birds, Part I. Slate Creek Press. Bolinas, CA.
56. MAIN, A.J., K.S. ANDERSON, H.K. MAXFIELD, et al. 1988. Duration of alphavirus neutralizing antibody in naturally infected birds. Am. J. Trop. Med. Hyg. 38: 208–217.
57. CRANS, W.J., D.F. CACCAMISE & J.R. MCNELLY. 1994. Eastern equine encephalomyelitis virus in relation to the avian community of a coastal cedar swamp. J. Med. Entomol. 31: 711–728.
58. GRUWELL, J.A., C.L. FOGARTY, S.G. BENNETT, et al. 2000. Role of peridomestic birds in the transmission of St. Louis encephalitis virus in southern California. J. Wildl. Dis. 36: 13–34.
59. STAMM, D.D. 1968. Arbovirus studies in birds in South Alabama, 1959–1960. Am. J. Epidemiol. 87: 127–137.
60. REISEN, W.K., J.O. LUNDSTROM, T.W. SCOTT, et al. 2000. Patterns of avian seroprevalence to western equine encephalomyelitis and Saint Louis encephalitis viruses in California, USA. J. Med. Entomol. 37: 507–527.
61. BIGLER, W.J., E. LASSING, E. BUFF, et al. 1975. Arbovirus surveillance in Florida: wild vertebrate studies 1965–1974. J. Wildl. Dis. 11: 348–356.
62. MCLEAN, R.G., J. MULLENIX, J. KERSCHNER & J. HAMM. The house sparrow (Passer domesticus) as a sentinel for St. Louis encephalitis virus. 1983. Am. J. Trop. Med. Hyg. 32: 1120–1129.

63. KOMAR, N., J. BURNS, C. DEAN, *et al.* 2001. Serologic evidence for West Nile virus infection in birds in Staten Island, New York, after an Outbreak in 2000. Vector-Borne Zoonotic Dis. **3.** In press.
64. REISEN, W.K., L.D. KRAMER, R.E. CHILES, *et al.* 2000. Response of house finches to infection with sympatric and allopatric strains of western equine encephalomyelitis and St. Louis encephalitis viruses from California. J. Med. Entomol. **7:** 259–264.
65. SWAYNE, D.E., J.R. BECK & S. ZAKI. 2000. Pathogenicity of West Nile virus for turkeys. Avian Dis. **44:** 932–937.
66. SWAYNE, D.E., J.R. BECK, C.S. SMITH, *et al.* 2001. Fatal encephalitis and myocarditis in young domestic geese (*Anser anser domesticus*) caused by West Nile virus. Emerg. Infect. Dis. **7:** 741–753.
67. CALISHER, C.H., N. KARABATSOS, J.M. DALRYMPLE, *et al.* 1989. Antigenic relationships between flaviviruses as determined by cross-neutralization tests with polyclonal antisera. J. Gen. Virol. **70:** 37–43.
68. INOUYE, S., S. MATSUNO & Y. TSURUKUBO. 1984. "Original antigenic sin" phenomenon in experimental flavivirus infections of guinea pigs: studies by enzyme-linked immunosorbent assay. Microbiol. Immunol. **28:** 569–574.

Vector Surveillance for West Nile Virus

DENNIS J. WHITE

Arthropod-Borne Disease Program, New York State Department of Health, Albany, New York 12237, USA

ABSTRACT: West Nile virus (WNV) was detected in the metropolitan New York City (NYC) area during the summer and fall of 1999. Sixty-two human cases, including seven fatalities, were documented. The New York State Department of Health (NYSDOH) initiated and implemented a statewide mosquito and WNV surveillance system. We developed a WNV response plan designed to provide local health departments (LHD) a standardized means to begin to assess basic mosquito population data and to detect WNV circulation in mosquito populations. During the 2000 arbovirus surveillance season, local health agencies collected 317,676 mosquitoes and submitted 9,952 pools for virus testing. NYSDOH polymerase chain reaction (PCR) testing detected 363 WNV-positive pools. Eight species of mosquitoes were found to be infected. Of the 26 counties conducting mosquito surveillance, WNV-positive mosquitoes were detected only in NYC, on Long Island, and in four counties in the lower Hudson River valley region. LHD larval surveillance provided initial or enhanced mosquito habitat location and characterization and mosquito species documentation. Adult mosquito surveillance provided LHD information on species' presence, density, seasonal fluctuations, virus infection, minimum infection ratios (MIR) and indirect data on mosquito control efficacy after larval or adult control interventions. Collective surveillance activities conducted during 1999 and 2000 suggest that WNV has dispersed throughout the state and may affect local health jurisdictions within NYS, adjacent states, and Canada in future years. Vector surveillance will remain a critical component of LHD programs addressing public health concerns related to WNV.

KEYWORDS: West Nile virus; mosquito; vector; arbovirus; surveillance

INTRODUCTION

West Nile virus (WNV) was detected initially in the metropolitan New York City (NYC) area during the summer and fall of 1999.[1] Sixty-two human cases, including seven fatalities, were documented. The New York State Department of Health (NYS-DOH) initiated an aggressive departmental effort to implement a statewide mosquito and virus surveillance system in concert with local and federal health agencies.[2] We developed a WNV response plan designed to provide local health departments (LHD) a standardized means to begin to assess basic mosquito population data and to detect WNV circulation in mosquito populations. During the 2000 arbovirus surveillance season, local health agencies collected 317,676 mosquitoes and submitted

Address for correspondence: Dennis J. White, Ph.D., Director, Arthropod-Borne Disease Program, New York State Department of Health, Corning Tower Building, Empire State Plaza, Albany, NY 12237. Voice: 518-474-4568; fax: 518-473-1708.

djw05@health.state.ny.us

9952 pools for virus testing. NYSDOH polymerase chain reaction (PCR) testing detected 363 WNV-positive pools. Eight species of mosquitoes were found infected. Of the 26 counties conducting mosquito surveillance, WNV-positive mosquitoes were detected only in NYC, on Long Island, and in four counties in the lower Hudson River valley region.

Larval surveillance conducted by LHDs allowed for initial or enhanced habitat location and characterization and mosquito species documentation. Adult mosquito surveillance provided LHD information on species' presence, density, seasonal fluctuations, virus infection, minimum infection ratios (MIR) and indirect data on mosquito control efficacy after larval or adult control interventions.

Larval mosquito surveillance will be an essential component of effective and efficient LHD mosquito intervention programs against WNV. Adult mosquito surveillance can provide extremely valuable data for a variety of purposes when performed in a standardized manner and may need to be tailored for certain LHDs according to their available resources. Collective surveillance activities conducted during 1999 and 2000 suggest that WNV may have dispersed throughout the state and may affect local health jurisdictions within NYS, adjacent states, and Canada in future years. However, larval and adult mosquito surveillance can be used to accomplish wide-ranging objectives. While adult mosquito surveillance will be used similarly in future years to identify vector species, enhanced larval and adult mosquito surveillance can also focus on other critical information that will allow us to better understand the ecology of this and other mosquito-borne zoonotic diseases. This paper will describe the range and application of these mosquito surveillance activities and discuss the value of the derived information.

SURVEILLANCE APPLICATIONS

Local, state, and federal public health agencies have a wide variety of tools and resources available to use in the assessment of mosquito population dynamics. Many of these tools have been available for almost one hundred years. In very general terms, surveillance includes the use of the appropriate tools in the appropriate locations to collect the widest variety of specimens of interest to one's particular objectives. For public health purposes, surveillance can be defined as the ongoing, systematic collection, analysis, and interpretation of data for the purpose of describing, monitoring, or controlling a health event. Technological applications for product improvement over time have continued to ensure the availability of effective tools to collect a wide range of data that can assist in the determination of public health threat assessments related to mosquito-borne problems, either as nuisance populations or as vectors of zoonotic disease. Public health–oriented agencies, academic institutions, public works agencies, and other agencies are often tasked with the responsibility to identify nuisance or disease risks associated with mosquito populations within their jurisdictions. These agencies must develop their priority objectives and then identify a protocol for surveillance that will allow them to reach these objectives.

In its simplest form, mosquito surveillance can be conducted to focus on immature or mature stages of mosquitoes, most commonly for larval or for adult female mosquitoes, respectively.[3–5] Depending on the tools used or the agency priorities, larval surveillance activities can provide information related to a wide variety of topics. Data related to, for example, habitat preference, species composition in their aquatic habitat, life-tables, population density, duration of larval and pupal stages, weather and precipitation factors, predictions for adult emergence, and effectiveness of immature mosquito population control interventions (larval control), may be derived from comprehensive immature mosquito surveillance activities.

Similarly, comprehensive adult mosquito surveillance can accomplish a wide variety of objectives.[3–5] In addition, several collection mechanisms exist to help sample a variety of physiological states of adult females, whether populations are host-seeking, ready for oviposition, diurnal resting, or hibernating, for example. Data can be developed, for example, related to species' diversity, species' abundance, population density, seasonal range of species' activity, physiological age, blood meal determination, control intervention assessment, flight range, virus infection, minimal infection ratios, and vector potential. Properly conducted adult mosquito surveillance activities can provide a wide range of integrated data that will assist in the understanding of the ecology and public health risks associated with local mosquito populations or mosquito-borne diseases they can transmit.

LARVAL SURVEILLANCE

Using nothing more than a white plastic or enamel dipper on the end of a 3–4 foot pole, an individual with good observational and data-recording skills, and some hiking endurance, can accomplish a great deal. Cumulated data related to standing water habitat sampling, characterization, and mapping will provide the basis for a comprehensive ecological database identifying mosquito breeding areas within the agency's jurisdiction.

A wide range of analysis and assessment can be generated from comprehensive larval surveillance. For example, larval surveillance can include a large-scale survey to identify habitat locations, an effort to characterize these habitats biologically, chemically, physically, or ecologically, or to assess the effectiveness of efforts taken to modify the mosquito-producing potential of these habitats.

Regularly repeated visits to existing sites and other newly identified areas will provide the long-term seasonal data that will be more easily subject to population trend and statistical analyses. Measures of species composition, species diversity, seasonal population fluctuations, population management, and other research studies can be accomplished using very simple larval surveillance protocols. This cumulative surveillance information will also provide the necessary biological data to make informed decisions related to control timing, duration, frequency, and effectiveness.

Mosquito surveillance activities focusing on West Nile virus adds a slightly different dimension for public health or public works agencies in the northeastern United States. St. Louis encephalitis (SLE) virus affected much of the eastern half of the United States in the mid-1970s. Since that outbreak, many agencies in the Northeast that have done any mosquito surveillance have concentrated on eastern equine encephalitis (EEE) virus or perhaps on California encephalitis (CE) virus and their associated vectors. Most primary or secondary mosquito vectors associated with these viruses will breed in natural permanent or temporary wetlands. The primary amplifying vectors associated with WNV (*Culex* species) are "container" breeders, taking advantage of man-made structures or objects in which water accumulates and can become rather putrid with decaying organic material, although it is not uncommon to find *Culex* immatures in habitats with relatively clear water. These "containers" may range in size from a discarded coffee cup or automobile tire, to bird baths, clogged rain gutters, abandoned swimming pools or pool covers, to sewage or wastewater treatment facilities, for example. As water in these containers becomes more organic (with algae, grass or leafy debris), it becomes more attractive as a place for gravid *Culex* females to oviposit eggs.

It is important to note that other potential bridge vectors capable of moving WNV from the amplifying bird hosts to mammals can also breed in containers (*Ochlerotatus japonicus*, *Oc. albopictus*, *Oc. triseriatus*, etc). These and other species of mosquitoes will need to be sampled (and controlled) in habitats other than containers when WNV is found to have breached the avian maintenance cycle. The ultimate control of WNV transmission may include larval control in a wide variety of natural and man-made habitats. For these reasons, it is extremely important to identify and characterize all significant mosquito breeding habitats in the affected jurisdiction. Certain habitats may not require any interventions, while others may require repeated comprehensive efforts to reduce or eliminate mosquito breeding. Without good, thorough immature mosquito surveillance, the responsible agency may not know the difference.

For these reasons, public health and public works agencies concerned with WNV may need to focus immature mosquito surveillance activities in more urban or suburban settings than is most often associated with surveillance activities for EEE or CE viruses.[5] Since these mosquitoes are associated with oviposition sites that are in proximity to human populations, risks associated with human disease exposure are likely to be greater in urban or suburban settings. This fact necessarily makes agency surveillance or control activities much more visible and accountable to the public they are serving.

Concerns regarding mosquito breeding, nuisance biting populations, disease risk determinations, and population intervention effectiveness will be constantly addressed by the general public, medical providers, and elected officials. Programs can begin to provide responsible answers to these questions through comprehensive and careful larval surveillance, as one component of the entire effort to identify the public health threats related to mosquitoes in their jurisdiction. In addition to the effort spent on immature mosquito ecology, proactive public health and public works agencies will also implement and maintain surveillance efforts focusing on adult mosquitoes. It is fairly safe to state that this is often the only stage of mosquito the majority of people ever see in their day-to-day activities. It is also the stage most people will complain about as the female mosquitoes seek a blood meal to produce the next generation of eggs and larvae.

ADULT SURVEILLANCE

A wealth of knowledge related to mosquito biology, ecology, nuisance status, and disease threat can be generated by agencies conducting comprehensive adult mosquito surveillance using very simple tools and concepts.[5–7] Adult mosquito surveillance complements immature mosquito surveillance in agency or institutional efforts to understand the full spectrum of disease threat assessment associated with mosquito-borne viruses, whether for WN, EEE, SLE, or CE viruses in the United States. The challenge for the responsible agencies, however, is associated with the establishment and implementation of a solid foundation of adult mosquito collections, maximizing the available human and equipment resources.

In simplest terms, since male mosquitoes do not feed on blood, public health and public works agencies (along with the general population) are concerned with adult female mosquitoes. In order for mosquitoes to generate a batch of eggs, the female mosquito must successfully feed on a host. The protein derived from this blood meal (whether from an amphibian, reptile, bird, or mammal) is converted through the physiological process of oogenesis to fully developed ovaries ready to lay a few hundred eggs within a week to ten days in most cases.

Female mosquitoes have few needs in life. Other than reasonable temperatures and humidity to sustain survival (as well as a few male mosquitoes of the same species), female mosquitoes exist only to seek blood meals, sites to rest and digest the blood meal, and sites where she can lay her eggs. A wide variety of tools are available to capitalize on these behaviors in order to conduct a comprehensive surveillance program. All one needs to do is to provide appropriate trapping methods to attract that portion of the adult mosquito population that is seeking a host, and the other components of the population that are seeking a place to rest and digest blood meals or seeking a suitable oviposition site. Several types of trapping methods exist that can provide surrogate sites capable of attracting adult mosquitoes in these differing physiological states.

While the collection methods are fairly simple in concept and relatively easy to employ, the outcome of these surveillance efforts can include very comprehensive data in efforts to identify public health issues related to nuisance or disease vector populations.[5–7] In order to generate mosquito population trend analyses, a significant effort should be employed in selecting appropriate surveillance sites and methods. In ideal situations, once adult surveillance sites are selected and found to be productive, the trap locations should not change. In this way, weekly population baseline data are collected and maintained throughout the entire season. Occasionally, trap sites may need to move through a target area. It is possible that it may take several potential sites before productive sites are located. Agencies that may not have full budget support for numerous trapping equipment may need to rotate trapping resources around the target area in order to get representative data from as wide an area as possible. However, this activity decreases the long-term value of population assessment or the ability to determine effectiveness of interventions, and decreases the power of statistical analyses used for other comprehensive surveillance purposes.

In addition to the typical adult mosquito population composition and diversity data, as well as seasonal fluctuation and duration of biting activity, important physiological assessments can be derived. This can include separate investigations of host-seeking activity, age composition and parity rates, host preference studies and oviposition behavior. All of this information, when properly analyzed spatially and temporally, can lead toward better understanding of species' infection rates, vector potential analysis, determination of intervention effectiveness, and other research studies.

Host-seeking females can be attracted successfully to traps, using one or a combination of light, heat, and carbon dioxide (usually as subliming dry ice or burning propane) as attractants. Several trap designs exist, but most employ these or similar attractants. Mosquitoes seeking a resting location (especially *Culiseta, Culex,* or *Anopheles*) can be attracted to dark painted wooden boxes open on one end in forested habitats providing a dark, humid, protected habitat in which blood meal digestion can occur. Mosquitoes seeking oviposition sites can be attracted to specially designed traps using clear or putrid water as an olfactory attractant mimicking other container breeding sites. As females are attracted to either the light traps or gravid traps, they are blown into a catch chamber by a battery-powered fan and subject to collection by surveillance staff the following day. Ovipositing females will deposit eggs on the surface of a wooden or fabric paddle kept moist by being partially submerged in the water in the container.

RESOURCE AND TRAINING REQUIREMENTS

In order to accomplish these multiple tasks over the wide geographic area that may be affected by WNV or other mosquito-borne diseases, agencies and institutions may require a wide variety of resources and training. Acquisition of the appropriate surveillance equipment and supplies, proper placement and timing of the surveillance tools, larval and female mosquito species' identification, habitat characterization, physiological and intervention assessments, and vector potential calculations will require internal staff development and training. Staff may also request assistance with methods to report the complex information obtained through these procedures within their own and other agencies. The NYSDOH will build upon initial training activities offered during 2000 and expand coverage into all these areas for LHDs and academic institutions requesting this assistance.

RESEARCH ACTIVITIES

These surveillance activities, when performed in a standardized, comprehensive fashion, can help answer significant questions related to WNV and other mosquito-borne disease or nuisance issues. Hypothesis generation related to the behavior and physiology of these mosquitoes can focus on a number of issues. Routine surveillance can identify mosquito population trends, intervention effectiveness, mosquito host preference studies, vertical transmission studies, insecticide bioassay, and resistance analysis and serve to answer questions related to apparently complex enzootic cycles in nature. As new data are obtained, investigators may derive related information on potential alternate vector species, mosquito flight ranges, surveillance trap model efficiencies, or even indicators of public satisfaction with agency activities in a prescribed area. Relationships among the presence of mosquito species and dead bird surveillance, or suspect equine or human case investigations can be better elucidated by close analysis of information derived from rather simple mosquito collection activities or specially designed research studies.

CALCULATIONS

The utility of surveillance data can be expanded even further through the use of relatively simple mathematical calculations. Graphical representation of daily or weekly surveillance data over the course of an entire season can be predictive and help to identify time periods of expected nuisance populations. Cumulative annual data can be manipulated to develop normalized representations of 3–5 year averages, against which current year surveillance data can be compared. The availability of related short-term weather and longer-term climate data, for example, overlapped onto the long-term seasonal summary data, can help agencies develop some predictive abilities for future mosquito population surges.

Species composition of adult collections can be determined by accurate mosquito identifications and categorization of specific species into primary, secondary (bridge vectors), or nuisance species, depending on the recognized contributions of that species to the mosquito-borne disease cycle. These data can be helpful to improve the ability to predict when secondary vectors may be in abundance and more likely to carry the virus out of the normal amplifying host cycle and increase risks to other susceptible ("dead-end") hosts.

In addition to the collection and processing of numbers of mosquitoes and species of mosquitoes in a surveillance program, agencies and institutions are often interested whether certain collections of adult mosquitoes are infected with viruses pathologic to birds or animals. Arbovirus surveillance systems can employ a number of surveillance components to include mosquitoes, birds, humans or other animals. By combining arbovirus surveillance efforts (using laboratory testing for viruses) with ongoing mosquito and vertebrate surveillance systems, the composite value of agency surveillance systems can be expanded greatly. Data related to public health threat assessments, minimum infection ratios, and vectorial capacity[8] determination can be generated through careful analysis of well-designed surveillance systems and laboratory data. Mosquito surveillance data then become more useful for predictive analysis of human health threat assessments. Increasing rates of infection in mosquito pools can be directly related to increased risks for human infection, as measured by vector potential analysis. Full determination of vector potential requires information related to mosquito species, current virus infection rate in that species, mosquito age structure (parity status), as well as human and mosquito population density in the area where the surveillance activity is taking place.

Similar data assessment can be extremely valuable to determine whether interventions (biological control, pesticide application, habitat modification, education, etc.) were effective in reducing the human health threat. It is very important for agencies or institutions to determine whether money spent on interventions resulted in decreased numbers of mosquitoes or in decreased risk of human exposure to infected mosquitoes. Simple percentage reduction calculations[9] can be developed from pre- and postintervention mosquito population counts in the area subject to the intervention (treatment area) as compared to the same pre- and postintervention data collected from a similar area not subject to the intervention (control area).

$$\% \text{ Control} = 100 - (T/U \times 100),$$

where T = posttreatment means divided by the pretreatment means in the area subject to the intervention, and U = posttreatment means divided by the pretreatment means in an area that was not subjected to the intervention.

More complex analyses, such as regression analysis or analysis of variance calculations can provide a more thorough understanding of the effect of other variables, such as, for example, trap types, temperature, humidity, and habitat as well as the actual duration of effective control. Staff in the Arthropod-Borne Disease Program is developing these programs. We will also try to make them available to local health department staff on the New York State Department of Health's Health Information Network (HIN) as a self-contained macroprogram for easy data entry and analysis.[10]

MAPPING

Agencies should take advantage of new technologies available for Geographic Position System (GPS) description of all sites used in mosquito surveillance systems. GPS satellite location data are now sufficiently accurate to provide reasonable latitude and longitude coordinates useful for repeated visits to surveillance sites within and among sequential surveillance seasons. These data fit into the full Geographical Information System (GIS) analyses that can help provide multidimensional descriptions of multilayered surveillance data. Immature mosquito breeding areas can be mapped and monitored, natural or man-made habitats can be pinpointed, and resulting seasonal mosquito data can be applied and analyzed over time. Seasonal or annual population trends, for example, spray zones and notification logs, can all be mapped and made available to the residents of the area, increasing the value of the surveillance system and demonstrating the scope of comprehensive data maintained for decision-making purposes.[11]

REPORTING

Comprehensive surveillance activities require comprehensive data analysis, interpretation, summarization, and prompt reporting in order to understand what the surveillance data mean and whether a response is required. All agencies involved in generating surveillance data need to develop a reliable reporting mechanism so that those individuals and agencies who are responsible for supporting the surveillance activities or for responding to the surveillance data (education campaigns, intervention programs, budgetary development, etc.) can base their actions on reliable, prompt data.

Reporting mechanisms can be custom-designed around the structure and scope of the surveillance program and range from weekly representations of graphic and tabular data to thorough complex electronic relational databases.[9] Through this range of reporting responses, staff responsible for surveillance programs will gain from the increased visibility and satisfy issues related to program accountability to those people supporting the program (administrative staff, political leaders, funding agencies, etc.). Surveillance data will also be valuable for staff in agencies in peripheral jurisdictions who may be extremely concerned about disease activity in the general area.

MINIMALLY ACCEPTABLE MOSQUITO SURVEILLANCE ACTIVITY

For agencies facing extremely austere fiscal conditions, LHDs may need to determine absolute priorities to be accomplished with existing resources. For example, if an LHD determined that virus testing of collected mosquitoes was the ultimate priority, their minimally acceptable surveillance system might include the following scenario: adult mosquito collections could be obtained by four gravid traps and four dry-ice baited light traps, set for two nights a week, one of each in four separate locations. The following week, four new locations could be sampled, again with one of each type of trap, until at the end of the first four-week cycle, traps would return to the original four sites for the second seasonal collection. In order to collect mosquitoes to the gravid traps in this scenario, it would be important to make up the gravid water suspension two to three days prior to their employment. Mosquitoes of the same species, collected in the same location during the same week, could then be combined in pools of 10–100 specimens and submitted to the appropriate laboratory for virus testing. This system would require staff provision of batteries and dry ice, along with mosquito recovery each morning for identification, enumerating, and reporting. Cooperating homeowners can be taught to set up the traps in the evenings by inserting the batteries in the traps at the appropriate time two nights a week.

Given additional support, LHDs should strongly consider conducting larval mosquito surveillance as well. As described earlier, mosquito habitat location, species' identification, and considerations for source reduction can be derived from very small financial investments.

These minimally acceptable surveillance activities may significantly decrease an agency's ability to accomplish other population or ecological objectives with any degree of scientific or statistical certainty, and does not allow for even basic surveillance trends or other investigational purposes.

SUMMARY

Mosquito surveillance activities imply much more than arbovirus testing. Larval and adult mosquito surveillance activities can provide LHDs with a wide spectrum of interrelated data, including assessment of species' composition, density, age determinations, vector potential, or intervention effectiveness, for example. The NYS-DOH Arthropod-Borne Disease Program has recently experienced programmatic expansion as a result of the WNV outbreak in the northeastern United States. We aim to assist LHDs struggling with their own infrastructure issues in order to provide surveillance activities commensurate with their individual available resources. Consultation and training will be available on a regular, continuous basis for LHDs or other related agencies and institutions requesting assistance.

REFERENCES AND RESOURCES

1. CDC. 1999. Update: West Nile virus encephalitis—New York, 1999. Morb. Mortal. Wkly. Rep. **48:** 944–946, 955.
2. CDC. 2000. Update: West Nile virus activity—Eastern United States, 2000. Morb. Mortal. Wkly. Rep. **49**(46): 1044–1047.

3. MEANS, R.G. 1979. Mosquitoes of New York. Part I. The Genus *Aedes* with Identification Keys to Genera of Culicidae. State Science Service, New York State Museum. Albany, NY.
4. MEANS, R.G. 1987. Mosquitoes of New York. Part II. Genera of Culicidae Other Than *Aedes* Occurring in New York. State Science Service, New York State Museum. Albany, NY.
5. MOORE, C.G., R.G. MCLEAN, C.J. MITCHELL, *et al.* 1993. Guidelines for arbovirus surveillance programs in the United States. CDC. Public Health Service. US Dept. of Health and Human Services.
6. GUBLER, D.J., G.L. CAMPBELL, R. NASCI, *et al.* 2000. West Nile virus in the United States: guidelines for detection, prevention, and control. Viral Immunol. **13:** 469–475.
7. CDC. 2000. Guidelines for surveillance, prevention, and control of West Nile virus infection—United States. Morb. Mortal. Wkly. Rep. **49:** 25–28.
8. SPIELMAN, A. & A.A. JAMES. 1990. Transmission of vector-borne disease. *In* Tropical and Geographical Medicine, 2nd edit. K.S. Warren & A.A.F. Mahmood, Eds.: 146–159. McGraw Hill. New York.
9. SCHULZE, T., G.C. TAYLOR, L.M. VASVARY, *et al.* 1992. Effectiveness of an aerial application of carbaryl in controlling *Ixodes dammini* (Acari: Ixodidae) adults in a high-use recreational area in New Jersey. J. Med. Entomol. **29**(3): 544–547.
10. GOTHAM, I.J., M. EIDSON, D.J. WHITE, *et al.* 2001. West Nile virus. a case study in how NY State Health information infrastructure facilitates preparation and response to disease outbreaks. J. Public Health Manag. Practice. In press.
11. HAY, S.I., S.E. RANDOLPH & D.J. ROGERS. 2000. Remote Sensing and Geographical Information Systems in Epidemiology. Advances in Parasitology, Vol. 47. Academic Press. New York.

Web site resources with extensive West Nile virus information:

New York State Department of Health: www.state.health.ny.us
Centers for Disease Control and Prevention: www.cdc.gov
American Mosquito Control Association: www.mosquito.org
New Jersey Mosquito Control Association: www.njmosquito.org
New York City Department of Health: www.health.nyc.gov
National Atlas: www.nationalatlas.gov/virusmap.html
Rockland County, NY (Use of GIS in WNV management): www.co.rockland.ny.us

West Nile Virus Infection in Birds and Mammals

LAURA D. KRAMER AND KRISTEN A. BERNARD

Arbovirus Laboratories, Wadsworth Center,
New York State Department of Health, Slingerlands, New York 12159, USA

ABSTRACT: West Nile virus (WNV) was found throughout New York State in year 2000. The epicenter was located in New York City with a high level of activity in the immediately surrounding counties, including Rockland, Westchester, Nassau, and Suffolk. During 2000, WNV testing was performed by the Wadsworth Center on 3,687 dead birds, representing 153 species, 46 families, and 18 orders. There were 1,203 WNV-positive birds, representing 63 species, 30 families and 14 orders. The percentage of WNV-positive birds was 33% for all birds tested throughout the state, with no significant difference in infection rates in migratory versus resident birds, although significantly more resident birds were submitted for testing. The highest apparent mortality for the entire season was observed in American crows in Staten Island, a location that also showed the highest minimal infection rate in *Culex pipiens* complex mosquitoes. Studies examining tissue tropism of WNV in corvids and noncorvids from the epicenter and from remote locations indicated that the kidney was the most consistently infected tissue in birds, regardless of level of infection. The brain was the next most consistently positive tissue. The differences in infection among the tissues were most apparent when low levels of virus were present. Experimental mouse inoculation demonstrated a classical flavivirus infection pattern.

KEYWORDS: West Nile virus; tissue tropism; birds; mammals

INTRODUCTION

West Nile virus (WNV) is a newly emerging mosquito-borne virus now found on four continents, Africa, Asia, Europe, and North America. The infection in humans has been characterized by a broad range of clinical symptoms, from asymptomatic infection to mild nonspecific symptoms, including fever and headache, to more serious cases with myocarditis and encephalitis.[1] In 1999, 62 cases of WNV were confirmed in New York City and in 2000, 14 cases. Serosurveys conducted in 1999 demonstrated that 2.6% of the population in an area of high viral activity had antibody to WNV,[2] and in 2000, approximately 1% of the population demonstrated seroconversion.[2]

The introduction of WNV to the northeastern United States in 1999 was accompanied by unprecedented mortality in indigenous and captive birds. This was unex-

Address for correspondence: Laura D. Kramer, Ph.D., Director, Arbovirus Laboratories, Wadsworth Center, New York State Department of Health, 5668 State Farm Road, Slingerlands, NY 12159. Voice: 518-869-4524; fax: 518-869-4530.

Kramer@wadsworth.org

pected since, historically, in countries where WNV is enzootic, the virus has led to minimal disease in avian species. WNV has been demonstrated to infect a wide variety of vertebrate species besides man and birds, as indicated by evidence of antibody to the virus and virus isolation.[3] Studies during the 1950s in Egypt indicated that the hooded crow and the house sparrow had antibody rates of 65 and 42%, respectively, and virus was isolated from the blood of an adult crow.[4]

The work presented here is aimed at elucidating WNV infection in vertebrates other than man. Data from 2000 in New York State were analyzed to determine which bird species were found infected most frequently with WNV in 2000, and which avian tissues were most often infected. Five out of 149 wild mammals were found to be infected with WNV in year 2000 in New York State. These included one little brown bat (*Myotis lucifugus*), one big brown bat (*Eptesicus fuscus*), one squirrel (*Sciurus carolinensis*), one domestic rabbit (*Oryctolagus cuniculus*), and one eastern chipmunk (*Tamias striatus*). A preliminary study delineating infection in white mice as a model for infection in mammals was undertaken to begin to define the pathogenesis of WNV.

MATERIAL AND METHODS

Tissue Submission and Processing

Dead birds and mammals were submitted for necropsy to the Department of Environmental Conservation, Wildlife Pathology Unit, New York State. Multiple tissues from suspect animals were forwarded to the Arbovirus Laboratories of the Wadsworth Center, New York State Department of Health, for viral assay. Protocols for handling tissues and for viral assays have been described previously.[5] Briefly, 50 mm^3 sections of tissue were excised and triturated directly in lysis buffer containing guanidium isothiocyanate (Qiagen, CA). RNA was extracted as per the manufacturer's instructions, and reverse transcription–polymerase chain reaction (RT-PCR) was conducted using an ABI Prism 7700 Sequence Detector using TaqMan One-Step RT-PCR master mix (Applied Biosystems, Foster City, CA). Two sets of primers/probes (1160; 3111) were used as described.[5,6] Ct values—the PCR cycle at which an increase in the fluorescence rises above the threshold value determined by the standard curve—were recorded; from this the TaqMan score was calculated, that is, + to ++++.

Determination of Minimum Infection Rate (MIR) in Mosquitoes

MIRs were calculated assuming one infected mosquito per pool per 1000 mosquitoes tested. Mosquito pools were processed as described.[5] Briefly, pools were triturated using SpexCertiPrep 8000-D mixer mill (Metuchen, NJ). A 350 µL aliquot was removed immediately for RNA extraction, which was conducted as described above for vertebrate tissue, as was RT-PCR. The remainder of the triturated pool was held for inoculation of cell culture to detect live infectious virus.

Cell Culture Assay

African green monkey kidney (Vero) cell cultures in 25-mm flasks were inoculated with 0.1 mL homogenized and clarified mosquito suspension. Monolayers were checked daily for seven days for evidence of cytopathology (cpe). After seven days or when cpe was observed, cells were spotted on slides, fixed and stained with primary antibody, H5.46 WNV monoclonal antibody, and secondarily with goat anti-mouse IgG fluorescein-conjugated antibody (Kirkegaard and Perry Laboratories, Gaithersburg, MD). Fluorescence was evaluated using an Olympus BH-2 microscope equipped with FITC filter set.

Plaque Assay

Cell culture plaque assays to quantitate infectious virus were conducted as previously described.[7] Briefly, six-well Costar plates with Vero cell monolayers were inoculated with homogenized and clarified tissue suspensions, 0.1 mL per well. A single overlay of 2.0% oxoid agar with 0.8 mL of 1.0% neutral red was added; plaques were read from day 3 to day 7.

Pathogenesis of West Nile Virus in Adult Mice

Female Balb/C mice, five weeks old, were inoculated intraperitoneally with 10^3 PFU WNV isolated from a pool of 50 *Cx. pipiens* mosquitoes from New York in 2000. Virus was diluted in low endotoxin phosphate-buffered saline containing 1% fetal bovine serum (diluent). Three control mice were inoculated with diluent alone, and three additional mice were not inoculated, but were housed with inoculated mice as contact controls. The mice were weighed and observed for clinical signs daily. Three mice each were sacrificed at 19 and 28 hours, days 2, 3, 4, 5, 8, and 9. Control mice were held for 24 days. Heart blood was collected, and the brain, liver, spleen, kidney, and heart were harvested for assay of infectious virus. All tissues were weighed, and diluent was added to make a 20% homogenate for brain or 10% homogenate for all other organs. The limit of detection was 250 PFU/g for brain and 500 PFU/g or mL for other organs and serum.

RESULTS

Avian Infection

A comparison of infection rates in year-round residents, migrants, mixed populations (in which only a portion of the population migrates), and captive birds indicated that the predominant number of birds that died and were tested for WNV were permanent residents (TABLE 1). However, there was no difference in the proportion of birds from all categories that were infected, 30 to 43%.

The proportion of American crows found infected with WNV was compared with the number of human[8] and equine[9] cases in the five boroughs of NYC, Long Island (Nassau and Suffolk counties), and two other locations within the epicenter, Westchester and Rockland counties (FIG. 1). Ten of 14 cases in humans in New York State were detected on Staten Island (SI), where more than 90% of the crows tested were infected, and the minimal infection rate in *Cx. pipiens* complex mosquitoes (*Cx. pipiens* and *Cx. pipiens-restuans* combined) was 10.9. Three other boroughs in NYC—Brooklyn, Manhattan, and Queens—had one to two human cases, and all other locations had none. The greatest numbers of dead crows were submitted by

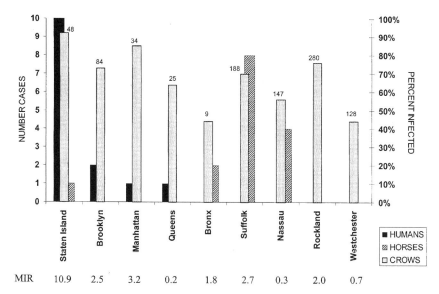

MIR   10.9   2.5   3.2   0.2   1.8   2.7   0.3   2.0   0.7

FIGURE 1. Relative infection rates of crows, humans, and equines by location in epicenter of WNV outbreak, 2000. MIR, minimal infection rate in *Culex pipiens* and *Culex pipiens-restuans* complex mosquitoes combined. Number of human and equine cases and percentage positive crows are reported. Numbers above bars represent number of crows tested.

TABLE 1. Infection in birds with different migration patterns

Behavior pattern	Number tested	Species	Positive Individuals	Percent
Year-round residents	2924	28	1116	38
True migrants	51	14	22	43
Mixed population	175	15	53	30
Captive birds	25	6	10	40

Rockland county, of which 75% were infected with WNV; the MIR in *Cx. pipiens* complex mosquitoes in Rockland was 2.0, but no human or horse cases were observed. Suffolk had the second highest number of dead crows submitted for testing and had the greatest number of equine cases in NYS (8), but infected horses also were detected in Staten Island, the Bronx, and Nassau. More detailed information on WNV infection in birds and mosquitoes can be found in Bernard *et al.*[10]

The MIRs of *Cx. pipiens* and *Cx. pipiens-restuans* complex mosquitoes were combined. Other *Culex* species were not included in this summary because of problems encountered with identification of other species of *Culex* mosquitoes (unpublished data, Kramer). Vero cell cultures inoculated with positive mosquito pools of all species indicated that infectious virus could be detected in 111/266 (41.7%)

TABLE 2. WNV cell culture results for mosquitoes collected in New York State during 2000

Mosquito species	No. positive pools by RT-PCR	No. positive pools by cell culture (*n* tested)
Ochlerotatus cantator	1	0 (1)
Oc. japonicus	5	0 (5)
Oc. triseriatus	3	1 (3)
Ae. vexans	10	1 (10)
Ae. species	1	0 (0)
An. punctipennis	1	0 (1)
Culex pipiens	79	25 (60)
Cx. pipiens-restuans	212	61 (146)
Cx. salinarius	31	13 (26)
Cx. species	19	9 (13)
Psorophora ferox	1	1 (1)

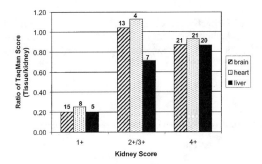

FIGURE 2. Relative TaqMan score of brain, heart, and liver compared to kidney. The numbers above the bars indicate the number of tissues compared in parallel with the kidney. 1+ represents Ct value 32–36; 2+ to 3+, 24–32; 4+, 14–25.

(TABLE 2). Passage through cell culture did not allow for amplification of initially undetectable levels of infectious virus.

Tissue Tropism in Birds

TaqMan RT-PCR results from kidney, heart and brain tissues from 49 crows were compared in order to determine tissue tropisms of WNV (FIG. 2). Birds found infected with low, medium, and high concentrations of viral WNV RNA during 2000 were selected. Multiple tissues from the crows were tested in parallel, but not all tissues were available from all birds. Each tissue was scored as its TaqMan score relative to the TaqMan score of the kidney of the same bird, and the mean was taken. Kidney was the most consistently positive tissue, regardless of the level of infection. The heart, brain and liver of birds with TaqMan scores of 3–4+ in the kidney had levels

KRAMER & BERNARD: WEST NILE VIRUS IN BIRDS AND MAMMALS

of viral RNA equal to that of the kidney, and these tissues therefore were equally good indicators of infection. Similarly, heart and brain of birds with TaqMan scores of 2+ in the kidneys were infected to an equal extent; liver, however, had 0.7 (70%) of the level of viral RNA. The heart, brain, and liver of birds with kidneys that were low positives (1+) had approximately 0.2 (20%) of the kidney's level of viral RNA.

Focal Infection of Tissues

A study was conducted to determine the uniformity of viral infection in various organs of crows. The level of viral RNA was determined in 8 to 15 separate sections excised from each of 12 individual paired crow brains and kidneys (TABLE 3). There was insufficient tissue available to excise 15 sections in every case. All but four positive tissues demonstrated variable levels of viral RNA (i.e., from Ct value 36 to 14, TaqMan score 1+ to 4+) in excised tissue sections. Four tissues demonstrated Ct values < 25 (i.e., 4+ levels of viral RNA in all sections: 3 brains, crows 10, 11, 12 and one kidney, crow 12). In two of the 12 crows (crows 1 and 3), brains were negative when the corresponding kidneys had several sections that were low positives (Ct 36 to 32); in one additional crow (crow 2), the brain was negative (- or ±) when the kidney was highly positive (Ct 29 to14). In one crow (crow 4), 13 of 15 brain sections were highly positive with Ct values < 29, but only one of 11 kidney sections was a low positive with a Ct value of 34. The variability observed among sections of both brain and kidney was more than 10-fold in some instances.

Tissue Tropism in Mammals

The WNV-inoculated mice appeared healthy until day 6 when mild clinical signs were evident in one mouse. Neurologic signs, ranging from ataxia and weakness to bilateral hindleg paralysis, were observed on days 7 through 9 in two of the six remaining mice. The maximum weight loss was 9%. No clinical signs were observed in the mock-inoculated or contact control mice. The following gross pathologic changes were observed in some, but not all mice: myocarditis (days 4, 5, 8, and 9); splenomegaly and lymphadenopathy (day 5); hemorrhagic meninges, hepatic lipidosis, lymphonecrosis of spleen and lymph nodes, reduced thymic size, and intestinal distention (days 8 and 9). Virus in the serum reached a peak of $10^{5.4}$ PFU/mL after three days and was cleared rapidly with only one mouse having a detectable viremia day 4 (FIG. 3). Infectious virus was also present early in the spleen of two mice at 19 h; one spleen contained 10^3 PFU/mL in the absence of detectable viremia. The titer in the spleen then increased to a peak at day 3 to 4. The heart was first positive at 28 h, and then increased in titer until day 4. On each of days 5, 8, 9, one heart was positive with low levels of virus, $10^{3.2}$–$10^{3.5}$ PFU/g. Virus was first detected in the kidney after 2 days. The level of infectious virus in this tissue increased slowly, reaching a peak on day 5, with $10^{5.2}$ PFU/g virus. The brain of one mouse was infected at 28 hours. The concentration of virus in the brain remained low until day 5, when one mouse had a significantly increased titer, $10^{4.8}$ PFU/g. By day 8, one mouse was very sick, with $10^{6.6}$ PFU/g virus in its brain, and $10^{3.2}$ PFU/g virus in its heart. Another mouse, which was mildly ill on day 8 with ruffled fur but no neurologic signs, was found dead on day 9. The kidney and brain of this mouse had detectable virus, but with titers below the peak, $10^{2.7}$ and $10^{4.9}$ PFU/g, respectively.

TABLE 3. Focus of West Nile virus in the brain and kidney of infected American crows

Crow	Brain							Kidney						
	N	\(TaqMan Score\)						N	\(TaqMan Score\)					
		-	+/-	1+	2+	3+	4+		-	+/-	1+	2+	3+	4+
1	15	100%						15	93%		7%			
2	15	100%						8					38%	63%
3	15	87%	13%					15	60%	20%	20%			
4	15	7%	7%			60%	27%	11	73%	18%	9%			
5	15	7%	7%	7%	13%	27%	47%	10			10%			90%
6	15			7%	20%	40%	33%	11					18%	82%
7	10				30%	40%	30%	8						88%
8	15				27%	40%	33%	9			11%	44%	22%	22%
9	12					67%	33%	15					13%	87%
10	15						100%	9			11%	44%		44%
11	15						100%	15					13%	87%
12	15						100%	11						100%
C_T range		40	40 - 36	36 - 32	32 - 29	29 - 24	25 - 14		40	40 - 36	36 - 32	32 - 29	29 - 24	25 - 14

N = Number of tissue samples per organ.

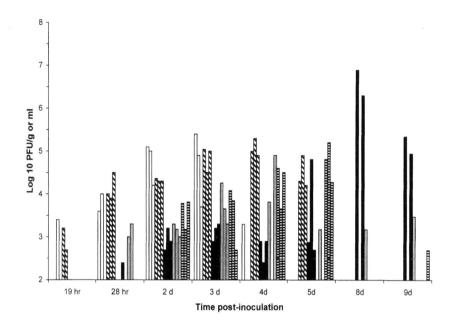

FIGURE 3. Experimental infection of Balb/C mice with WNV. Mice were inoculated intraperitoneally with 10^3 PFU WNV isolated from a pool of *Culex pipiens* in NY, 2000. Each bar represents results for a tissue from an individual mouse. White bar=serum; diagonally hatched bar=spleen; black bar=brain; stippled bar=heart; horizontally hatched bar=kidney. No bar indicates that the sample was below the limit of detection (250 to 500 PFU/g or mL).

DISCUSSION

WNV has a very broad host range. In 2000 in the northeastern US, more than 60 species of birds became infected and died from this virus. This is in sharp contrast to the biology of WNV in Europe, Asia and Africa, where there are few reports of bird mortality. Laboratory experiments with Hooded Crows demonstrated a high mortality in young birds and development of immunity in adult birds.[11] Fourteen orders of birds were found infected with WNV in New York State in 2000.[10] The predominant number of dead birds tested were members of the Order Passeriformes, followed by Galliformes, Columbiformes, and Charadriiformes. When species that had a minimum of 10 individuals tested were compared, the percent of positive birds ranged from 15% (Ciconiformes) to 44% (Psittaciformes).[10]

In New York State, within the epicenter of viral activity—the five boroughs of NYC, Long Island (Nassau and Suffolk counties), Rockland and Westchester counties—American crows demonstrated significantly greater mortality from WNV than did other species of birds.[10] In other locations in the state, no difference in infectivity was observed among bird species found dead. A sharp increase in sightings of dead crows preceded the first human case detected in NYC,[12] possibly providing an early warning of increased risk to man. The highest MIR in mosquitoes on Staten Island correlated with the greatest proportion of infected crows and the greatest number of human cases. Other locations had lower MIRs, but five of eight had MIRs greater than 1. An MIR of 1 with St. Louis encephalitis virus, a related flavivirus, in Florida has been understood to signify increased risk to humans.[13] It is important to recognize, however, that the WNV MIRs reported here are a measure of the number of mosquitoes with detectable viral RNA and not in many cases, infectious virus. This is not surprising since the limit of detection of the TaqMan RT-PCR assay was determined to be 0.08 PFU or $10^{-1.1}$ $\log_{10}$ PFU.[5] Thus the significance of the MIRs must be interpreted with caution. Mosquitoes that have evidence of viral RNA only and no infectious virus represent incompetent vectors, but theoretically they might have become competent with an increased extrinsic incubation period had they lived out their lifespan. Calculation of MIRs for each species also is dependent on correct identification of mosquitoes, which in some cases was problematic in 2000 (unpublished data, Kramer).

Although the greatest number of birds submitted for testing were year-round residents of New York State, there was no difference in infection rates among birds with different breeding behavior. Viremic migratory birds are suspected to contribute to the movement of WNV in southern Europe.[14] Similarly, migrating species on the East Coast of the US may provide a mechanism of viral transport over distance and thereby a means of viral spread to new areas throughout both temperate and tropical regions of the Western Hemisphere. However, the true likelihood that this would happen is unclear because the length of time that birds have viremic titers sufficient to infect vector mosquitoes may be short in duration. Birds that will be most important to the transmission cycle probably gather in large groups in locations with high numbers of ornithophilic mosquitoes.

The analysis of RNA levels in brain, heart, kidney and liver indicated that the kidney, and secondarily the brain, was the avian tissue most consistently infected with WNV. These results confirmed those of Steele et al.[15] They examined birds infected with WNV in 1999, following introduction of the virus into New York, and found that the kidney was the tissue most frequently infected, but that the brains of most birds were also infected with WNV. Furthermore, the examination of the focal infection within the kidney and brain, as determined by TaqMan assay of multiple sections, suggests that the kidney displays consistently higher levels of viral antigen than does the brain. This observation is further supported by immunofluorescent staining of frozen tissue sections of the brain and kidney (unpublished data). WNV antigen appears much more focal in the brain than in the kidney, which showed evidence of staining throughout.

The experimental infection in mice demonstrated a classical flavivirus pattern of infection. After peripheral inoculation, virus was found in lymphoid tissues, followed by the heart and kidney. Peak viremia occurred on day 2 to 3. Virus was found in the brain as early as 28 h and consistently on days 2 and 3. It is important to note that the viremia was high for all three of these time points; therefore, the virus measured in the brain may represent virus in the blood. By day 4, virus unambiguously had invaded the brain. Thus, the NY strain of WNV was neuroinvasive in adult mice. Using three-week-old outbred mice, Halevy et al. found similar results after peripheral inoculation using an Israeli strain of WNV.[16]

ACKNOWLEDGMENTS

We would like to acknowledge the considerable contributions of the Arbovirus Laboratories' staff, including Elizabeth B. Kauffman, Susan A. Jones, Alan P. Dupuis II, Kiet A. Ngo, Greg D. Ebel, Donna M. Young, and David Nicholas. We thank Ward Stone and the Wildlife Pathology Unit of the Department of Environmental Conservation, the Division of Epidemiology of the New York State Department of Health, the New York City Department of Health, and the Centers for Disease Control and Prevention.

REFERENCES

1. SAMPSON, B.A., C. AMBROSI, A. CHARLOT, *et al.* 2000. The pathology of human West Nile Virus infection. Hum. Pathol. **31:** 527–531.
2. CDC. 2001. Serosurveys for West Nile virus infection—New York and Connecticut counties, 2000. Morb. Mortal. Wkly. Rep. **50:** 37-39.
3. HAYES, C.G. 2000. West Nile Fever. *In* The Arboviruses: Epidemiology and Ecology, Vol. V. T.P. Monath, Ed.: 59–88. CRC Press, Inc. Boca Raton, FL.
4. TAYLOR, R.M., T.H. WORK, H.S. HURLBUT & F. RIZK. 1956. A study of the ecology of West Nile virus in Egypt. Am. J. Trop. Med. Hyg. **5:** 579.
5. SHI, P-Y., E.B. KAUFFMAN, P. REN, *et al.* 2001. High throughput detection of West Nile virus RNA. J. Clin. Microbiol. **39:** 1264–1271.
6. LANCIOTTI, R.S., A.J. KERST, R.S. NASCI, *et al.* 2000. Rapid detection of west nile virus from human clinical specimens, field-collected mosquitoes, and avian samples by a TaqMan reverse transcriptase-PCR assay. J. Clin. Microbiol. **38:** 4066–4071.
7. REISEN, W.K., R.P. MEYER, S.B. PRESSER & J.L. HARDY. 1993. Effect of temperature on the transmission of western equine encephalomyelitis and St. Louis encephalitis viruses by *Culex tarsalis* (Diptera:Culicadae). J. Med. Entomol. **30:** 151–160.
8. CDC. 2000. Update: West Nile Virus activity—Eastern United States, 2000. Morb. Mortal. Wkly. Rep. **49:** 1044–1047.
9. TROCK, S.C., B. MEADE, A.L. GLASER, *et al.* 2001. West Nile outbreak among horses in New York State, 1999 and 2000. Emerg. Infect. Dis. In press.
10. BERNARD, K.A., J.G. MAFFEI, S.A. JONES, *et al.* 2001. Comparison of West Nile virus infection in birds and mosquitoes in New York State in 2000. Emerg. Infect. Dis. **7:** 679–685.
11. WORK, T.H., H.S. HURLBUT & R.M. TAYLOR. 1953. Isolation of West Nile virus from hooded crow and rock pigeon in the Nile Delta. Proc. Soc. Exp. Biol. Med. **84:** 719–722.
12. EIDSON, M., L.D. KRAMER, W. STONE & I. GOTHAM. 2001. Dead bird surveillance as an early warning system for West Nile virus. Emerg. Infect. Dis. **7:** 631–635.
13. DAY, J.F. & L.M. STARK. 1996. Transmission patterns of St. Louis encephalitis and eastern equine encephalitis viruses in Florida: 1978–1993. J. Med. Entomol. **33:** 132–139.
14. RAPPOLE, J.H., S.R. DERRICKSON & Z. HUBALEK. 2000. Migratory birds and spread of West Nile virus in the Western Hemisphere. Emerg. Infect. Dis. **6:** 319–328.
15. STEELE, K.E., M.J. LINN, R.J. SCHOEPP, *et al.* 2000. Pathology of fatal West Nile virus infections in native and exotic birds during the 1999 outbreak in New York City, New York. Vet. Pathol. **37:** 208–224.
16. HALEVY, M., Y. AKOV, D. BEN-NATHAN, *et al.* 1994. Loss of active neuroinvasion of West Nile virus: pathogenicity in immunocompetent and SCID mice. Arch. Virol. **137:** 355–370.

Epidemic West Nile Encephalitis in Romania

Waiting for History to Repeat Itself

GRANT L. CAMPBELL,[a] CORNELIA S. CEIANU,[b] AND HARRY M. SAVAGE[a]

[a]*Division of Vector-Borne Infectious Diseases, National Center for Infectious Diseases, Centers for Disease Control and Prevention, Public Health Service, U. S. Department of Health and Human Services, Fort Collins, Colorado 80522-2087, USA*

[b]*Institute Cantacuzino, Bucharest, Romania*

ABSTRACT: Seroprevalence data suggest that West Nile virus activity in southern Romania dates to the 1960s or earlier. In the summer of 1996, southeastern Romania and especially Bucharest experienced an unprecedented epidemic of West Nile encephalitis/meningitis, with at least 393 hospitalized cases and 17 deaths. Contributing factors included a susceptible avian population and urban/suburban infrastructural conditions that favored the production of large numbers of *Culex pipiens pipiens*. The epidemic ended spontaneously in early autumn. Results of serosurveys conducted as the epidemic waned pointed to the recent, novel introduction of West Nile virus to Bucharest. During 1997–2000, 39 scattered human cases of clinical West Nile virus infection (mean, 10 per year; range, 5–14 per year)—including 5 (13%) fatal cases—were diagnosed serologically throughout the region, but epidemic disease did not recur. Results of limited ecologic surveillance efforts during 1997–2000 suggested the existence of numerous focal areas of enzootic West Nile virus activity within the region. The authors explore the possible factors that led to the 1996 epidemic, review the ecologic and human data gathered during the postepidemic period of 1997–2000, summarize the public health lessons offered by the epidemic and its aftermath, and speculate on the future of epidemic West Nile virus activity in southeastern Romania.

KEYWORDS: West Nile virus; West Nile fever; flavivirus; epidemiology; Romania; *Culex pipiens*; encephalitis; meningitis; meningoencephalitis

The 1996 epidemic of West Nile (WN) meningoencephalitis in Romania was significant for a variety of reasons.[1] Although previous seroprevalence studies in humans and other species and anecdotal human case reports indicate that WN virus (WNV) activity in southern Romania has occurred since at least the 1960s,[2] the 1996 epidemic produced the country's first well-documented human WN viral disease cases and its first WNV isolate.[1,3] This epidemic was among the largest WN viral disease epidemics ever recognized and only the second such epidemic ever recognized in Europe.[1,4] In previous large epidemics of WN viral disease, most clinically apparent

Address for correspondence: Grant L. Campbell, M.D., Ph.D., Division of Vector-Borne Infectious Diseases, CDC, P.O. Box 2087, Fort Collins, CO 80522-2087; Voice: 970-221-6459; fax (970) 221-6476.

GLCampbell@cdc.gov

cases were of classic WN fever, a nonspecific febrile illness often accompanied by skin rash and lymphadenopathy but without neurologic involvement.[5,6] By contrast, the 1996 Romanian epidemic was the first documented large epidemic of WN viral disease in which the preponderance of clinically apparent cases involved the central nervous system (CNS). This preponderance of neurologic disease cases, which is characteristic of North American epidemics caused by the closely related St. Louis encephalitis (SLE) virus,[7] was subsequently seen in epidemics of WN viral disease in Russia, the United States, and Israel during 1999–2000.[8–11]

OVERVIEW OF THE 1996 EPIDEMIC

The 1996 Romanian epidemic of WN viral disease has been previously described.[1,3] Briefly, hospital-based surveillance identified nearly 400 cases of WN encephalitis (16%), meningitis (40%), or meningoencephalitis (44%), including 17 (4%) fatal cases in persons aged > 50 years, with onset dates ranging from July 15 to October 12 with a peak in early September.[1] The true totals of cases and fatalities were almost certainly higher because implementation of national surveillance was delayed and because, in some clinically suspected cases, including many fatal cases, optimal specimens were unavailable for laboratory testing. Clinical incidence and case-fatality rates increased significantly with age but were not related to gender. The epidemic was confined to 15 districts in the Danube plain of southeastern Romania, with an overall clinical incidence rate of 4 per 100,000 population. Sixty-one percent of case-patients were urban residents, and Bucharest itself had the highest clinical incidence rate (12 per 100,000).[1]

On the basis of the results of a seroprevalence survey conducted as the epidemic waned, the overall WN viral infection rate in Bucharest during the epidemic was estimated to have been about 4%, without significant variation related to age, gender, or geographic region of the city.[1] The essentially flat distribution of age-specific infection rates among Bucharest residents is evidence that WNV had rarely, if ever, infected this population before 1996. The results of a second seroprevalence survey indicated that the estimated WN viral infection rate in seven non-Bucharest districts had been about 1%, which argues against recent widespread endemicity of WNV in those areas. Extrapolation of these serosurvey results to the general population gave estimates of up to 96,000 infections among 2.3 million Bucharest residents, and 31,000 infections among 3.4 million residents of the seven non-Bucharest districts. Based on Bucharest data, the estimated clinical-to-subclinical infection ratio was between 1:140 and 1:320.[1] A retrospective case-control study found that having seen mosquitoes in one's home (odds ratio = 14; $P < 0.01$) and having lived in an apartment building with a flooded basement (odds ratio = 4; $P = 0.01$) were significantly associated with WNV seropositivity.[12]

A concurrent epidemic of milder clinical WN viral infections (WN fever cases) was neither reported to public health authorities by the medical community during the epidemic, nor retrospectively identified during the Bucharest seroprevalence survey. In the latter, 31 seropositive and 37 seronegative persons were questioned about the frequencies of minor illness symptoms recalled in the recent past, and differences were not significant.[1] However, this small study may have lacked sufficient statistical power to detect modest differences in the frequencies of symptoms between the two groups. In addition to the problem of small sample sizes, seronegatives (like seropositives) were persons sampled at outpatient specialty clinics (polyclinics) and therefore may have been more likely than the average Bucharest resident to have had recent illnesses with mild symptoms such as fever, headache, joint pain, and rash, making them a less-than ideal comparison group. It is possible, therefore, that an epidemic of milder clinical WN viral infections did in fact occur in the region but was lost in the general background of nonspecific febrile illnesses. In large measure, the striking predominance of neurologic manifestations among reported cases probably reflected hospital-based surveillance, as well as the absence of case-finding efforts in outpatient clinics.[1]

A retrospective case series of 160 serologically confirmed WN viral disease patients hospitalized during the epidemic included 121 (76%) encephalitis patients, 30 (19%) meningitis patients, and 9 (6%) "acute febrile disease" patients.[13] On the average, patients with encephalitis (58 years) were older than those with meningitis (36 years) or "acute febrile disease" (41 years). Although some of the latter cases may have represented classic WN fever cases, those classified as "acute febrile illness with meningeal reaction" probably were mild aseptic meningitis cases. As described, the clinical features of the WN encephalitis and meningitis cases in Romania[13–15] seem typical of those seen with other neurotropic arboviruses, especially SLE virus.[16] Compared to nonfatal WN encephalitis cases, Cernescu and colleagues[15] observed that fatal cases were more likely to have been in older individuals and associated with higher cerebrospinal fluid (CSF) white blood cell counts and protein concentrations, hyponatremia, and the presence of anti-WN viral IgM antibody in CSF in the absence of IgG antibody. Notably, although weakness or paralysis was reported in about 15% of WN encephalitis cases,[13] diffuse flaccid paralysis and axonal polyneuropathy (i.e., a Guillain-Barrè-like syndrome) was not described. In New York in 1999, such a syndrome was seen in 6 (16%) of 37 WN encephalitis cases,[9] a distinguishing feature that led to the recognition of the epidemic.[14]

Neutralizing antibody to WNV was found in 1 of 12 (8%) wild birds and 30 of 73 (41%) domestic fowl, including 19 of 52 (37%) chickens, sampled in the greater Bucharest area during early October 1996.[3] During the same time period, nearly 6000 individual mosquitoes were collected, mainly from Bucharest and mostly by aspiration; 96% were *Culex pipiens pipiens*. Houses, poultry sheds, and apartment complexes ("blockhouses") were routinely found to be infested with this species. Leaking pipes, standing water, raw sewage, and *Cx. p. pipiens* larvae were common in blockhouse basements.[3] A strain (RO97-50) of WNV was isolated from a pool of *Cx. p. pipiens* aspirated from the walls and ceiling of a blockhouse in central Bucharest. The minimum infection ratio in this species was 0.2 per 1000. Genetic characterization of strain RO97-50 showed it to be most closely related to WNV strains from sub-Saharan Africa.[3,17] Although the epidemic investigation reportedly yielded a second strain of WNV, strain 96-1030 from human CSF,[1,15,17] unfortunately this strain has not been fully characterized.

FACTORS CONTRIBUTING TO THE 1996 EPIDEMIC

Many diverse and complex factors—some readily apparent and others that remain obscure—undoubtedly contributed to the epidemic. The poverty and deteriorated urban/suburban infrastructure that resulted in abundant *Cx. p. pipiens* larval habitat within the region was a major factor. During the epidemic investigation in Bucharest, blockhouses were commonly found to be in poor general condition, often with basements flooded with drinking water or raw sewage.[3] Public corridors commonly harbored large resting populations of adult *Cx. p. pipiens*.[1] Single family homes that are interspersed with blockhouses in some parts of the city were commonly found to possess abundant *Cx. p. pipiens* larval habitat (e.g., rain water collection barrels), adult resting places (e.g., poultry sheds), and amplifying hosts (e.g., domestic fowl).[3] Individual apartments and single family homes often lacked window and door screens, and those screens that were present were often in disrepair.

Weather almost certainly contributed to the epidemic, especially the relative lack of precipitation in Bucharest during late spring and early summer of 1996.[3] This pattern has been observed in a number of urban SLE epidemics[18] and in the 1999 WN encephalitis epidemic in New York City (University of Nebraska, National Drought Mitigation Center web site, http://enso.unl.edu/ndmc/impacts/us/usjuly99.htm. Assessed October 20, 2001), all of which involved *Cx. pipiens*. The production of this species is enhanced by summer drought conditions, presumably through the concentration of organic material in standing water sources.[3]

The human population of Bucharest and surrounding areas was apparently highly susceptible to WN viral infection. Among serum samples collected during 1993–1996 for influenza serology and banked, IgG antibody to WNV was detected in none of 151 samples from Bucharest and 4 of 71 (6%) samples from surrounding areas.[1] More importantly, the preepidemic bird population in Bucharest must have been both ample in size and highly susceptible, although the preepidemic avian seroprevalence is unknown. The bulk of the evidence suggests that, during or only shortly before 1996, one or more WN viral strains were introduced to Bucharest, either for the first time ever or after a lengthy absence. Migratory birds are the most likely vehicle of such an introduction and sub-Saharan Africa is the most likely distant origin.[3] The more proximate origin, however, is unknown. Possibilities include the Danube River basin and delta of southeastern Romania, where enzootic bird–mosquito transmission cycles of WNV could exist.[1,3]

The contribution of autogenous (form molestus) *Cx. p. pipiens* populations to the Romanian epidemic and other urban SLE and WNV epidemics is unknown, but this is an important issue that deserves further study. Unpublished observations suggested that autogenous and anautogenous *Cx. p. pipiens* populations filled different ecological niches within Bucharest, that autogenous populations were more common in urban blockhouses but virtually absent in nearby agricultural villages, and that autogenous and anautogenous populations commonly overlapped in areas of single-family homes within the city.[3] Although *Cx. p. pipiens* clearly plays a crucial role in the amplification of SLE and WN viruses within avian populations in urban areas, its role in the actual transmission of these viruses to humans is less clear. Typical (i.e., anautogenous) *Cx. p.pipiens* populations are highly ornithophilic and rarely if ever feed on humans.[19] One hypothesis states that SLE and WN viruses are transmitted to humans by autogenous *Cx. p. pipiens* populations, which are thought to more readily feed on humans,[20] while another states that transmission to humans is by hybrid females that result from the interbreeding of autogenous and anautogenous populations.[21] The role of "bridge" vectors—mosquito species that more readily feed on both birds and mammals (e.g., certain *Aedes* species and *Culex* species other than *Cx. p. pipiens*)—in the transmission of WNV to humans in southeastern Romania is also unknown.

EVIDENCE FOR CONTINUED TRANSMISSION DURING 1997–2000

Following the 1996 epidemic, Romania implemented a modest surveillance program for continued WN viral circulation and human disease.[22,23] During 1997–2000, "enhanced" passive surveillance (passive surveillance augmented by alerts to district health departments) for human cases of WN encephalitis and meningitis was conducted in Bucharest and elsewhere in southeastern Romania. Serologic tests of serum, CSF, or both were employed. A total of 39 cases including 5 fatalities (13%) were diagnosed: 14 in 1997, 5 in 1998, 7 in 1999, and 13 in 2000.[23] Cases occurred from May to September; 82% occurred in August or September. The median age of case-patients was 45 years (range, 8–76 years); 62% of case-patients were male. Fourteen cases were in rural residents and 25 were in urban or suburban residents, including 7 cases in Bucharest. In 37 of the 39 cases, the reported predominant clinical manifestations were CNS disease: meningitis (24 cases), meningoencephalitis (12 cases), and encephalitis (1 case). The remaining two cases were WN fever with exanthem but without neurologic involvement and were diagnosed in hospitalized patients who were initially suspected of having measles.[22]

In 1997 and 1999, limited mosquito collections were made in southeastern Romania, mainly using gravid traps and aspirators.[23] During May–October 1997, collections at 25 Bucharest sites and 8 non-Bucharest sites yielded more than 16,000 mosquitoes (87% *Cx. p. pipiens*), 88% of which were from Bucharest. During July–September 1999, more than 7,000 mosquitoes (80% *Cx. p. pipiens*) were collected in Teleorman and Tulcea districts. Mosquitoes were tested for WNV variously by suckling mouse brain assay, plaque assay, or antigen-capture immunoassay (EIA), with negative results.

In 1997, sentinel chickens were used to detect WNV activity in Bucharest. In early May, four flocks of approximately 20 four-week-old chickens each were placed at each of two sites, for a total of approximately 160 birds (C. Cernescu, Institute of Virology, Bucharest, personal communication, 2001).[22] Testing for antibody to WNV was by IgG EIA. Chickens were bled biweekly from late June through mid-August, and again in mid-October. Although birds found to be newly seropositive at each interval were not replaced, they were excluded from seroprevalence calculations at subsequent bleedings. Seroconversions among previously seronegative chickens at each interval were 23%, 26%, 40%, 16%, and 13%, respectively.[22] Because seroconversions were not confirmed by neutralization tests, these rather striking results should be interpreted cautiously. Financial constraints precluded the use of sentinel chickens in subsequent years (C. Cernescu, personal communication).

During 1997–2000, domestic fowl (including chickens, ducks, geese, and turkeys) were bled between July and September in Bucharest and three other districts in southeastern Romania, and tested for antibody to WNV by neutralization or IgG EIA or both. The overall seroprevalence was 34 of 447 (8%), including at least 7 seropositives among 34 young-of-the-year.[23] During July-September 1999, 152 wild birds of 22 species and 6 orders were sampled in the Teleorman and Tulcea districts. Of these, 95% were passerines and 70% were tree sparrows (*Passer montanus*). A total of 12 birds (8%) had neutralizing antibody to WNV, including 7 seropositives among 12 young-of-the-year; all seropositives were nonmigratory species.

PUBLIC HEALTH LESSONS

Recognition of the etiology of the Romanian WN encephalitis epidemic of 1996 was significantly delayed. Initially suspected to be an epidemic of enteroviral disease, the true cause was not suspected until early September[1] and not confirmed until the third week in September as the epidemic was ending. There were at least two reasons for this delay. First, because WN encephalitis had not been seen in Europe since the early 1960s, and because CNS disease was not a prominent feature of previous large epidemics of WN viral disease, clinicians and public health officials in Romania understandably had a low index of suspicion for this disease. It seems likely that, in the foreseeable future, a higher index of suspicion will exist concerning any European summertime epidemic of encephalitis that primarily involves elderly patients. In fact, this seems to have been the case with the 1999 Russian epidemic.[8] Second, because state-of-the-art laboratory testing for WN viral infection was unavailable in Romania, confirmation of the true cause of the epidemic was delayed while samples were sent to France for reference testing.[1] This problem has since been addressed in Romania, but it persists in many other countries in Europe and elsewhere that are at risk for epidemic WN encephalitis. As the Romanian epidemic dramatically demonstrated, the absence of a public health infrastructure to monitor and respond to arboviral diseases and their vectors can exact a high price in terms of human morbidity and mortality.

This epidemic added WN encephalitis to the long list of diseases associated with deteriorated urban infrastructure, which is reminiscent of some SLE epidemics in the United States.[18,24] The dynamics of WNV transmission in urban areas are poorly understood. A better understanding of the biology, bionomics, and feeding patterns of *Cx. pipiens* and other urban ornithophilic mosquito species, and potential bridge vectors, is essential. The postepidemic Romanian data suggest that intense urban epizootic WNV activity does not necessarily result in intense epidemic activity.[22,23] A similar phenomenon was observed in the eastern United States in 2000,[25] but it remains poorly understood. Virtually nothing is known of the enzootic cycles of WNV transmission that may exist in the Danube delta and other rural areas of the Danube basin.

Notably, neither WNV-associated avian mortality nor equine WN viral disease cases were reported during the Romanian epidemic (or to date in the postepidemic era). Widespread avian mortality (especially among crows and other members of Corvidae) has been an apparently unique and unprecedented feature of WNV transmission in North America.[26] In recent years, significant numbers of equine WN encephalitis cases have been documented in Europe, Africa, and the United States.[26–28] The reasons for the apparent absence of both equine WN encephalitis cases in Romania and widespread WNV-associated avian mortality in the Eastern Hemisphere remain obscure. Although the former could well be a surveillance artifact, the latter seems more likely to be due to either increased virulence of the North American epidemic/epizootic strain, increased susceptibility of at least some avian species in the Western Hemisphere, or a combination. In any event, these observations emphasize that a given arbovirus may not behave identically in different hemispheres or on different continents.

SPECULATION ON THE FUTURE

Clearly, upgrading and maintaining the urban infrastructure in Bucharest—including the elimination of mosquito breeding sources from blockhouses and single-family homes—will depend on major economic development and take many years or decades. Meanwhile, to prevent a recurrence of the 1996 epidemic, the establishment of better arboviral surveillance and a long-term, sustained, organized, urban *Culex* control program that focuses on source reduction and larval control, continues to be essential. That this has not occurred, due to a shortage of political will, funds, or both, is proof that the central lesson of this epidemic has yet to be learned. *Cx. p. pipiens* remains abundant in urban and suburban areas of southeastern Romania, as do susceptible avian and human hosts, and WNV continues to circulate in the region.[22,23] Thus, the current situation in the region seems ripe for a recurrence of a major epidemic of WN encephalitis.

Other urban areas of Eastern Europe are also at risk for epidemic WN encephalitis. The conditions necessary for the initiation of epidemic transmission of neurotropic flaviviruses are numerous and complex,[29] and only minimal or no arboviral surveillance is being conducted in most of those areas. Thus, the timing of such an epidemic is unpredictable. To some extent, the situation can be viewed as a race between economic development and the convergence of a number of poorly understood natural phenomena.

REFERENCES

1. Tsai, T.F., F. Popovici, C. Cernescu, et al. 1998. West Nile encephalitis epidemic in southeastern Romania. Lancet **352:** 767–771.
2. Hubalek, Z. 2000. European experience with the West Nile virus ecology and epidemiology: could it be relevant for the New World? Viral Immunol. **13:** 415–426.
3. Savage, H.M., C. Ceianu, G. Nicolescu, et al. 1999. Entomologic and avian investigations of an epidemic of West Nile fever in Romania in 1996, with serologic and molecular characterization of a virus isolate from mosquitoes. Am. J. Trop. Med. Hyg. **61:** 600–611.
4. Hayes, C.G. 1989. West Nile fever. In The Arboviruses: Epidemiology and Ecology, Vol. V: 59–88. T.P. Monath, Ed. CRC Press. Boca Raton, FL.
5. Marberg, K., N. Goldblum, V.V. Sterk, et al. 1956. The natural history of West Nile fever. I. Clinical observations during an epidemic in Israel. Am. J. Hyg. **64:** 259–269.
6. McIntosh, B.M., P.G. Jupp, I. Dos Santos, et al. 1976. Epidemics of West Nile and Sindbis viruses in South Africa with *Culex* (*Culex*) *univittatus* Theobald as vector. S. Afr. J. Sci. **72:** 295–300.
7. Tsai, T.F. & C.J. Mitchell. 1989. St. Louis encephalitis. In The Arboviruses: Epidemiology and Ecology, Vol. IV: 113–143. T.P. Monath, Ed. CRC Press. Boca Raton, FL.
8. Platonov, A.E., G.A. Shipulin, O.Y. Shipulina, et al. 2001. Outbreak of West Nile virus infection, Volgograd Region, Russia, 1999. Emerg. Infect. Dis. **7:** 128–132.
9. Nash, D., F. Mostashari, A. Fine, et al. 2001. The outbreak of West Nile virus infection in the New York City area in 1999. N. Engl. J. Med. **344:** 1807–1813.
10. Centers for Disease Control and Prevention. 2001. Serosurveys for West Nile virus infection—New York and Connecticut counties, 2000. Morb. Mortal. Wkly. Rep. **50:** 37–39.

11. BIN, H., Z. GROSSMAN, S. POKUMUNSKI, *et al.* 2001. West Nile fever in Israel, 1999–2000: from goose to human. Ann. N.Y. Acad. Sci. **951**. This volume.
12. HAN, L.L., F. POPOVICI, J.P. ALEXANDER JR., *et al.* 1999. Risk factors for West Nile virus infection and meningoencephalitis, Romania, 1996. J. Infect. Dis. **179:** 230–233.
13. CEAUSU, E., S. ERSCOIU, P. CALISTRU, *et al.* 1997. Clinical manifestations in the West Nile virus outbreak. Rom. J. Virol. **48:** 3–11.
14. ASNIS, D.S., R. CONETTA, A.A. TEIXEIRA, *et al.* 2000. The West Nile virus outbreak of 1999 in New York: the Flushing Hospital experience. Clin. Infect. Dis. **30:** 413–418.
15. CERNESCU, C., S.M. RUTA, G. TARDEI, *et al.* 1997. A high number of severe neurologic clinical forms during an epidemic of West Nile virus infection. Rom. J. Virol. **48:** 13–25.
16. BRINKER, K R. & T.P. MONATH. 1980. The acute disease. *In* St. Louis Encephalitis. T.P. Monath, Ed.: 503–534. American Public Health Association. Washington, DC.
17. LANCIOTTI, R.S., J.T. ROEHRIG, V. DEUBEL, *et al.* 1999. Origin of the West Nile virus responsible for an outbreak of encephalitis in the northeastern United States. Science **286:** 2333–2337.
18. MONATH, T.P. 1980. Epidemiology. *In* St. Louis Encephalitis. T.P. Monath, Ed.: 239–312. American Public Health Association. Washington, DC.
19. TEMPELIS, C.H. 1975. Host-feeding patterns of mosquitoes, with a review of advances in analysis of blood meals by serology. J. Med. Entomol. **11:** 635–653.
20. BARR, A.R. 1967. Occurrence and distribution of the *Culex pipiens* complex. Bull. World Health Org. **37:** 293–296.
21. SPIELMAN, A. 2001. Structure and seasonality of neartic *Culex pipiens* populations. Ann. N.Y. Acad. Sci. **951**. This volume.
22. CERNESCU, C., N.I. NEDELCU, G. TARDEI, *et al.* 2000. Continued transmission of West Nile virus to humans in southeastern Romania, 1997–1998. J. Infect. Dis. **181:** 710–712.
23. CEIANU, C.S., A. UNGUREANU, G. NICOLESCU, *et al.* 2001. West Nile virus surveillance in Romania, 1997–2000. Viral Immunol. **14:** 251–262.
24. LOUISIANA DEPARTMENT OF HEALTH. 1995. Update: St. Louis encephalitis outbreak, 1994. Louisiana Morb. Rep. **6:** 4.
25. CENTERS FOR DISEASE CONTROL AND PREVENTION. 2000. Update: West Nile Virus activity—Northeastern United States, 2000. Morb. Mortal. Wkly. Rep. **49:** 820–822.
26. KOMAR, N. 2000. West Nile viral encephalitis. Rev. Sci. Tech. **19:** 166–176.
27. CANTILE, C., G. DI GUARDO, C. ELENI, *et al.* 2000. Clinical and neuropathological features of West Nile virus equine encephalomyelitis in Italy. Equine Vet. J. **32:** 31–35.
28. OSTLUND, E.N., R.L. CROM, D.D. PEDERSEN, *et al.* 2001. Equine West Nile encephalitis, United States. Emerg. Infect. Dis. **7:** 665–669.
29. DAY, J.F. 2001. Predicting St. Louis encephalitis virus epidemics: lessons from recent, and not so recent, outbreaks. Annu. Rev. Entomol. **46:** 111–138.

West Nile Encephalitis in Russia 1999–2001

Were We Ready? Are We Ready?

ALEXANDER E. PLATONOV

Central Research Institute of Epidemiology, Moscow, Russia

ABSTRACT: In 1963–1993, several strains of West Nile virus (WNV) were isolated from ticks, birds, and mosquitoes in the southern area of European Russia and western Siberia. In the same regions, anti-WNV antibody was found in
0.4–8% of healthy adult donors.[7] Sporadic human clinical cases were observed
in the delta of the Volga River. In spite of this, WNV infection was not considered by the health authorities as a potentially emerging infection, and the large
WNV outbreak in southern Russia, started in late July 1999, was not recognized in a timely fashion. First evidence suggesting a WNV etiology of the outbreak was obtained by IgM ELISA on September 9.[12,14] Two weeks later, the
specific WNV RT-PCR was developed and WNV disease was confirmed in all
14 nonsurvivors from whom brain tissue samples were available. Retrospective
studies of serum samples by IgM ELISA indicated WNV etiology in 326 of 463
survivors with aseptic meningitis or encephalitis.[14] Moreover, 35 of 56 patients
who contracted aseptic meningitis in 1998 had a high titer of WNV IgG antibody,[14] so the WNV infection seems to have been introduced into the Volgograd
region before 1999. A complete sequence (AF317203) of WN viral RNA, isolated from the brain of one Volgograd fatality, and partial sequences of an envelope E gene from other nonsurvivors showed that the Volgograd isolate had the
greatest homology (99.6%) with WN-Romania-1996 mosquito strain RO97-50.

KEYWORDS: West Nile virus; Russia; Volgograd Region

ARBOVIRAL DISEASES AND WEST NILE VIRUS INFECTION: BACKGROUND

Vector-borne infectious diseases were responsible for more human disease and
death in the seventeenth through the early twentieth centuries than all other causes
combined.[1] A substantial portion of these diseases were caused by viruses that are
vectored by arthropods (arboviruses) such as dengue and yellow fever in tropical areas and, in more temperate climates, tick-borne encephalitis, Japanese encephalitis,
Congo-Crimean hemorrhagic fever, West Nile fever, St. Louis encephalitis, and
Western and Eastern equine encephalitis, for example. During the 1940s, the arthropod-borne diseases of public health importance were controlled in part by the use of
DDT and related pesticides. Unfortunately, there has been a significant emergence
of epidemic arboviral disease worldwide in the past 20 years.[1,2] Major global demographic and societal changes, namely population growth, urbanization, environmen-

Address for correspondence: A.E. Platonov, D.Sc., Central Institute of Epidemiology, Novo-
gireevskaya St. 3A, Moscow 111123, Russia. Voice: 7-095-3651528; fax: 7-095-3055423.
platonov@pcr.ru

tal pollution, and modern agricultural practices, have directly affected the resurgence of mosquito-borne and tick-borne infections. The jet airplane has provided the ideal mechanism for transporting pathogens among population centers, covering large distance in a very short time.

A number of severe arboviral infections are caused by viruses belonging to the genus *Flavivirus*, family Flaviviridae, for example, dengue and yellow fever, tick-borne encephalitis, Japanese encephalitis (JE), West Nile (WN) fever, St. Louis encephalitis, etc. WN virus (WNV) is a member of the JE antigenic complex. Mosquito-borne WN fever is an endemic febrile illness in Africa, the Middle East and Southwest Asia. Kunjin virus, a subtype of WNV, is a WN counterpart in Australia and Southeast Asia.

Several vector-borne infections caused by flaviviruses are endemic in the territory of the Russian Federation. The most important one was probably tick-borne spring-summer encephalitis causing from 5000 to 10,000 cases per year, mainly in the Ural and Siberian regions, such as Republic Udmurtia, with a case fatality rate about 1.5%.[3] Mosquito-borne Japanese encephalitis was sporadically diagnosed in the Russian Far East. Another example of flaviviral human disease is zoonotic Omsk hemorrhagic fever (OHF). The peak of annual incidence, reaching 4000 cases per 100,000 population, was observed in 1945–1949 in Omsk Region (province) in Siberia. During the past 10 years, from 2 to 40 OHF cases have been reported in Novosibirsk Region.[4]

In 1963–1993, several strains of WNV were isolated from ticks, birds, and mosquitoes in the southern area of European Russia and western Siberia, and in the adjacent republics of the former USSR (FIG. 1).[2,5,6] In the same regions, anti-WN IgG antibody was found in 0.4–4% of healthy adult donors (FIG. 2). The Astrakhan Region was the most affected area; up to 8% of the healthy human population were WN-seropositive and sporadic human clinical cases were observed.[7] Southern areas of Russia have a climate consistent with successful mosquito-to-vertebrate transmission of WNV, at least in some hot summers.[2,6,8,9]

In spite of this, WNV infection was not considered by the health authorities as a potentially emerging infection. Regional virological laboratories were not supplied with WNV diagnostic tools and regional epidemiologists and clinicians were not proficient in control and treatment of WNV disease.[3] Specialists from the Ivanovsky Institute of Virology, Moscow, Russia, however, had expertise in both fundamental research and surveillance of arboviral infections. The WN-IgM ELISA was developed at the Institute of Virology for research purposes, but was not officially approved for diagnostic purposes owing to financial constraints.

WEST NILE FEVER/ENCEPHALITIS OUTBREAK IN 1999

The large WN outbreak in southern Russia started in late July 1999 and was not promptly recognized.[10,11] It was not until at September 9, when more than 400 patients were hospitalized in Volgograd Region with acute neuroinfection, that first data were obtained by IgM ELISA in the Ivanovsky Institute of Virology, suggesting a WN-etiology of the outbreak.[12] Two weeks later, the specific WN RT-PCR was developed in the Central Research Institute of Epidemiology and WN disease was confirmed in all 14 nonsurvivors from whom the brain tissue samples were

TABLE 1. West Nile virus infection in Volgograd Region in 1999

Diagnosis[a]	Number of patients (total)	Patients investigated for the presence of WN-IgM in serum samples[b]	Patients positive for WN-IgM antibody, titer > 1:800[c]	Estimated number of patients with WN infection[d]
Encephalitis	92	65 (71%)[e]	44 (68%)[e]	68
Serous meningitis	422	398 (94%)	288 (72%)	305
Fever	428	153 (36%)	48 (31%)	134
Any of above	942	616 (65%)	380 (61%)	507

[a]Clinical diagnosis. The patients hospitalized from July 25, 1999 to September 27, 1999.
[b]Absolute number and percentage of total number of patients (column 2).
[c]Absolute number and percentage of number of investigated patients (column 3).
[d]If all patients would be investigated for WN infection.
[e]Brain tissue samples from additional 14 nonsurvivors, included in column 2 but not in columns 3 and 4, were studied by RT-PCR and were positive for the presence of WN RNA.

available.[10,11] The WN strain was isolated later from one of these brain samples; another WN strain was isolated from the blood of a patient who contracted the disease in Astrakhan (FIG.1).[13]

Retrospective studies of serum samples by IgM ELISA indicated WNV etiology in 326 of 463 survivors with serous meningitis or encephalitis.[14] In total, 394 cases of clinical WNV infection were confirmed and at least 100 additional clinical WNV cases were suspected among more 900 patients hospitalized in Volgograd Region with a diagnosis of aseptic meningoencephalitis, aseptic meningitis, or acute viral infection with fever (TABLE 1). Ninety-five percent of clinical WNV cases occurred either in Volgograd City (about 1,000,000 inhabitants) or in Volzskii City (about 300,000 inhabitants). Volgograd is located on the right bank (West) of great Volga River and Volzskii City is on the opposite bank. The attack rate for clinical illness in these cities was about 40/100,000 people. The number of affected persons with milder disease is thought to have been at least a hundred times greater than the number of clinical cases in WN fever epidemics,[15] so up to 5% of Volgograd population might have been infected with WNV during July–September 1999.

Forty patients with acute aseptic meningoencephalitis died as a result of the development of pathological cerebral symptoms, coma and respiratory failure.[9,10,14] Seventy-six percent of the nonsurvivors were older than 60 years of age. Death did not occur during first 3 days of the disease; in 50% of the cases the lethal outcome was observed 10 or more days after the WN encephalitis onset. Clinical presentation of WN disease in Russia during 1999 was discussed elsewhere; it is noteworthy that such "classical" signs of WN infection as lymphadenopathy, splenomegaly, skin rash or exanthema were rare or absent.[9,10,14,16–19] High fever (up to 39–40°C), prolonged asthenia (up to 20 days) and headache (up to 30 days) were observed in all patients. The central nervous system was usually involved; paresis and/or paralysis was observed in 15–20% of cases.

During the same July–September 1999 period, 89 WNV cases with 5 deaths in Astrakhan Region and at least 38 WNV cases with 3 deaths in Krasnodar Region were reported.[3,18] In another publication, 85 cases of serous meningitis or encepha-

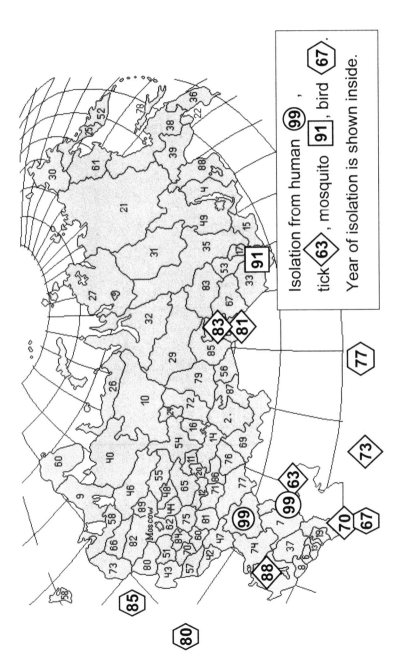

FIGURE 1. **The map of places and years of West Nile virus isolation.** Each symbol represents one WNV strain. Year of isolation is shown inside and a symbol shape codes the source of isolation. The territory of the Russian Federation is shown in gray. The boundaries of large administrative districts (republics, territories, and regions) are shown. Small numbers inside the region's area mean the number of districts in the statistical registry.

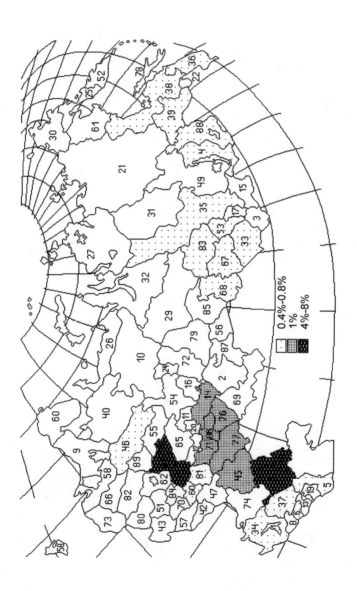

FIGURE 2. Seroprevalence of antibodies to West Nile fever virus in healthy adults in the Russian Federation. Pattern fills code the prevalence of antibodies (%) in a region; white areas correspond to the regions where the investigation was not done.

0.4%–0.8%
1%
4%–8%

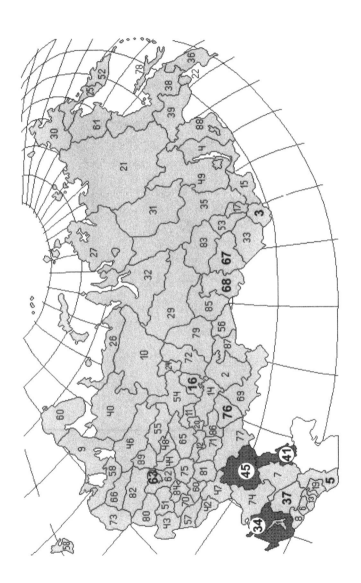

FIGURE 3. The map of administrative districts of the Russian Federation. All regions are enumerated. The number of regions, discussed in the text and tables, are given in **bold** letters. The regions where human WN fever cases occurred in 1999 are *shaded.* 45–Volgograd Region; 41–Astrakhan Region; 34–Krasnodar Region. 3–Republic of Altai; 5–Republic of Dagestan; 16–Republic of Udmurtia; 37–Stavropol Region; 67–Novosibirsk Region; 68–Omsk Region; 76–Samara Region; 63–Moscow City.

litis were reported in Krasnodar Region in August–September 1999, for which diagnostic high titers of anti-WN IgM were found in patients' serum.[20] Most human cases occurred in the regional capitals, Astrakhan City and Krasnodar City. The former is located in the delta area of the great Volga River and the latter is located near the delta area of the large Kuban River (FIG. 3).

Several publications noted the findings of WN antigen and WN RNA in the samples of mosquitoes, ticks, and vertebrates collected in 1999 in Volgograd and Astrakhan Regions, so the potential for WNV circulation was demonstrated.[14,21,22]

WEST NILE DISEASE IN THE 1990s: EARLY WARNING FOR AND PREDISPOSITION TO THE OUTBREAK IN 1999

Could this outbreak of human WNV infection in Russia have been predicted and prevented? Neither the large outbreak of WN fever in Romania in 1996 (more than 400 clinical cases),[16,23] nor the outbreak in New York in 1999 (>60 clinical cases),[24,25] nor any other large WNV outbreak in the temperate climate zone was expected.[26] Nevertheless, some warning signs might have been present.

Retrospective review of hospital records and official medical statistics from Volgograd reveals a high number of cases and deaths clinically diagnosed as meningococcal meningitis during the summers of 1997 and 1998, whereas the seasonal peak

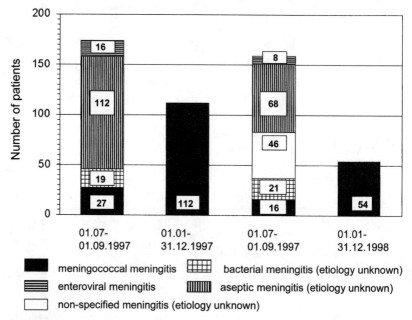

FIGURE 4. Number of patients hospitalized with suspected meningitis in Volgograd Region in 1997–1998. Some cases of aseptic meningitis were retrospectively diagnosed as WN meningitis (see text). Only meningococcal meningitis is shown for the whole years 1997 and 1998. Most cases, reported as meningococcal meningitis, were diagnosed according to clinical presentation without positive laboratory findings.

TABLE 2. Meningococcal disease. Age distribution of lethal cases (absolute number and %)

Territory and year	0–4 y n (%)	5–19 y n (%)	20–39 y n (%)	40–59 y n (%)	60+ n (%)	Overall n (%)
Russia, 1998	322 (62)	61 (12)	37 (7)	58 (11)	43 (8)	521 (100)
Volgograd Region, 1997–1998	11 (46)	3 (13)	1 (4)	2 (8)	6 (25)	24 (100)
Volgograd Region, 1990–1996	61 (66)	7 (8)	6 (7)	9 (10)	9 (10)	92 (100)
Astrakhan Region, 1993–1998	21 (48)	4 (9)	3 (7)	6 (14)	10 (21)	44 (100)
Astrakhan Region, 1990–1992	19 (83)	2 (9)	0 (0)	0 (0)	2 (9)	23 (100)
Krasnodar Region, 1996–1998	33 (72)	7 (15)	3 (7)	3 (7)	0 (0)	46 (100)
Stavropol Region, 1996–1998	32 (63)	6 (12)	1 (2)	9 (18)	3 (6)	51 (100)

of meningococcal incidence occurs usually in February–March in Russia (FIG. 4). In addition, the age distribution of "meningococcal" lethal cases in the Volgograd Region in 1997–1998 was unusual. In Russia more than 60% of meningococcal deaths are observed in children less than 5 years of age, whereas only 6–10% are observed in patients older than 60 years (TABLE 2). However, in the Volgograd Region in 1997–1998 and in Astrakhan Region in 1993–1998, the percentage of lethal cases observed in patients older than 60 years exceeded 20%. At least a portion of these "meningococcal meningitis" cases may represent WNV infection, indicating that the virus may also have been frequently introduced into or persistent in the Volgograd Region since 1997 and in the Astrakhan Region since 1993. By contrast, the meningococcal mortality in the older population was normal during 1990–1999 in the near regions of Krasnodar, Stavropol, and Samara and the Republic of Dagestan as well as in the Volgograd Region during 1990–1996 and in the Astrakhan Region during 1990–1992 (TABLE 2 and data not shown).

Moreover, in July-August 1997 128 cases of acute serous meningitis were registered in the Volgograd Region.[14] Sixteen of 128 cases were caused either by enteroviruses or herpes viruses; 112 cases remained without laboratory diagnosis. There were 68 cases of unknown serous meningitis in August 1998 (FIG. 4). When these patients were studied retrospectively in January 2000, 35 of 56 patients, who contracted serous meningitis during the summer of 1998, had a high titer of WNV IgG antibody.[14] A high titer of WNV IgG antibody was found in serum samples from 5 of 111 patients, who had been diagnosed with serous meningitis during the summer of 1997. Thus, the WNV infection seems to have been introduced into the Volgograd Region before 1999.

In the Romanian 1996 outbreak, Han et al. found WNV infection to be associated with the presence of mosquitoes indoors and flooded apartment building basements.[9] These features suggested a peridomestic route of transmission consistent with the ecology and breeding habits of *Culex pipiens*. A similar study has not yet been done in Russia, but antimosquito control efforts were obviously constrained during recent years of economic shortage. In Astrakhan City in 1999, only 6% of building basements were treated with insecticides, whereas previously this figure often reached 97%.[3] From 1995 to 1998, the area of building basements subjected to anti-mosquito chemical measures decreased at least twice in Volgograd City. Mosquito surveys indicated that mosquitoes colonized up to 85% apartment buildings. Entomological observations demonstrated that about 30% of open water areas in the Volgograd Region might support larval mosquito development. However, during the last 15 years, mosquito larvicides were applied only to the open water areas nearby some summer recreation places (less than 0.5 km^2 annually).[3,14]

The dry summer in Romania during 1996 has been reported. Dry summers have also been associated with epidemics of St. Louis encephalitis in urban areas of the USA.[9] Dry summers are believed to provide conditions that support larval habitat for *Culex* mosquitoes and to increase oviposition by *Cx. pipiens* in flooded basements. The summer 1999 was similarly dry and hot in southern Russia.

WEST NILE VIRUS MOLECULAR GENETICS: ENDEMIC OR IMPORTED STRAINS?

Complete sequence (AF317203) of WN viral RNA, isolated from the brain of a dead Volgograd patient,[27] and partial sequences of envelope E gene from other non-survivors and Russian WNV strains,[10] showed that the Volgograd isolate had the greatest homology with the WN-Romania-1996 mosquito strain RO97-50 (99.8% for complete amino acid (aa) sequence of polyprotein and 99.6% for nucleotide complete (nt) sequence). Nearly the same level of homology was observed within the WNVs isolated at the same time and at the same place, namely in New York during 1999, that is from 99.8% to 99.9% for aa or nt sequences. The isolates, which were epidemiologically unrelated but belonged to the same genetic WNV lineage 1, for example, WN-Romania-1996M and WN-Eg101 strains, differed in 0.35–0.55% of aa sequence and 3.3–4.6% of nt sequence. Most strains of lineage 1 differed from the strain Kunjin-MRM61C and the strain WN-Nigeria (belonging to lineage 2) in more than 2% of aa sequence and more than 12% of nt sequence. A complete sequence of E gene (1503 nt) was also known for the WNV strain isolated in Kenya 1998 from a mosquito [GenBank # AF146082]. The similarity with WN-Volgograd-1999 E gene was 99.4% for aa and 98.9% for nt. In spite of the similarity of the Russian, Romanian, and Kenya strains, the exact mode of strain introduction remains unclear. Migratory birds may act as introductory hosts and then as amplifying hosts.[28] South Russia, Romania and Kenya are connected with intensive bird migration pathways.

The recent WNV epidemics were characterized by the high rate of neurological disorders and mortality (5–10%).[10,17,24] Whether the high pathogenicity is defined by the genetic peculiarities of new WNV strains remains to be elucidated. Of note, the Volgograd isolate lacked a potential glycosylation site in E protein. In animal models there is some evidence that the glycosylation attenuates the virulence of WNV and other flaviviruses.[29,30]

WEST NILE DISEASE IN 1997–1999: DID WE DO OUR BEST?

"People have studied St. Louis encephalitis for 50 years, and outbreaks are still unpredictable."[26] Despite the apparent presence of some warnings in 1997–1998, the medical community was not ready for the outbreak in 1999. Retrospectively, one could say that the severe cases of viral encephalitis affecting elderly persons in summer or early autumn suggested an investigation for WNV infection. If such an investigation had given positive results, this should have led to intensive vector and bird studies.

There was a serious gap in time between the onset of the WNV epidemic and the correct laboratory diagnosis in 1999. Patients were admitted to and even discharged from hospitals with the diagnosis of, for example, acute viral respiratory infection, pneumonia, and presumably bacterial meningitis.[14,16,19] The most frequent diagnosis was serous meningitis but enteroviral etiology was suspected. As a result, the health authorities enhanced the control of water supply quality but did not address mosquito control. The intensive use of insecticides was started only in mid-September 1999 when the epidemic began to wane. To date, there is no specific treatment for flaviviral infection,[31] so the treatment of WNV meningitis and encephalitis was symptomatic and generally correct. However, several cases of WNV meningitis, with the prevalence of polymorphonuclear leukocytes in the cerebrospinal fluid at an early stage of disease, were misdiagnosed as suspect bacterial meningitis and treated by antibiotics.

Given the increased associated social and medical concerns, additional funds were allocated promptly to treat patients and to provide additional medical personnel. The Russian Ministry of Health and Regional governments cooperated in these efforts. When the clinical samples became available in Moscow, the basic research institutes were able to diagnose WNV infection promptly. The D.I. Ivanovsky Institute of Virology used the already developed IgM-ELISA, and the Central Institute of Epidemiology developed specific RT-PCR tests immediately. In general, the history of the 1999 WNV outbreak demonstrated clearly that an adequate response to newly emerging or reemerging infections requires preexisting structures, diagnostic and treatment facilities, as well as education of the regional physicians and epidemiologists who meet an infection first.

WEST NILE DISEASE IN 2000: EVOLUTION AND CONTROL

There was no official report of WNV morbidity or control measures from the Astrakhan and Krasnodar Regions in 2000. During the summer and autumn of 2000, Astrakhan physicians treated 14 patients with febrile illness who had diagnostic titers of serum anti-WN IgM (K.M. Galimzyanov, personal communication).

The Volgograd health authorities reported 11 WNV cases in Volgograd, 14 cases in Volzskii City, and 5 cases in other smaller settlements in 2000. The cases occurred from August 1 to September 30 with a maximum during the week of August 28 to September 3, 2000 (5 cases). More than 50% of patients were 60 years of age or older (age range from 21 to 73 years). There were 4 cases of encephalitis, 18 cases of meningitis, and 7 cases of fever. Laboratory diagnosis was based on IgM-capture ELISA, revealing the high titer of WN antibody in patient serum samples.

Continued transmission of WNV to humans in the years after the initial large outbreak was observed also in Romania in 1997–1998 and in the northeastern USA in
2000,[32,33] but the number of cases decreased in subsequent years. Probably, in temperate climate zones, a human WNV epidemic requires several conditions to coin-
cide, such as high number of mosquitoes, high temperature, and concurrent epizootic
in birds. The relative importance of preventive measures remains to be evaluated.
The use of insecticides for treatment of apartment basements was increased 20-fold
in Volgograd in 2000 in comparison to 1997–1998. Regional entomologists estimated that the population of *Culex* mosquitoes had decreased threefold in 2000 whereas
the number of *Aedes* and *Anopheles* mosquitoes was about the same.

WEST NILE DISEASE IN THE FUTURE:
PROSPECTS AND PLANS IN RUSSIA

The basic principles for surveillance, prevention, and control of WNV infection
are the same in any country.[2,3,7,34,35] Nevertheless the ecological and social peculiarities of the Russian Federation may require some adjustment of the ideal strategy. According to CDC guidelines, **surveillance activities** include the following (in italics):

1. *Active mosquito surveillance to monitor WN virus activity and to identify potential vectors* (CDC). Several WNV strains were isolated from ticks in Russia (FIG.
1). This may be the mechanism of WNV persistence in Russian conditions.[2,6,7]
Therefore, tick surveillance is also desirable.

2. *Active bird surveillance to monitor WN virus activity in both wild and sentinel
bird populations, and, in particular, surveillance for dead crows* (CDC). Sentinel
chicken surveillance was not effective in the USA in 2000[26] and would be unlikely
to be established in Russia. Possibly, this may be substituted by surveillance in domestic bird populations, which were widely infected in Romania in 1996.[9,15,23]
There were no reports of intensive bird deaths in Southern Russia in 1999. Does this
result from the lack of surveillance or does it reflect a difference between the Volgograd and New York strains? Additional studies are necessary to evaluate the benefits
of bird surveillance in Russia. D.K. Lvov suggested decreasing bird populations in
urban environments as a control strategy.[7]

3. *Enhanced passive veterinary surveillance, with emphasis on horses* (CDC).
Veterinary WNV cases were not reported in Russia, although some horses and, especially, camels had anti-WN antibody in the Astrakhan Region.[7] The importance of
veterinary surveillance has to be evaluated.

4. *Enhanced passive human surveillance to report viral encephalitis and aseptic
meningitis* (CDC). Meningitis, with the exception of meningococcal meningitis, is
not a notifiable disease in Russia, so sporadic cases of meningitis would not be reported. Active surveillance is necessary in potentially endemic regions. Outbreaks
of aseptic meningitis/encephalitis should be reported and controlled. Severe cases of
viral encephalitis affecting older persons in summer or early autumn should alert the
medical and public health communities.

Surveillance requires the following minimal **diagnostic support**[34]:

1. *The IgM and IgG ELISAs to provide initial testing for human and animal specimens; neutralization tests to identify specific flavivirus antibodies;*

2. *RT-PCR capability to detect viral RNA. Antigen-capture ELISA to detect WN and other arboviruses in mosquito pools. Immunohistochemistry to detect virus in autopsy tissue. Virus isolation and identification capability (CDC).*
In our experience, RT-PCR has become a more sensitive and reliable, less expensive and laborious tool to diagnose many viral infections than antigen-capture ELISA and immunohistochemistry. The diagnostic triad may include:

(1) The IgM and IgG ELISAs for anti-WNV antibodies available for regional laboratories and used for initial diagnostic and screening purposes;

(2) RT-PCR assays for WN and other important arboviruses to detect viral RNA, in particular in pathologic materials (autopsy tissues, dead animals) and in mosquito pools;

(3) Virus isolation and identification capability, neutralization tests to identify specific flavivirus antibodies available in basic institutions, such as the Ivanovsky Institute of Virology.

In addition, the capability to sequence flaviviruses and clinical isolates is highly desirable for fine typing of WNV and other arboviruses. The official trials and approval of ELISA and RT-PCR assays for WN will require state financial and organizational support.

Prevention and Control

Mosquito control is the most effective and economical way to prevent transmission of WN to humans (CDC).[34] Russian specialists emphasize the importance of mosquito control programs in urban environments and near large cities.[3,7] It is necessary to kill both larvae and adults. Administrative efforts and public education to diminish the number of breeding places, such as flooded building basements, legal and illegal dumps, are required. Ecologically safe insecticides should be applied.[3]

Public Health Infrastructure and Development

The Russian health system has the capability of establishing adequate WNV surveillance and control. There are Regional Centers for Sanitary and Epidemic Control as well as the Anti-Plague Institutes or Anti-Plague Stations in the regions endemic for severe zoonotic diseases. These Centers and Stations may conduct a part of the above-mentioned surveillance and diagnostic activity, if the necessary equipment and assays are provided.[3,14] The practitioners and hospital medical personnel, and intensive case units in particular, should be educated in clinical diagnosis and treatment of arboviral fever, meningitis, and encephalitis.[11,16]

International Collaboration

Hopefully, the joint project entitled "The development and application of methods to control emergent/reemergent vector-borne diseases in Russia and the USA with special attention to West Nile encephalitis" will start this year. The participants of the project are the D.I. Ivanovsky Institute of Virology, the Central Research Institute of Epidemiology, and the State Research Center of Virology and Biotechnology "VECTOR" from Russia and the Division of Vector-Borne Infectious Diseases, CDC from the USA.

The project will include the following parts.

(1) Field research in areas potentially endemic for WNV infection in Russia, particularly in the Astrakhan Region, which has a long history of sporadic human WN fever cases, and also in the Volgograd and Krasnodar Regions, which experienced recent WNV epidemics. Collection of arthropod vectors, blood and tissue samples from birds and mammals, and biological samples from patients with suspected viral fever and encephalitis.

(2) Virus isolation from arthropod, human, and vertebrate samples; identification and genetic typing of these isolates.

(3) The development and application of nucleic acid techniques to detect and identify a range of arboviruses in human samples, and primary host and vector samples. Production of monoclonal antibodies and development of ELISA test systems for WNV and other arboviruses, using monoclonal antibodies and recombinant antigens.

(4) Estimation of antibody prevalence in vertebrates (particularly birds) and serological investigations of human serum samples collected in endemic areas.

As a result the epidemiology of WNV infection in the population and the full clinical spectrum of illness will be evaluated, such as estimating the ratio of clinically apparent to inapparent infection. Depending on the serologic study results or whether the WNV epidemic recurs in the study areas, additional case-control studies will help to determine risk factors for acquiring WNV infection. Taken together, the implementation of these tasks will clarify the distribution of WNV and other arboviruses in Russia, the relationships among WNV genotypes, the role of particular vector species, the transmission cycle of WNV in vectors and vertebrate hosts, and the incidence of human infection with WNV. Such knowledge will be essential for eventual development of effective surveillance, diagnosis, and control strategies for this important human pathogen.

REFERENCES

1. GUBLER, D.J. 1998. Resurgent vector-borne diseases as a global health problem. Emerg. Infect. Dis. **4:** 442–450.
2. LVOV, D.K., S.M. KLIMENKO & S.Y. GAIDAMOVICH. 1989. [Arboviruses and Arboviral Infections.] Meditsina. Moscow. (In Russian)
3. ONISHENKO, G.G. 2000. [Natural foci of infections in the Russian Federation and their prophylaxis.] Epidemiol. Infect. Dis. **4:** 4–8. (In Russian)
4. NETESOV, S.V. & J.L. CONRAD. 2001. Emerging infectious diseases in Russia, 1990–1999. Emerg. Infect. Dis. **7:** 1–5.
5. BUTENKO, A.M., M.P. CHUMAKOV & D.N. STOLBOV. 1967. [Serological and virological examinations in a natural focus of West Nile fever in the Astrakhan region]. Vopr. Med. Virusol. **1:** 208–211. (In Russian)
6. LVOV, D., A. AVERSHIN, A. ANDREEV, et al. 1990. Surveillance for arboviruses in the Soviet Union: relationships between ecology zones and viruses distribution. Arch. Virol. Suppl. **1:** 259–266.

Notes to Reference List: Russian titles of articles and books are given in our own translation in brackets. If the Russian journal volume was absent or not informative, it was substituted or supplemented by the journal number. The editors were not indicated for some Russian books.

7. LVOV, D.K. 2000. [West Nile fever.] Vopr. Virusol. **45**(2): 4–9. (In Russian)

8. CORNEL, A.J., P.G. JUPP & N.K. BLACKBURN. 1993. Environmental temperature on the vector competence of *Culex univittatus* (Diptera: Culicidae) for West Nile virus. J. Med. Entomol. **30:** 449–456.

9. HAN, L.L., F. POPOVICI, J.P. ALEXANDER JR., *et al.* 1999. Risk factors for West Nile Virus infection and meningoencephalitis, Romania, 1996. J. Infect. Dis. **179:** 230–233.

10. PLATONOV, A.E., G.A. SHIPULIN, O. YU. SHIPULINA, *et al.* 2001. Outbreak of West Nile infection, Volgograd region, Russia, 1999. Emerg. Infect. Dis. **7:** 128–132.

11. VENGEROV, YU.YA., T.I. FROLOCHKINA, A.N. ZHUKOV, *et al.* 2000. [West Nile virus infection as clinical and epidemiological problem.] Epidemiol. Infect. Dis. **4:** 27–31. (In Russian)

12. LVOV, D.K., A.M. BUTENKO, S.I. GAIDAMOVICH, *et al.* 2000. [Epidemic outbreak of meningitis and meningoencephalitis, caused by West Nile virus, in Krasnodar territory and Volgograd region.] Vopr. Virusol. **45**(1): 37–38. (In Russian)

13. LVOV, D.K., A.M. BUTENKO, V.I. GROMASHEVSKY, *et al.* 2000. Isolation of two strains of West Nile virus during an outbreak in Southern Russia, 1999. Emerg. Infect. Dis. **6:** 373–376.

14. ONISHENKO, G.G., N.G. TIKHONOV, A.N. ZHUKOV, *et al.* 2000. [West Nile fever in Volgograd region] *In* [Natural Foci of Infections in Low Volga Region.] N.G. Tikhonov, Ed.: 158–163. Print, Volgograd. (In Russian)

15. TSAI, T.F., F. POPOVICI, C. CERNESCU, *et al.* 1998. West Nile encephalitis epidemic in southeastern Romania. Lancet **352:** 767–771.

16. VENGEROV, YU.YA. & A.E. PLATONOV. 2000. [West Nile fever.] The Practitioner **10:** 56–60. (In Russian)

17. CEAUSU, E., S. ERSCOIU, P. CALISTRU, *et al.* 1997. Clinical manifestations in the West Nile virus outbreak. Rom. J. Virol. **48:** 3–11.

18. GALIMZYANOV, H.M., A.E. PLATONOV, G.A. SHIPULIN, *et al.* 2000. [West Nile fever in Russia.] *In* [Infectious Diseases: Diagnosis, Treatment, Prophylaxis.], p. 58. St. Petersburg. (In Russian)

19. STRIKHANOV, S.N., A.M. BUTENKO & E.O. SHISHKINA. 2000. [Clinical course of West Nile fever.] *In* [Infectious Diseases at the XXI Century, Part II.], p. 52. Ministry of Health. Moscow. (In Russian)

20. STRIKHANOV, S.N., A.M. BUTENKO, M.O. MKRTCHAN, *et al.* 2000. [Cases of West Nile fever in Krasnodar Region.] *In* [Infectious Diseases at the XXI Century, Part II.] pp. 52–53. Ministry of Health. Moscow. (In Russian)

21. TIKHONOV, S.N., V.A. ANTONOV, V.S. ZAMARAEV, *et al.* 2000. [The use of PCR for detection of West Nile fever virus RNA.] *In* [Genetic Diagnosis of Extremely Dangerous Infections.] V.V. Kutyrev, Ed.: 60–61. Slovo. Saratov. (In Russian)

22. GARANINA, S.B., A.K. ROGATKIN, S.A. SHERBAKOVA, *et al.* 2000. [Comparative efficiency of PCR and ELISA to detect West Nile and Crimean hemorrhagic fever viruses in field and clinical samples.] *In* [Genetic Diagnosis of Extremely Dangerous Infections.] V.V. Kutyrev, Ed.: 56–57. Slovo. Saratov. (In Russian)

23. SAVAGE, H.M., C. CEIANU, G. NICOLESCU, *et al.* 1999. Entomologic and avian investigations of an epidemic of West Nile fever in Romania in 1996, with serologic and molecular characterization of a virus isolate from mosquitoes. Am. J. Trop. Med. Hyg. **61:** 600–611.

24. ANONYMOUS. 1999. Update: West Nile-like viral encephalitis—New York, 1999. Morb. Mortal. Wkly. Rep. **48:** 890–892.

25. LANCIOTTI, R.S., J.T. ROEHRIG, V. DEUBEL, *et al.* 1999. Origin of the West Nile virus responsible for an outbreak of encephalitis in the northeastern U.S. Science **286:** 2333–2337.

26. ENSERINK, M. 2000. Infectious disease. The enigma of West Nile. Science **290:** 1482–1484.

27. PLATONOV, A.E., G.A. SHIPULIN, L. KARAN, *et al.* 2000. [Genetic and epidemiological relations of West Nile virus variants caused the epidemic outbreaks in 1996–1999.] *In* [Infectious Diseases: Diagnosis, Treatment, Prophylaxis.] p. 197. St. Petersburg. (In Russian)

28. RAPPOLE, J.H., S.R. DERRICKSON & Z. HUBALEK. 2000. Migratory birds and spread of West Nile virus in the Western Hemisphere. Emerg. Infect. Dis. **6:** 319–328.
29. CHAMBERS, T.J., M. HALEVY, A. NESTOROWICZ, *et al.* 1998. West Nile virus envelope proteins: nucleotide sequence analysis of strains differing in mouse neuroinvasiveness. J. Gen. Virol. **79:** 2375–2380.
30. MCMINN, P.C. 1997. The molecular basis of virulence of the encephalogenic flaviviruses. J. Gen. Virol. **78:** 2711–2722.
31. LEYSSEN, P., E. DE CLERCQ & J. NEYTS. 2000. Perspectives for the treatment of infections with Flaviviridae. Clin. Microbiol. Rev. **13:** 67–82.
32. CERNESCU, C., N.I. NEDELCU, G. TARDEI, *et al.* 2000. Continued transmission of West Nile virus to humans in southeastern Romania, 1997–1998. J. Infect. Dis. **181:** 710–712.
33. ANONYMOUS. 2000. Update: West Nile Virus activity—Eastern United States, 2000. Morb. Mortal. Wkly. Rep. **49:** 1044–1047.
34. ANONYMOUS. 2000. Guidelines for surveillance, prevention, and control of West Nile virus infection—United States. Morb. Mortal. Wkly. Rep. **49:** 25–28.
35. GUBLER, D.J., G.L. CAMPBELL, R. NASCI, *et al.* 2000. West Nile virus in the United States: guidelines for detection, prevention, and control. Viral Immunol. **13:** 469–475.

West Nile in the Mediterranean Basin: 1950–2000

B. MURGUE,[a] S. MURRI,[a] H. TRIKI,[b] V. DEUBEL,[c] AND H. G. ZELLER[a]

[a]Centre National de Référence des Arbovirus et des Fièvres hémorragiques virales, Institut Pasteur, Paris, France

[b]Institut Pasteur de Tunis, Tunis, Tunisia

[c]Centre de Recherche Mérieux Pasteur à Lyon, Lyon, France

ABSTRACT: Recent West Nile virus (WNV) outbreaks have occurred in the Mediterranean basin. In Algeria in 1994, about 50 human cases of WN encephalitis were suspected, including 8 fatal cases. In Morocco in 1996, 94 equines were affected of which 42 died. In Tunisia in 1997, 173 patients were hospitalized for encephalitis or meningoencephalitis. West Nile serology performed on 129 patients was positive in 111 cases (87%) including 5 fatal cases. In Italy in 1998, 14 horses located in Tuscany were laboratory confirmed for WNV infection; 6 animals died. In Israel in 1998, serum samples from horses suffering from encephalomyelitis had WNV antibodies and virus was isolated from the brain of a stork; in 1999 WNV was identified in commercial geese flocks, and in 2000 hundreds of human cases have been reported. In September 2000, WNV infection was detected in horses located in southern France, close to the Camargue National Park where a WNV outbreak occurred in 1962. By November 30, 76 cases were laboratory confirmed among 131 equines presenting with neurological disorders. No human case has been laboratory confirmed among clinically suspect patients. The virus isolated from a brain biopsy is closely related to the Morocco-1996 and Italy-1998 isolates from horses, to the Senegal-1993 and Kenya-1998 isolates from mosquitoes, and to the human isolate from Volgograd-1999. It is distinguishable from the group including the Israel-1998 and New York-1999 isolates, as well as the Tunisia-1997 human isolate.

KEYWORDS: West Nile virus; Mediterranean Basin

INTRODUCTION

West Nile fever is caused by a mosquito-borne flavivirus transmitted in natural cycles between birds and mosquitoes, particularly *Culex* species mosquitoes. West Nile virus (WNV) was first discovered in 1937 in the blood of a native woman of the West Nile province of Uganda who at that time was suffering from a mild febrile illness.[1] Since then, both sporadic cases and major outbreaks of West Nile fever have been reported in Africa, the Middle East, Europe, and Asia,[2] and many aspects of West Nile infection have been well documented since the early 1950s in Egypt and

Address for correspondence: Bernadette Murgue, M.D., Ph.D., CNR des Arbovirus et des Fièvres hémorragiques virales, Institut Pasteur, 25, rue du Dr-Roux, F-75724 Paris cedex 15 France. Voice: +33-(0)1 40 61 38 87; fax: +33-(0)1 40 61 31 51.
bmurgue@pasteur.fr

in Israel, the 1960s in France, and the 1970s in South Africa. However, during the last five years many reports about WNV have been published because of outbreaks occurring in Romania, Morocco, Italy, Russia and Israel but more especially with the discovery of the virus in North America in 1999.

In humans, West Nile infection is a nonsymptomatic or a mild febrile illness; however, encephalitis cases are reported with some fatalities particularly in older patients. WNV is also a cause of animal disease, especially in horses.

In Europe, no large outbreak of WNV infection was reported until the 1996 epidemic in Bucharest, which was the first to occur predominantly in an urban setting. Between July 15 and October 12, among 835 patients hospitalized with suspected central nervous system infection, 509 patients had appropriate blood samples, and 393 (77%) were laboratory confirmed, including 17 fatal cases.[3] Another large outbreak occurred in the Volgograd region in Russia between August and September 1999. Among 826 patients admitted during this period with suspected central nervous infection, serum samples were obtained from 318 patients, of whom 183 (58%) were laboratory confirmed, including 40 fatal cases.[4]

WEST NILE VIRUS IN THE MEDITERRANEAN BASIN (FIGURE 1)

Egypt 1951–1954

The first reported epidemics were described in 1951 in Israel[5] and the question at that time was whether WNV infection was of more than academic interest. The improvement of knowledge about WNV infection came from studies performed in Egypt. Indeed, the discovery in July 1950 of WNV in the blood of 3 children and WNV antibodies in a high percentage of the inhabitants in a village located in the north of Cairo,[6] led the NAMRU to conduct a four-year program for the study of West Nile virus beginning in the fall of 1951.[7]

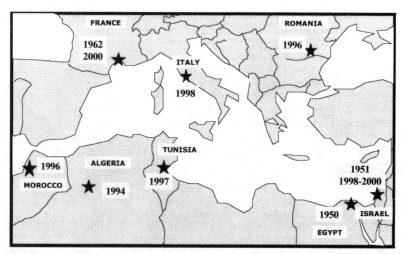

FIGURE 1. Major outbreaks reported in the Mediterranean basin: 1950–2000.

The investigations were carried out mostly in a restricted area in the upper Nile Delta, including (i) serological surveys studies in humans, mammals and birds, (ii) isolation of virus from naturally infected hosts and vectors, (iii) experimental infection in humans, equines, birds and arthropods, and (iv) ecological studies. Altogether, the results of these studies demonstrated that the main cycle of the virus involved mosquitoes and birds; humans and equines could be infected in this cycle. This conclusion paralleled the results of Reeves[8] on the primary avian-mosquito-avian cycle of viruses causing Western equine encephalitis in North America, with occasional tangential infection resulting in outbreaks in man and other animals.

In humans, serological surveys demonstrated that WNV was endemic along the Egyptian Nile with WNV antibodies reported in more than 60% of the population.[7] This percentage varied according to the age of children (44% < 15 years to 72% ≥ 15 years).

Although no suspected epidemics were reported during the surveys, WNV was isolated from the blood of children with an acute undiagnosed febrile illness and the occurrence of serological conversions from negative to positive were reported, mainly between August and November. These results suggested that in an endemic area, WN is essentially an infection of early childhood, taking place mainly during the summer months. Infection was mostly a self-limited, nonfatal febrile disease rarely associated with manifestations of encephalitis. These data were compatible with the results of experimental infections conducted with high doses of WNV (intramuscular or intravenously) in humans (21 and 78 patients) with incurable cancers in hopes of inhibiting the neoplasms.[9,10] In the great majority of the patients, there was no clinical sign or symptom other than fever. The remaining patients showed definite or suggestive clinical signs of diffuse encephalitis. From these data, it was suspected that humans could only be infected incidentally and were only partially involved in a broader cycle of the virus.

These experimental infections also demonstrated that, for most of the patients, virus was detected in blood as soon as 24 hours after inoculation and for 6 days or more (10% had viremia longer than 12 days). There was a direct correlation between persistence of viremia and severity of clinical illness. Virus was recovered from CSF but not in feces, urine or throat washings. The virus was frequently demonstrated in tumoral tissue and also was isolated in normal tissues: lymph nodes, spleen, lung and liver. WN antibodies were detected in most patients from at least three weeks following virus inoculation[10] by complement fixation and neutralization tests.

In mammal hosts other than humans, the results of serological surveys indicated that the virus was infectious to a rather wide range of animals, especially domestic quadrupeds with the exception of goats. By contrast, WNV could not be isolated from the brain of any of 22 mammals suspected of having central nervous system involvement.[7] Later on in 1959, a serological survey conducted on more than 400 equines demonstrated the presence of WNV antibodies in 54% of the animals. One suspected case was fatal and confirmed by viral isolation from the brain.[11]

Experimental infections of equines were conducted in order to study the role of equines as reservoirs of WNV. Animals infected through bites of infected mosquitoes developed neutralizing antibodies but failed to circulate virus.[7] Only two among nine equines inoculated peripherally (iv or sc) with WNV developed detectable but low and very short-term viremia. Low levels of neutralizing antibodies were detected in eight animals except after repeated antigenic stimulations that elicited neutralizing antibody levels comparable to those found in naturally infected animals.[11] These data suggested that although equines were natural hosts of WNV, they were probably dead-end hosts.

Among 78,067 arthropods (fleas, flies, ticks, lice, mites, and mosquitoes) collected, WNV was isolated only from mosquitoes (17 among 1003 pools): *Culex antennatus, C. univittatus,* and *C. pipiens.*[7] Experimentally WNV had been previously demonstrated to be transmitted by mosquitoes (*Aedes* and *Culex* species).[12,13]

In birds, among 420 animals tested, WNV neutralizing antibodies were frequently found in crows (65%) and sparrows (42%) and the virus was isolated from the blood of two pigeons (one of which was sick) and a crow.[7] Experimental infection of birds (hooded crows, house sparrows, and kestrels) by bite of WNV-infected mosquitoes demonstrated a high mortality rate of crows which had high circulating virus titers.[14]

Experimentally active vector cycle (infection through feeding followed by transmission through bite) was demonstrated only in mosquitoes. None of the soft ticks (*Ochlerotatus savignyi* and *O. erraticus*) tested could transmit the infection by feeding, although they could acquire infection from feeding on infected mice.[7]

The ecological studies demonstrated that, in a specific area, the percentage of humans with WNV antibodies was correlated with the percentage of crows with WNV antibodies. This observation led to the concept of nonendemic, transitional and endemic zones.[14] The study of the environment in these zones revealed differences—in the density of the human population and the intensity of land cultivation as well as the prevalence of mosquitoes and birds—which in combination could account for the persistence and activity of the virus. By contrast, climatic conditions did not appear to be a significant factor. The persistence of WNV during the three-year study in Egypt was explained by mosquitoes that remained active throughout the colder months.

Israel 1951–1952

During this four-year program, no epidemic was reported in Egypt. The first reported epidemic occurred in Israel in 1951–1952,[5] and cases were also recorded in 1957.[15] During the 1951 outbreak, 30 km south of Haifa, detailed clinical and biological characteristics of the disease were obtained. A total of 123 cases, without fatalities, occurred among 303 inhabitants. Children < 6 years represented 52% of the patients. The highest morbidity rate was among young children < 3 years old. After an incubation period of approximately 3 days, the main symptoms were fever (2 to 3 days), exanthem, headache, myalgia, anorexia, abdominal pain, and vomiting. Enlarged lymph nodes, angina, and diarrhea were less common. Recovery was quick in children but slow in adults; there were no sequelae. Virus was isolated from the blood of a patient after intracerebral inoculation in mice and WNV antibodies could be retrospectively demonstrated by complement fixation test in 54% of the patients. Cases were also reported in 1952 in the same area,[5] and cases with severe neurological manifestations were reported for the first time in 1957, as well as in 1962.[15]

France 1962–1965

In France, the 1962 WNV outbreak was reported during the summer in the Camargue region including the Rhône Delta. During this period, about 80 horses had neurological disorders characterized by ataxia and weakness; 25 to 30% of them died.[16]

Several human cases of encephalitis were also reported during the same period and some of them had antibodies against group B arboviruses.[17] However, WNV infection could only be confirmed in 1964 when the virus was isolated from *Culex modestus* mosquitoes and from the blood of two entomologists working in the field in September 1964.[18] Subsequently, 13 human patients have been reported with laboratory tests compatible with WNV infection[19] including one fatal case. In August 1965, a few cases of equine encephalitis were reported and in September, virus was also isolated from the spinal cord of a horse and from *Culex molestus* mosquitoes.[20]

Since 1965 there has been no real evidence for WNV infection, either in humans or in animals. During a serosurvey conducted in Camargue between 1975 and 1979, a low frequency of antibody response against WNV was observed among human (4.9%) and horse (2%) samples.[21] By contrast, a high frequency was observed against Tahyna virus (31% in human and 9% in horse), a Bunyavirus belonging to the California group, which induces febrile illness with central nervous system signs and which has been recorded in many countries in Europe as well as in Africa and Asia.[22] In May–July 2000, WNV antibodies were not detected in 46 horses located in the same area: Bouches du Rhône and Gard (J.P. Durand, unpublished data).

Recent Outbreaks

WNV epidemics were reported in South Africa in 1974[23] and 1983–1984[24] and sporadic cases were also reported in Russia, Romania, Spain,[25] and India, where virus was isolated from the brains of children who died from encephalitis.[26] No large and severe outbreak of WNV infection was reported in Europe until the 1996 epidemic in Bucharest, which was the first to occur predominantly in an urban setting,[3] with more than 800 suspected cases. In the Mediterranean basin, recent outbreaks occurred in Algeria in 1994, Morocco in 1996, Tunisia in 1997, Italy in 1998, Israel in 1998 and 2000 and in France in 2000.

Algeria 1994

In Algeria an epidemic occurred between August and September 1994 in the Timimoun oasis in the central Sahara. About 50 cases presented with high fever and neurological signs; among them 20 were clinical cases of encephalitis of whom 8 died. West Nile serology performed for 18 cases (14 clinical cases and 4 probable) was positive for 17 of them. Fifteen patients (including two fatal cases) had IgM antibodies with or without IgG and two patients had only IgG. All the 14 clinical cases were IgM-positive and 13 of them were children of 10 months to 9 years.[27]

Morocco 1996

In Morocco (provinces of Kenitra and Larache), from August to mid-October 1996, 94 equines were affected 42 of which died, and the disease was reported in all age categories.[28] Virus was isolated from a brain biopsy. A human encephalitis case was confirmed to be due to WNV.[29]

Tunisia 1997

In Tunisia, between September 7 and December 12 1997, 173 patients of whom 8 died, were hospitalized for meningitis or meningoencephalitis in two coastal districts: Sfax and Mahdia. The epidemic peak was reached between the last week of

October and the second week of November. Among 129 patients tested, WNV IgM ELISA was positive for 111 cases (86%) including 5 fatal cases (4.5%). The remaining 18 negative patients included 4 patients for whom ELISA was performed only in cerebro spinal fluid (CSF). Among positive cases, WNV IgM ELISA was performed in the CSF of 23 patients and was positive for 9 cases including 6 (3 fatal cases) for whom only CSF could be obtained.[30]

Detailed data could be obtained for the 31 positive patients located in Sfax.[31] The mean age of the patients was 52 (12 to 85), and 50% were more than 60 years old. The male to female ratio was 0.86. Mean hospitalization time was 10 days (3 to 30 days). The disease was always characterized by a high fever associated with asthenia (30%), arthralgia (17%), myalgia (10%), and a sore throat (30%). Three patients had a cutaneous eruption. All of the patients had signs of meningitis or meningoencephalitis. The clinical course of the disease was good for 26 patients, and for most of them apyrexia was noted at day 4 of hospitalization and neurological signs disappeared at day 6.

Three patients died: two 60-year-old men and one 62-year-old woman. At admission they showed altered states of consciousness. The disease was rapidly progressive during the first three days after admission with coma and respiratory signs followed by a cardiovascular shock leading to death. WNV was recently isolated in our lab from a brain biopsy.

A 27-year-old patient had a transient aggravation characterized by an aggravation of neurological signs, urinary retention, and respiratory manifestations. Two patients had sequelae such as chronic headache and tremor. Among the 44 patients for whom a serological diagnosis was not performed, three —aged 69, 78, and 90—died.

Italy 1998

In Italy, from August to early October 1998, 14 horses located in Tuscany were laboratory confirmed to have WNV infection; 6 animals died.[32] Virus was isolated from a brain biopsy (unpublished data).

Israel 1998–2000

In Israel in 1998, 18 serum samples from horses suffering from encephalomyelitis had West Nile neutralizing antibodies and virus was isolated from the brain of a stork.[33] In 1999, thousands of geese were destroyed when WNV was identified in commercial flocks.[34] An epidemic occurred in 2000[35] with more than 400 patients with encephalitis of whom 28 died (Malkinson, personal data).

France 2000

In southern France between September 6 and November 30, 2000, WNV was laboratory confirmed in 76 equines (21 fatalities) among 131 equines with neurological disorders. The last confirmed case was on November 3. All but three cases were located in a region called "la petite Camargue" (Herault and Gard provinces) harboring several large ponds and numerous colonies of migratory and settled birds as well as large mosquito populations.[36]

No human case of WNV has been laboratory confirmed among 51 suspected cases including 33 patients hospitalized with signs of encephalitis or meningoencephalitis, and 18 other cases with fever. By contrast, WNV antibodies were detected by neutralization test in 2 out of 33 gamekeepers working in this area; one of them had

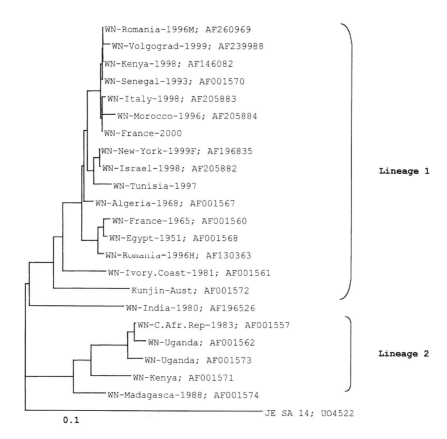

FIGURE 2. Phylogenetic trees based on nucleic sequence data of E-glycoprotein gene fragment of 254 bp. GenBank accession numbers for the sequences included in the tree are indicated. (From Murgue *et al.*[36])

a history of traveling in tropical countries, but the other one, who had a low but detectable IgM antibodies level, did not travel at all. Thus human transmission occurred during this outbreak; unfortunately, in the absence of a serological survey, it was impossible to evaluate the level of human infection among persons living in the infected area.

A serosurvey study has been undertaken in horses located within a radius of 10 km around confirmed cases. A total of 5133 horse sera were collected between September and November 2000 from the three different provinces where cases were reported. ELISA IgG was positive for 428 (8.3%) of these samples of which 248 (41.4%) were also IgM positive. There was a direct relationship between the number of positive clinical cases in an area, and the number of positive cases included in the serosurvey study (S. Zientara, personal data).

No abnormal mortality was reported in birds. WNV-neutralizing antibodies have been found in the sera of a few ducks and magpies collected in November and December 2000 (results to be published). None of the 37 mosquito pools, collected in September and October 2000 in a few areas where cases were confirmed, were positive for WNV (*C. pipiens, C. molestus, Ochlerotatus caspius* and *detritus* and *Anopheles maculipenis/hyrcanus*).

West Nile virus was isolated from a horse brain biopsy, and nucleic acid sequences was obtained from a RT-PCR reaction performed using primers located in the envelope gene fragment.[36] The phylogenetic analysis of this region showed (FIG. 2) that the West Nile France-2000 isolate belongs to lineage 1 and is closely related to both Morocco-1996 and Italy-1998 horse isolates. It is also very close to Senegal-1993 and Kenya-1998 mosquito isolates, as well as to the Volgograd-1999 human isolate. It is distinguishable from the group including both the New York-1999 and Israel-1998 isolates, as well as the Tunisian-1997 human isolate.[37]

DISCUSSION

West Nile virus infection is well known in the Mediterranean basin, where the first reported epidemic occurred in Israel in 1951. Until the beginning of the 1990s, epidemics or sporadic cases have been regularly reported in the Old World, however the number of encephalitis cases were usually limited as well as the number of fatal cases. Recent outbreaks involving humans and/or equines occurred in North Africa, the Middle East, and Europe, where the largest outbreaks occurred in 1996 in Bucharest and in 1999 in Volgograd. In the Mediterranean basin during the same period two large epidemics occurred—in Tunisia and in Israel. In Algeria, Morocco, Tunisia, and Italy, no further outbreak was reported the following years.

The transmission cycle of WNV is rather complex and not fully understood. It implies a chain of events that allows the amplification of the virus and in some undetermined circumstances further transmission to mammals. Many factors have been suggested to be involved in the occurrence of WNV in mammals, including density in birds and mosquito populations, land cultivation, and climatic conditions. However, WNV outbreaks are erratic and spatiotemporally limited phenomena, occurring quite unpredictably even if all conditions appear to be present in a definite place.

A lot of questions remain regarding WNV infection. Does it actually represent a major public health threat? Taking into account the number of cases reported all over the world during the last 10 years, it is unlikely that WNV infection now represents such a problem. For the future the answer is uncertain. What is the possibility that WNV infection will become a health risk for humans and/or equines? How can we predict the probability of occurrence of the disease in a specific place? Thus another main question is: What kinds of surveillance systems should be established and what should their objectives be?

ACKNOWLEDGMENTS

We thank all the partners involved in the management of the West Nile virus outbreak in France.

REFERENCES

1. SMITHBURN, K.C. et al. 1940. A neurotropic virus isolated from the blood of a native of Uganda. Am. J. Trop. Med. **20:** 471–492.
2. ZELLER, H. 1999. West Nile: une arbovirose migrante d'actualité. Med. Trop. **59:** 490–494.
3. TSAI, T.F. et al. 1998. West Nile encephalitis in southeastern Romania. Lancet **352:** 767–771.
4. PLATONOV, A.E. et al. 2001. Outbreak of West Nile virus infection, Volgograd region, Russia, 1999. Emerg. Infect. Dis. **7:** 128–132.
5. BERNKOPF, H., S. LEVINE & R. NERSON. 1953. Isolation of West Nile virus in Israel. J. Infect. Dis. **93:** 207–218.
6. MELNICK, J.L. et al. 1951. Isolation from human sera in Egypt of a virus apparently identical to West Nile virus. Proc. Soc. Exp. Biol. Med. **77:** 661–665.
7. TAYLOR, R.M. et al. 1956. A study of the ecology of West Nile virus in Egypt. Am. J. Trop. Med. **5:** 579–620.
8. REEVES, W.C. 1945. Observations on the natural history of western equine encephalomyelitis. Proceedings of the 49th annual meeting of the U.S. Livestock Sanitary Association, pp. 150–158.
9. SOUTHAM, C.M. & A.E. MOORE. 1951. West Nile, Ilheus, and Bunyamwera virus infections in man. Am. J. Trop. Med. Hyg. **31:** 724–741.
10. SOUTHAM, C.M. & A.E. MOORE. 1954. Induced virus infections in man by the Egypt isolates of West Nile virus. Am. J. Trop. Med. Hyg. **3:** 19–50.
11. SCHMIDT, J.R. & H.K. EL MANSOURY. 1963. Natural and experimental infection of Egyptian equine with West Nile virus. Ann. Trop. Med. Parasitol. **57:** 415–427.
12. PHILIP, C.B. & J.E. SMADEL. 1943. Transmission of West Nile virus by infected *Aedes albopictus*. Proc. Soc. Exp. Biol. Med. **53:** 49–50.
13. KITAOKA, M. 1950. Experimental transmission of the West Nile virus by the mosquito. Jpn. Med. J. **3:** 77–81.
14. WORK, T.H., H.S. HURLBUT & R.M. TAYLOR. 1955. Indigenous wild birds of the Nile Delta as potential West Nile virus circulating reservoirs. Am. J. Trop. Med. Hyg. **4:** 872–888.
15. HAYES, C.G. 1989. West Nile Fever. *In* The Arboviruses: Epidemiology and Ecology. T.P. Monath, Ed. Vol. V: 59–88.
16. JOUBERT, L. et al. 1970. Epidémiologie du virus West Nile: étude d'un foyer en Camargue. IV. La méningo-encéphalomyélite du cheval. Ann. Inst. Pasteur **118:** 239–247.
17. PANTHIER, R. 1968. Epidémiologie du virus West Nile: étude d'un foyer en Camargue. I. Introduction. Ann. Inst. Pasteur **114:** 519–520.
18. HANNOUN, C. et al. 1964. Isolement en France du virus West Nil à partir de malades et du vecteur *Culex modestus* Ficalbi. C. R. Acad. Sc. Paris. **259:** 4170–4172.
19. PANTHIER, R. et al. 1968. Epidémiologie du virus West Nile: étude d'un foyer en Camargue. III. Les maladies humaines. Ann. Inst. Pasteur **115:** 435–445.
20. PANTHIER, R. et al. 1966. Isolement du virus West Nile chez un cheval de Camargue atteint d'encéphalomyélite. C. R. Acad. Sc. Paris. **262:** 1308–1310.
21. ROLLIN, P.E. et al. 1982. Résultats d'enquêtes séroépidémiologiques récentes sur les arboviroses en Camargue: populations humaines, equines, bovines et aviaries. Med. Mal. Infect. **12:** 77–80.
22. KARABATSOS, N. 1985. *In* International Catalogue of Arboviruses, Including Certain Other Viruses of Vertebrates, 3rd edit., and Supplements 1986–98. American Society of Tropical Medicine and Hygiene. San Antonio, TX.
23. MCINTOSH, B.M. et al. 1976. Epidemics of West Nile and Sindbis viruses in South Africa with *Culex (Culex) univittatus* Theobald as vector. S. Afr. J. Sci. **72:** 295–300.
24. JUPP, P.G. et al. 1986. Sindbis and West Nile virus infections in the Witwatersrand-Pretoria region. S. Afr. Med. J. **70:** 218–220.
25. HUBALEK, Z. & J. HALOUZKA. 1999. West Nile fever—a reemerging mosquito-borne viral disease in Europe. Emerg. Infect Dis. **5:** 643–648.
26. GEORGES, A.J. et al. 1987. Fatal hepatitis from West Nile virus. Ann. Inst. Pasteur **138:** 237–244.

27. LE GUENNO, B. *et al.* 1996. West Nile: a deadly virus? Lancet **348:** 1315.
28. TBER. ABDELHAQ, A. 1996. West Nile fever in horses in Morocco. Bull. O.I.E. **11:** 867–869.
29. EL HARRACK, M., B. LE GUENNO & P. GOUNON. 1997. Isolement du virus West Nile au Maroc. Virologie. **1:** 248–249.
30. TRIKI, II. Epidémie de méningo-encéphalite à virus West Nile en Tunisie. Submitted to Trop. Med. Date of application: March 2001.
31. MARRAKCHI, C. 1998. Les manifestations neurologiques liées à l'infection par le virus West Nile. M.D. Thesis, Sfax University, 1998, Tunisia.
32. CANTILE, C. *et al.* 2000. Clinical and neuropathological features of West Nile virus equine encephalomyelitis in Italy. Equine Vet. J. **32:** 31–35.
33. MALKINSON, M., C. BANET & Y. WEISMAN. 1998. Intercontinental spread of West Nile virus by wild birds—recent epidemiological findings in Israeli livestock and birds. *In* Proceedings of the 2nd International Conference on Emerging Zoonoses, Strasbourg, France.
34. OFFICE INTERNATIONAL DES EPIZOOTIES. 1999. West Nile fever in Israel in geese. Dis. Info. **12**(45): 166.
35. SIEGEL-ITZKOVICH, J. 2000. Twelve die of West Nile virus in Israel. Br. Med. J. **321:** 724.
36. BERTHET, F.X., H.G. ZELLER, *et al.* 1997. V. Extensive nucleotide changes and deletions within the envelope glycoprotein gene of Euro-African West Nile viruses. J. Gen. Virol. **78:** 2293–2297.
37. MURGUE, B. *et al.* 2001. West Nile outbreak in horses in Southern France (2000): the return 35 years later. Emerg. Infect. Dis. **7:** 692–696.

West Nile Fever in Israel 1999–2000

From Geese to Humans

H. BIN,[a,b] Z. GROSSMAN,[a] S. POKAMUNSKI,[c] M. MALKINSON,[d] L. WEISS,[a] P. DUVDEVANI,[a] C. BANET,[d] Y. WEISMAN,[d] E. ANNIS,[e] D. GANDAKU,[e] V. YAHALOM,[f] M. HINDYIEH,[a,e] L. SHULMAN,[a] AND E. MENDELSON[a]

[a]Central Virology Laboratory, Public Health Services, Ministry of Health, Chaim Sheba Medical Center, Tel Hashomer, Israel

[b]Wadsworth Center, New York State Department of Health, Slingerlands, New York 12159, USA

[c]Veterinary Services, Ministry of Agriculture, Israel

[d]Kimron Vetererinary Institute, Ministry of Agriculture, Beit Dagan, Israel

[e]Department of Epidemiology and Infectious Diseases, Public Health Services, Ministry of Health, Israel

[f]MDA, National Blood Services, Tel Hashomer, Israel

ABSTRACT: West Nile virus (WNV) caused disease outbreaks in Israel in the 1950s and the late 1970s. In 1998 an outbreak of WNV in goose farms and evidence of infection in dead migratory birds were reported. Consequently, human diagnostic services for WNV were resumed, including virus isolation, serology, and RT-PCR. Risk factors for infection were assessed by a serological survey in 1999, which revealed a seroprevalence of (a) 86% in people who had close contact with sick geese, (b) 28% in people in areas along bird migration routes, and (c) 27% in the general population. Following two fatal cases in Tel Aviv in September 1999 and one encephalitis case in the southern Eilot region, a regional serological survey was initiated there. The survey revealed two more WNV-associated acute encephalitis cases, an IgG seroprevalence of 51%, and an IgM seroprevalence of 22%. In the summer of 2000, acute cases of WN disease were identified in the central and northern parts of Israel, involving 439 people. The outbreak started in mid-August, peaked in September, and declined in October, with 29 fatal cases, primarily in the elderly. During the outbreak, diagnosis was based on IgM detection. Four virus isolates were subsequently obtained from preseroconverted frozen sera. Sequence and phylogenetic analysis of 1662 bases covering the PreM, M, and part of the E genes revealed two lineages. One lineage was closely related to a 1999 Israeli bird (gull) isolate and to a 1999 New York bird (flamingo) isolate, and the other lineage was closely related to a 1997 Romanian mosquito isolate and to a 1999 Russian human brain isolate.

KEYWORDS: West Nile virus; West Nile fever; Israel; geese

Address for correspondence: Hanna Bin, Ph.D., Head, Arboviruses and Hemorrhagic Diseases Section, Central Viroloy Laboratory, Public Health Services, Ministry of Health, Chaim Sheba Medical Center, Tel- Hashomer, 52621, Israel. Voice: +972-3-530-5268; fax: +972-3-530-2457.
hanna@sheba.health.gov.il

INTRODUCTION

West Nile fever (WNF) is caused by a flavivirus and is mainly transmitted by *Culex* mosquitoes. The virus circulates in nature through a zoonotic cycle. It is capable of infecting many species, including amphibians and reptiles,[1] with birds being the most efficient host for virus amplification. Humans and horses are considered dead-end hosts and are equally susceptible to the virus.

In most cases WN virus (WNV) causes a subclinical or influenza-like disease[2] except for the cases where epidemic outbreaks have been described. In these cases the virus has caused acute encephalitis or meningoencephalitis. The disease is characterized by high fever, rash, swollen glands, sore throat, conjunctivitis, muscle aches, weakness, disorientation, and stiff neck;[3,4] pancreatitis[5,6] and myocarditis[7] have also been associated with WNF. The disease has different manifestations in different age groups;[5,8] its incidence increases with age, and may have a fatal outcome in the elderly.[3,9]

WNF was first described in 1937 in Uganda, Africa.[10] The virus is endemic in Africa and Asia, and is characterized by epidemic outbreaks every few years during the late summer/fall. The first descriptions of the disease in Israel, which is located on the migratory route of many bird species from Europe to Africa, dates back to the 1940s.[11] Repeated outbreaks occurred in the central and northern part of the country during the 1950s,[12] when hundreds of cases were recorded, among them encephalitis and meningoencephalitis cases, mainly among the elderly.[5] The Central Virology Laboratory (CVL, Ministry of Health) records showed continuous diagnosis of WNF between 1974 and 1982 (N. Varsano, personal communication). In 1979 and 1980 there were two WNF episodes in the Negev (southern Israel) among soldiers, some with encephalitis,[13,14] for which WNV was confirmed at the CVL. A serosurvey among army personnel during 1982–1989 showed that immunity increased with age. Thus, groups of 18–20, 21–30, and 40–55 years had 7%, 10.5%, and 42% IgG seroprevalence, respectively.[15,16]

A cohort study performed in 1989–1990, on hospitalized children aged <1 y–17 y with unexplained encephalitis, meningitis or rash showed evidence of recent exposure to WNV (9.5% had IgM antibodies), The overall seroprevalence was 34% (by either IgG or IgM), with a rate of 20% in the <1 y age group and 45% in the rest of the cohort (Varsano, N., B-E. Lachmi & S. Lustig, 1990, unpublished data).

After 1990, no clinical cases, seroepidemiological studies, or bird and mosquito isolations were reported until 1998 when Malkinson *et al.*[17] reported WNV isolation from domestic geese, and migratory and local bird populations. High morbidity in goose flocks was associated with clinical symptoms in goose farmers while the reports of outbreaks in Romania in 1996[3] and in southern Russia in 1999[18] which were characterized by high case-fatality rates, prompted us to investigate human infections in Israel, and to prepare for a possible outbreak in humans. This report describes the course of human infections in Israel prior to the outbreak in 2000, and the main features of the 2000 outbreak, including isolation and molecular analysis of four WN viruses from human sera.

MATERIAL AND METHODS

Patients and Sera

Blood samples for seroprevalence studies were collected from volunteers with their informed consent. The volunteers filled out a questionnaire to provide information about their profession, recent clinical symptoms, and contact with sick birds. Additional samples were taken from the CVL serum bank. Preseroconversion sera from patients submitted for diagnosis of WNF just after onset of clinical symptoms, were used for virus isolation, identification and genetic analysis.

WNV Strains

Two Israeli WNV isolates were propagated in Vero cells (ATCC CCL-81). They were derived from a domestic goose in 1998[19] and from a white-eyed gull in 1999. Both isolations were performed at the Kimron Veterinary Institute (KVI) and their identities confirmed by RT-PCR at the Institut Pasteur (Dr. Deubel, paper in preparation). Virus was grown for 5 days and harvested after showing CPE of 90%.

Antigens for ELISA

Antigen was prepared from the goose or gull WNV isolates. The infected cell slurry was precipitated with polyethyleneglycol 6000.[20] We used the current WNV circulating in Israel rather than other strains, in order to improve the sensitivity and specificity of the ELISA for human serology. Uninfected Vero cells were processed in parallel, and were used as mock-infected control antigen.

Serology

Microneutralization Assay

Sera were first analyzed using microneutralization CPE reduction assay.[21] The challenge virus used was the 1998 goose isolate. This assay was used in the early serological surveys and clinical diagnoses and later helped to establish and validate the ELISA assays, with modifications.[22] We found a 96% agreement between the two tests, allowing us to adopt the ELISA as our test of choice for determination of the immune status of humans.

IgG ELISA

The assay consists of five steps starting with coating microtiter plate wells with viral antigen or mock antigen in carbonate-bicarbonate buffer pH 9.6, then blocking with 5% skim milk in phosphate-buffered saline containing Tween 20 (SM-PT). This was followed by incubation with dilutions of human sera and then with horseradish peroxidase (HRP)–conjugated anti-human IgG antibody, both diluted in 3% skim milk in SM-PT. Finally, the substrate O-Phenylenediamine dihydrochloride (OPD, Sigma) was added and the reaction stopped with 1M H_2SO_4 and the optical density (O.D.) at 492 nm was read. The background of nonspecific reactions presented as readings with the control mock antigen and subtracted from the readings of the viral antigen. The cutoff was determined as the average of many negative neutralizing antibody samples plus three standard deviations.

IgM-Capture (CAP) ELISA

The IgM antibody-capture ELISA developed at CVL in 1999, is based on the method described by Tsai *et al.* (1998), with modifications in the antigen source, and the anti-flavivirus monoclonal antibody, which reacted with Kunjin (KUN) and WN viruses (JCU/KUN/2B2, TropBio, James Cook University, Townsville, Qld, Australia). This antibody targets an epitope in the E protein that is common to both viruses.[23,24] KUNV has been recently classified as a subtype of WN virus by the International Committee for the taxonomy of viruses.[25,26]

During the outbreak, adjustments had to be made to cope with the massive demand for daily testing. Since this test was rapid and sensitive it enabled us to report results within 24 to 48 hours. Patients' sera or CSF were diluted at 1:100 and 1:2000, or 1:10, and 1:100, respectively. Control mock-antigens were omitted, because the background readings were very low. Nonetheless, the cutoff was adjusted to a point higher than 3 SD above the mean of the negative controls to prevent detection of false positives. An equivocal zone ("gray-zone") was defined at 20% above and below the mean O.D. values of the negative controls.

Virus Isolation and Identification

Virus isolation was performed on Vero cell monolayers using the tube method. Infected cells that showed CPE were evaluated with RT-PCR and a sample of the supernatant was passed on another Vero cell monolayer to confirm the presence of WNV. In addition, infected cells that showed CPE were also evaluated by indirect immunofluorescent assay (IFA) using the monoclonal antibody JCU/KUN/2B2. Cells from monolayers that did not show CPE were passed onto fresh Vero cell monolayers and monitored for another 7 days. Cells that did not show CPE after a total of 14 days incubation were reported as negative for WNV only after confirmation that the cells were also negative by IFA.

Phylogenetic Analysis of WNV Isolates from Humans

Patient samples were analyzed for WNV by RT-PCR using primer sequences for the envelope gene generously provided by Drs. L. Kramer, K. Bernard, and P-y. Shi from the Wadsworth Center, Arbovirus Laboratories, New York State Department of Health, Slingerlands, as described by Lanciotti *et al.* and Shi *et al.*[27,41] The primers Kun 108, Kun 848, Kun 998c and Kun 1830c were used in RT-PCR for sequence analysis.[28] Sequence analysis was performed on a 1662bp fragment of the WN virus genome encoding 309 nt upstream from the premembrane protein (prM), the entire prM and membrane protein (M) genes and 855 nt of the 5' portion of the envelope glycoprotein (E) gene. Purification of the RT-PCR product and sequence and phylogenetic analyses were as described.[29] Both strands of the amplified PCR products were sequenced.[30]

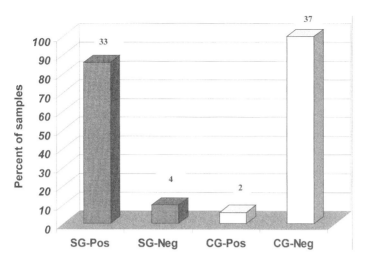

FIGURE 1. Seroprevalence of antibodies to WNV in goose farmers and veterinarians. SG–study group, farmers and veterinarians who worked with sick goose flocks, $N = 37$. CG–control group, farmers and veterinarians who worked with healthy geese or poultry. Veterinarians, $N = 39$.

RESULTS

Early Serological Surveys in 1998–1999

Morbidity in domestic geese due to WNV was reported in 1998 by the veterinary services, Ministry of Agriculture. Thereafter we initiated a study among goose farmers and poultry veterinarians to detect human infections following contact with sick geese. Sera were collected from volunteer goose farmers and veterinarians working with sick geese (study group, $N = 37$) or healthy geese (control group, $N = 39$), between December 1998 and October 1999. The sera were tested initially by neutralization assays and later by IgG ELISA for antibodies to WNV. The results shown in FIGURE 1 indicated a strong association between positive serology and contact with flocks of sick geese. Several farmers reported having a flu-like illness when their geese were sick. Interestingly, although sick and healthy flocks of geese were almost always found in different villages, in one village both sick and healthy flocks were found concomitantly. The veterinarians and farmers working with these flocks presented with correlated serological status. This finding is of particular interest because whether bird to bird or bird to human transmission of WNV occurs is still an open question.

Study in Rural Populations Living along Bird Migration Routes

During 1998, WNV was isolated from different bird species, in particular migratory storks, near Eilot, in the most southern part of Israel.[31] The birds were reported to be sick or dead. By contrast, storks captured in northeast Israel were seropositive,

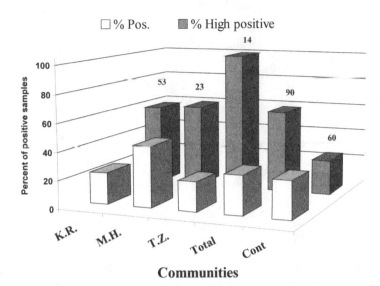

FIGURE 2. Seroprevalence of antibodies to WNV and percent of high positive in three communities in the Jordan Valley, along bird migration route. K.R., M.H. & T.Z. are abbreviated names of the communities. Cont: age matched controls from other regions of Israel, not along bird migration routes. % positive: percent of positive sera in each group. % high positive: percent of high positives among the positive sera in each group.

but WNV was not isolated from them. To study whether human infections were associated with the infected birds without reports of unusual morbidity in the general population, we conducted a serological survey in northern communities located along bird migration routes and feeding areas. Fish farming in open ponds near these communities attract hundreds of migratory birds during migration. Sera were collected from 90 volunteers from three communities in the Jordan Valley and were tested for WNV IgG by ELISA. Sixty serum samples from the CVL bank, collected in the summer of 1998 from males and females aged 30–50 years in other parts of the country (unconnected with migration) were used as controls. The seroprevalence found in the rural communities in the Jordan Valley was 28% (average of the three communities) ranging from 21–43% (FIG. 2), whereas the prevalence in the control group was 22%. However, 58–100% of the individuals in the three rural communities had high antibody titers (1:6400–1:48,000) whereas in the control group only 25% of the positives had high antibody titers; mostly the titers were less than 1:6400. These findings suggest that individuals in the rural communities may have been repeatedly exposed to WNV, apparently owing to their residence and work in close proximity to large numbers of migratory birds.

Seroprevalence by Age in a Control Group

To assess the seroprevalence of WNV IgG in different age groups in Israel we used sera from the CVL bank (kindly provided by N. Varsano and R. Handcher). Sera from 56 infants aged 12–18 months and 33 serum samples from 14-year-old

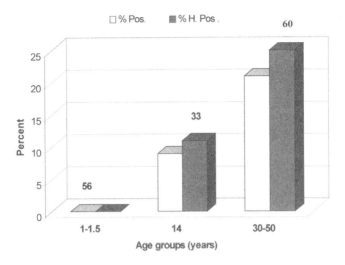

FIGURE 3. Seroprevalence of antibodies to WNV in the general population according to age. Sera were collected in 1998 and chosen from areas with no reports of WNV. Screening was done by IgG ELISA.

children collected in 1998 were tested alongside the adult group described above. The results depicted in FIGURE 3 show that the seroprevalence increases with age from 0% in the age group 12–18 months, to 7% in 14-year-olds, to 22% in the age group 30–50.

The First Human Clinical Cases in Urban Areas

In August 1999, a married couple (75/76 years old) from Tel Aviv were hospitalized with high fever and respiratory distress. Both patients later developed encephalitis and coma. The wife died three weeks after hospitalization and the husband survived for six months and died of multiorgan failure. Both tested positive for IgG and IgM in the serum and CSF. The initial diagnosis was done by Dr. R. Swanepoel, National Institute for Virology, South Africa, and later confirmed by Dr. Grant L. Campbell, CDC, Fort Collins, CO (Prof. S. Berger, Tel Aviv Medical Center, personal communication).

Morbidity in Rural Eilot District

In December 1999, a 34-year-old female from a southern rural community was hospitalized in the Chaim Sheba Medical Center Tel-Hashomer with neurological symptoms compatible with encephalitis. In view of concurrent reports on WNF in Tel Aviv and the lack of any other diagnosis of the causative agent, the patient's serum was tested for WNV IgG and were found to be high positive (>1:48,000) and IgM positive. The patient's residence in the Eilot region, where birds infected with WNV were previously found, suggested that human infections might be prevalent in

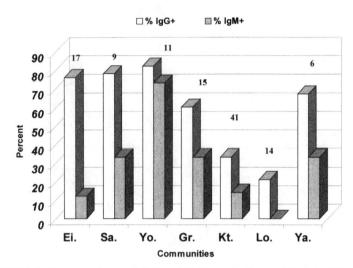

FIGURE 4. Seroprevalence of IgG and IgM antibodies to WNV in Eilot region. Mixed population, by age and health condition located at the southern part of Israel, $N = 113$. % IgG$^+$ and % IgM$^+$: Percent of positive immunoglobulins. Ei., Sa., Yo. etc., are abbreviated names of the kibbutzim.

the area. The patient's community physician and nurse were then contacted for information on unusual morbidity in the area and for collection of serum specimens. Of 37 sera collected in the patient's community (Ktura), 33% were positive for WNV IgG, half of them with high titers (>1:6400). Some of the people reported having recent clinical symptoms resembling WNF. An expanded serosurvey which included most of the rural communities in the Eilot district is shown in FIGURE 4. The IgG prevalence ranged from 21% to 82%. The IgM prevalence ranged from 0% to 73% with direct correlation to the IgG prevalence. Since this small cohort comprised various age groups and a mixture of healthy and symptomatic individuals, a thorough epidemiological analysis was not pursued. However, the average 67% IgG prevalence and 30% IgM prevalence in the Eilot district were strong indications of active WNV circulation in this region during and preceding the study period (January–April, 2000). A retrospective investigation revealed two cases of encephalitis and meningoencephalitis in young adults from two adjacent communities, whose IgM were positive and IgG titers were 1:12,000 and 1:100,000. These data suggest that an outbreak in the Eilot district preceded by several months the outbreak in the central and northern regions of Israel.

WNF Outbreak, August–October 2000

Starting in mid-August and lasting until the end of October high morbidity from WNF was recorded throughout the entire country (FIG. 5). The total number of cases, including sporadic cases in July and November 2000, was 439, with 29 fatal cases (4 additional patients with WNV IgM died from complications of other diseases). The outbreak started in central Israel and spread north and south. The highest attack

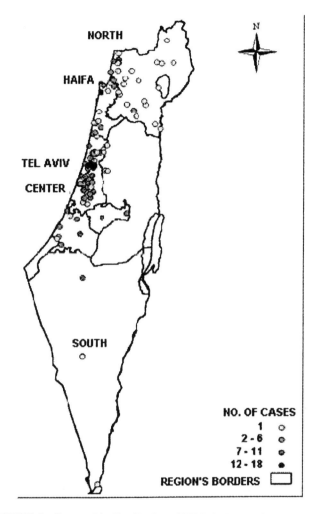

FIGURE 5. Geographic distribution of WNF in Israel, October 2000.

rates were in the center and the lowest were in the South.[32] During the outbreak, laboratory diagnosis was based on the capture IgM ELISA assay, which was done at 1:100 and 1:2000 serum dilutions and 1:10 and 1:100 in CSF samples. The turnaround time for reporting results to physicians and to the Epidemiology Department of the Ministry of Health was 24–48 hours. The outbreak dynamics, reflected by the weekly cases tested and the percentage of positive patients, are shown in FIGURE 6. Interestingly, the percentage of positive cases was the highest at the beginning of the outbreak and declined gradually. This reflects the increasing awareness of physicians and perhaps also the public panic, which was augmented by media reports.

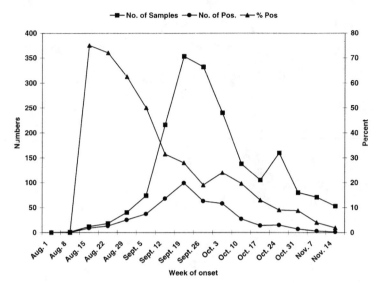

FIGURE 6. WNF weekly distribution during the outbreak, Aug.–Oct. 2000. Assayed by CAP-IgM ELISA.

Clinical data available for 233 hospitalized and 37 ambulatory patients revealed that 73% of the hospitalized patients had some form of CNS involvement, while only 8% of the ambulatory patients had mild encephalitis.[32,33] Morbidity increased significantly over age 45 (69% of the cases, FIG. 7) and mortality increased dramatically over age 65 (96%) as shown in FIGURE 8. Morbidity and mortality rates in males and females of all ages were almost identical (data not shown).

Virus Isolation and Phylogenetic Analysis

During the outbreak no attempts were made to isolate virus or diagnose cases by molecular assays (RT-PCR). After the outbreak, specimens stored at −70°C were used for virus isolation. Virus isolation from serum was successful from four living WNV IgM-negative patients. Patient 1(WN_0043) was a 51-year-old female from the central region. Patient 2 (WN_0233) was a 20-year-old male from the north-central region. Patient 3 (WN_0247) was a 5-year-old male with encephalitis residing in the center. Patient 4 (WN_0304) was a 55-year-old female from the north. Only the 5-year-old patient developed meningoencephalitis, while the others did not develop a CNS disease. All four virus isolates were confirmed as WNV by IFA. The WNV isolates derived from patients 3 and 4 had grown faster on Vero cells than those isolated from patients 1 and 2 (4 days versus 7 days, respectively). Isolates from patients 3 and 4 were positive by RT-PCR directly from serum; positive RT-PCR results from all 4 isolates could be achieved after culture amplification. The analysis of the four isolates is presented in FIGURE 9.

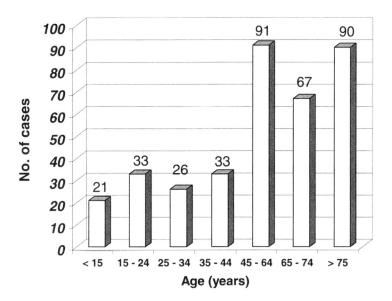

FIGURE 7. WNF cases in different age groups, during the outbreak, Aug.–Oct. 2000. Assayed by CAP-IgM ELISA.

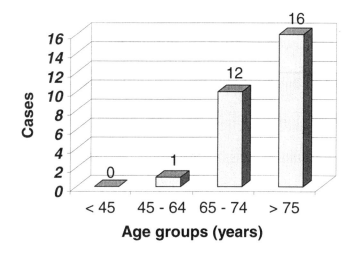

FIGURE 8. Mortality rate during the WNF outbreak in humans. Morbidity by age.

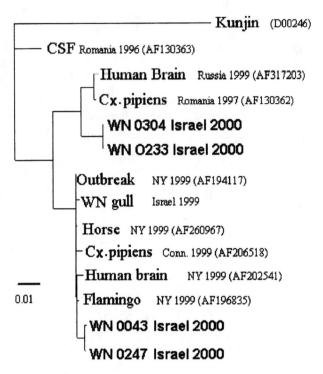

FIGURE 9. Phylogenetic analysis of four human islolates during the outbreak. Molecular identification was performed on preseroconverted frozen serum. 407 bp were amplified from WNV primers specific to the E gene. Sequencing of 1662 nt from the PreM, M, and E gene was performed with KUN primers.

RT-PCR, sequencing and phylogenetic analysis of a region encompassing 1662 nucleotides of the PrM, M, and partial 5' E genes revealed two lineages. One lineage comprised two identical isolates from central Israel and was most closely related (99.7% homology) to flamingo, mosquito, and horse isolates from New York, 1999, or Israeli gull, 1999. The other lineage, comprising two isolates from the north and north-central regions of Israel was most closely related (98% homology) to an avian isolate from northern Israel, 2000, a mosquito isolate from Romania, 1997, and to a Russian isolate from the 1999 outbreak in Volgograd. The presence of two lineages is compatible with an endemic situation or with repeated introductions.

DISCUSSION

WNF is not a reportable disease in Israel, but several outbreaks and clinical cases were documented between 1951 and 1982. The last outbreak in Israel was in 1980[13] and the last three encephalitis cases were reported in 1981.[14] The large outbreaks in Romania in 1996 and in southern Russia in 1999, and the reappearance of WNV in migratory and domestic birds in Israel, presaged the reemergence of the disease in humans, potentially on a large scale, in Israel. To investigate the extent of human infections by assessing the population immunity and tracing human cases, we have reestablished diagnostic abilities in the CVL. New and improved ELISA methods for detection of IgG and IgM antibodies were developed during 1998–1999 and virus isolation, neutralization, immunofluorescence and RT-PCR assays were established. Concomitantly, serum specimens were collected from volunteers in communities considered to be at high risk of infection (goose farmers and veterinarians and residents of communities located along bird migration routes). Control sera from the general population were collected in 1998 from the CVL serum bank. We found that the seroprevalence in the general population in 1998 (22% in adults) was lower than the seroprevalence reported during the 1980s,[16] which reached 42%. However, our sample size was small (60 adult control sera) and cannot support any final conclusion. Studies with much larger samples are under way, with special attention to new immigrants and their place of birth.

By following the flyways of sick birds, we detected recent human infections in two population groups: (a) goose farmers and veterinarians residing in the central region of Israel who came in close contact with sick geese, and (b) members of rural communities in the southernmost region of Israel (Eilot district). In both groups we found high IgG prevalence and high IgG titers, and a high rate of IgM positivity in the Eilot district population. All these are markers of recent WNV infection. Reports from many of the volunteers from these two groups describing a recent WNF-like illness and the three encephalitis cases in the Eilot district were compatible with the laboratory data. The data collected by our investigations prior to the outbreak confirmed that WNV was active in recent years and human infections were very common around goose farms in 1998 and 1999 and in Eilot in 1999.

The two fatal human cases, which occurred in Tel Aviv in the late summer of 1999, were a clear indication that the virus spread was not limited to rural areas. Repeated alerts issued by the Ministry of Health to all health-care providers in Israel prompted infectious disease specialists to include WNF in the differential diagnosis of high fever and encephalitis cases. This resulted in a large number of laboratory-confirmed cases which were identified during the late summer and fall of 2000, forming an outbreak-like epidemiological curve. An unusual feature of this outbreak was the spread of the disease in almost all highly populated areas of Israel, including primarily the central and northern regions. This is in contrast to previous outbreaks which were more localized[5,12,13] and were reported in one region only each time. Viruses isolated from four patients' sera were sequenced and showed two clusters. Of particular interest is that these two lineages corresponded to the lineages found in birds in Israel, presenting a similar geographic distribution: a strain most similar to the Romanian-1997 strain was found in patients residing in the north, and a strain most similar to the New York-1999 strain was found in patients residing in the central region. Although the number of human isolates is too small to draw any conclusions regarding the routes by which the virus spreads or any association of virus strain with the severity of the clinical symptoms, the finding of two lineages suggests either that the virus has been endemic for many years (supported by the high prevalence of antibodies in sera from 1998) or that migrating birds have introduced several virus strains concomitantly in recent years.

Alternatively, one can hypothesize, based on the early signs of disease in geese in 1997, that after the 1996 outbreak in Romania, a new strain with a modified genome was introduced into Israel's local birds via migratory birds. By finding geese as new, highly susceptible hosts the WN virus was amplified and might have changed further and passed on to other birds, mosquitoes and, with the overflow, to humans. Changes in the viral genome could have happened in recent years via a dynamic process in Africa, Europe,[18,28,34–36] the Middle-East or Israel.[19,37] Isolation and phylogenetic analysis of viruses from many birds, mosquitoes, and humans, and comparisons to isolates from other countries, may provide more clues to the virus zoonotic cycles and routes of spread.

The conditions that allowed the development of such a widespread morbidity are complicated and include in addition to the virus also environmental and host-related factors which require further investigation. The increased morbidity could be attributed to the following promoting factors (as recently suggested by Lustig *et al.*[38]): (a) climatic factors—consecutive warmer-than-usual summers for the last three years in Israel (Israel Meteorological Service, personal communication) might have forced the bird population to congregate at diminishing water sources, increasing the bird to bird transmission via mosquitos carrying more virus particles than usual, and finally leading to transmission to humans. Similar climatic descriptions were observed in Romania, Russia and the northeastern United States.[18,39,40] (b) Demographic changes—in the early 1990s approximately one million people from Russia moved to Israel as did immigrants from other countries and foreign workers who most likely had not been previously exposed to WN virus. These immigration waves apparently increased the size of the population susceptible to WNV infection.

ACKNOWLEDGMENTS

We are most grateful to Prof. R. Swanepoel and Dr. F. Burt, from the Special Pathogens Unit, National Institute for Virology, Johannesburg, South Africa, who helped in confirming the first cases of WNF, while we developed the diagnostic assays. We thank Prof. S. Berger and Dr. M. Weinberg, from Tel Aviv Medical Center, Tel Aviv, Israel, for being the first to suspect WN disease in the two patients from Tel Aviv. We also thank Dr. D. Gubler, from the Division of Vector-Borne Infectious Disease, CDC, Fort Collins, CO, USA, for helping out during the establishment of the Arboviruses laboratory in the CVL by supplying bioreagents. Thanks go to B-E. Lachmi and S. Lustig from the Israel Institute for Biological Research, for helping with expert advice and bioreagents. We thank Drs. V. Deubel and L. Fiette, from Institut Pasteur, Paris, France, for being involved in further molecular and histopathology diagnosis of the first clinical case of WN fever. We also thank our Central Virology Laboratory virologists for helping with their vast expertise, in particular N. Varsano, R. Handcher, Dr. Z. Smetana, M. Vax, Z. Cohen, and Z. Sofiyev. Special thanks go to all those who worked relentlessly, jointly with our staff, during the outbreak, namely, Drs. D. Sofer and F. Mileguir, and R. Pavel and N. Stern. Special thanks go also to D. Glasner, from Kfar Ruppin, Nurse Sigal and E. Usha, Chief Epidemiological Nurse from Eilot region, and Prof. Y. Harishano, Neurology Department in Soroka Medical Center, Beer-Sheba and Yoseftal Medical Center, Eilat. Thanks are also due to Drs. H. Penner, from the Entomological Laboratory, Central

Public Health Laboratories, Ministry of Health, Jerusalem, and U. Shalom and L. Orshan, from the Ministry of the Environment, Pesticide Unit, Jerusalem, for help in collecting, and species identification of mosquito pools, before and during the outbreak, although the data were not included in this article.

The pilot study "West Nile virus—the causative agent for West Nile fever in humans in Israel" was partially supported by a research grant from the Ministry of Health Chief Scientist, Jerusalem.

REFERENCES

1. NIR, A., A. AVIVI, Y. LASOWSKI, *et al.* 1972. Arbovirus activity in Israel. Israel J. Med. Sci. **8:** 1695–1701.
2. HAYES, C.G. 1989. West Nile fever. *In* The Arboviruses: Epidemiology and Ecology. T.P. Monath, Ed.: Vol. 7: 59-88. CRC Press. Boca Raton, FL.
3. TSAI, T.F., F. POPOVICI, C. CERNESCU, *et al.* 1998. West Nile encephalitis epidemic in southeastern Romania. Lancet **352:** 767–771.
4. HOEY, J. 2000. West Nile fever in New York City. Can. Med. Assoc. J. **162:** 1036.
5. SPIGLAND, I., W. JASINSKA-KLINGBERG, E. JOFSHI & N. GOLDBLUM. 1958. Clinical and laboratory observations in an outbreak of West Nile fever in Israel. Harefuah **54:** 275–281.
6. PERLMAN A. & J. STERN. 1974. Acute pancreatitis in West Nile fever. Am. J. Trop. Med. Hyg. **23:** 1150–1152.
7. HUBÁLEK, Z. & J. HALOUZKA. 1999. West Nile fever a reemerging mosquito-borne viral disease in Europe. Emerg. Infect. Dis. **5:** 1–16.
8. TAYLOR R.M., T.A. WORK, H.S. HURLBUT & F. RIZK. 1956. A study of the ecology of West Nile virus in Egypt. Am. J. Trop. Med. Hyg. **5:** 579–620.
9. U.S. DEPARTMENT OF HEALTH, EDUCATION AND WELFARE, PUBLIC HEALTH SERVICE, CENTER FOR DISEASE CONTROL. 1999. West Nile-like viral encephalitis—New York, 1999. CDC Morb. Mortal. Wkly. Rep. **48:** 845–849.
10. SMITHBURN, K.C., T.P. HUGES, A.W. BRUKE & J.H. PAUL. 1940. Neutrotophic virus isolated from blood of native of Uganda. Am. J. Trop. Med. **20:** 471–492.
11. LEFFKOWITZ, M. 1942. On the frequent appearance of an unclear infectious disease. Harefuah **22:** 3–4.
12. BERNKOPF, H., S. LEVINE & R. NERSON. 1953. Isolation of West Nile virus in Israel. J. Infect. Dis. **93:** 207–218.
13. KATZ, G., E. NILI, L. RANNON & Y.L. DANON. 1989. West Nile Fever—occurrence in a new endemic site in the Negev. Isr. J. Med. Sci. **25:** 39–41.
14. FLATAU, E., D. KOHN, O. DAHER & N. VARSANO. 1981. West Nile fever encephalitis. Isr. J. Med. Sci. **17:** 1057–1059.
15. ZAIDE, Y., M. SCHWARZ, R. SLEPON, *et al.* 1990. Prevalence of antibodies to West Nile virus among various Israeli military populations. Presented at the Annual Meeting of the Israeli Society for Microbiology, Haifa, Israel.
16. COHEN, D., Y. ZAIDE, E. KARASENTY, *et al.* 1999. Prevalence of antibodies to West Nile fever, sandfly fever Sicilian, and sandfly fever Naples viruses in healthy adults in Israel. Public Health Rev. **27:** 217–230.
17. MALKINSON, M., C. BANET, J. WEISMAN, *et al.* 1999. West Nile fever: recent evidence for intercontinental dispersion of the virus by migratory birds. Presented at the 11th International Congress of Virology, Sydney, Australia.
18. PLATONOV, A E., G.A. SHIPULIN, O.YU. SHIPULINA, *et al.* 2001. Outbreak of West Nile virus infection, Volgograd region, Russia, 1999. Emerg. Infect. Dis. **7:** 1–7.
19. LANCIOTTI, R.S., J.T. ROEHRIG, V. DEUBEL, *et al.* 1999. Origin of the West Nile virus responsible for an outbreak of encephalitis in the northeastern United States. Science **286:** 2333–2337.
20. GOULD, E.A. & J.C.S. CLEGG. 1985. Growth, titration and purification of Togaviruses. *In* Virology, a Practical Approach. B.W.J. Mahy, Ed.: 343–374. IRL Press. Oxford, England.

21. LIDSEY, H.S., C.H. CALISHER & J.H. MATHEWS. 1976. Serum dilution neutralization test for California group virus identification and serology. J. Clin. Microbiol. **4:** 503–510.
22. FEINSTEIN, S., Y. AKOV, B-E. LACHMI, *et al.* 1985. Determination of human IgG and IgM class antibodies to West Nile virus by enzyme linked immunosorbent assay (ELISA). J. Med. Virol. **17:** 63–72.
23. BLITVITCH, B.J., J.C. MACKENZIE, R.J. CHOEN, *et al.* 1995. A novel complex formed between the flavivirus E and NS1 proteins: analysis of its structure and function. Arch. Virol. **140:** 145–156.
24. HALL, R.A., B.H. KAY, G.W. BURGESS, *et al.* 1990. Epitope analysis of the envelope and non-structural lipoproteins of Marry Valley encephalitis virus. J. Gen. Virol. **70:** 2923–2930.
25. HALL, R.A. 2000. Kunjin Virus—Australia. ProMED, Mar 13.
26. MACKENZIE, J.S. 2001. Kunjin Virus—Australia (NT): Alert. ProMED, Feb. 6.
27. LANCIOTTI, R.S., A.J. KERST, R.S. NASCI, *et al.* 2000. Rapid detection of West Nile virus from human clinical specimens, field-collected mosquitoes, and avian samples by TaqMan reverse transcriptase-PCR assay J. Clin. Microbiol. **38:** 4066–4071.
28. SAVAGE, H.M., C. CEIANU, G. NICOLESCU, *et al.* 1999. Entomologic and avian investigations of an epidemic of West Nile fever in Romania in 1996, with serologic and molecular characterization of a virus isolate from mosquitoes. Am. J. Trop. Med. Hyg. **61:** 600–611.
29. SHULMAN, L.M., R. HANDSHER, C.F. YANG, *et al.* 2000. Resolution of the pathways of poliovirus Type 1 transmission during an outbreak. J. Clin. Microbiol. **38:** 945–952.
30. HINDIYEH, M., L.M. SHULMAN, E. MENDELSON, *et al.* Isolation and characterization of West Nile virus from the blood of viremic patients during the 2000 outbreak in Israel. Emerg. Infect. Dis. **7:** 748–750.
31. MALKINSON, M., C. BANET & J. WEISSMAN. 1998. Intercontinental spread of West Nile virus by wild birds—recent epidemiological findings in Israeli livestock and birds. Presented at the 2nd International Conference on Emerging Zoonoses, Strasbourg, France, November 5–9.
32. CHOWERS, M.Y., R. LANG, F. NASSER, *et al.* Part II. Clinical characteristics. Emerg. Infect. Dis. **7:** 675–678.
33. WEINBERGER, M., S.D. PITLIK, D. GANDACU, *et al.* West Nile outbreak, Israel 2000. Part I. Epidemiologic aspects. Emerg. Infect. Dis. **7:** 686–691.
34. BERTHET, F.X., H.G. ZELLER, M.T. DROUET, *et al.* 1997. Extensive nucleotide changes and deletions within the envelope glycoprotein gene of Euro-African West Nile viruses. J. Gen. Virol. **78:** 2293–2297.
35. DEUBEL, V. 1998. West Nile virus encephalitis, equides—Italy. ProMED, Dec.
36. HUBÁLEK, Z., J. HALOUZKA & Z. JURICOV. 1999. West Nile fever in Czechland. Emerg. Infect. Dis. **5:** 2–5.
37. JIA, X-Y., T. BRIESE, I. JORDAN, *et al.* 1999. Genetic analysis of West Nile New York 1999 encephalitis. Lancet **354:** 1971–1972.
38. LUSTIG, S., M. HALEVY, P. FUCHS, *et al.* 2000. Can West Nile virus outbreaks be controlled? Isr. Med. Assoc. J. **2:** 733–737.
39. HAN, L.L., F. POPOVICI Jr. J.P. ALEXANDER, *et al.* 1999. Risk factors for West Nile virus infection and meningoencephalitis, Romania, 1996. J. Infect. Dis. **179:** 230–233.
40. EPSTEIN, P.R. 2000. Global warming: the hidden health risk. Sci. Am. **283:** 36–43.
41. SHI, P-Y., E.B. KAUFFMAN, P. REN, *et al.* 2001. High-throughput detection of West Nile Virus RNA. J. Clin. Microbiol. **39:** 1264–1271.

The Ecology of West Nile Virus in South Africa and the Occurrence of Outbreaks in Humans

PETER G. JUPP

Special Pathogens Unit, National Institute for Virology and Department of Virology, University of the Witwatersrand, Private Bag X4, Sandringham 2131, South Africa

ABSTRACT: This paper reviews studies done on West Nile virus (WNV) in South Africa, mainly between 1962 and 1980 on the temperate inland plateau (Highveld and Karoo). The virus is maintained in an enzootic transmission cycle between feral birds and the ornithophilic mosquito *Culex univittatus*. About 30 avian species have been shown to be involved without mortality. Humans, and other mammals, although they may have antibodies, are considered blind-alleys in the transmission cycle except perhaps some dogs. *Cx. univittatus* also transfers infection to humans, almost invariably causing only a mild illness. Its usually low anthropophilism may explain why annual human infection on the Highveld is limited to sporadic cases. Besides multiple isolations from field collections of *Cx. univittatus*, this mosquito is both highly susceptible to the virus and an efficient transmitter. *Culex theileri* is a minor vector. In the summer of 1974 there was a large epidemic in the dry Karoo after unusual rains: there were many human cases, the infection rate in *Cx. univittatus* was 39.0/1000, and postepidemic immune rates in humans and birds were high. In 1984 there was an epizootic in Gauteng Province in the Highveld with an infection rate in *Cx. univittatus* reaching 9.6/1000 and more human infections than usual. The much lower immune rates in the KwaZulu-Natal coastal lowlands than on the plateau and the single isolation from *Cx. neavei*, which replaces *Cx. univittatus* in the lowlands, are explained by the low susceptibility of *Cx. neavei* to the virus. Genetic relatedness of isolates from different countries showed two lineages, with one lineage comprising only African isolates, including 25 South African strains, which had a sequence homology of 86.3–100%. This suggests that the viral enzooticity does not depend on annual importation of virus in migrant birds.

KEYWORDS: West Nile virus; South Africa; ecology; human outbreaks

INTRODUCTION

This paper reviews the studies done on West Nile virus (WNV) in South Africa, mainly between 1962 and 1980, but also some work done before and after this period. Most of the studies were carried out in the inland plateau region (FIG. 1). This is an area with a temperate climate 400–2000 meters above sea level comprising the Karoo (the western two-thirds) and the Highveld (the eastern third). The Karoo is

Address for correspondence: Peter G. Jupp, Ph.D., D.Sc., Special Pathogens Unit, National Institute for Virology and Department of Virology, University of the Witwatersrand, Private Bag X4, Sandringham 2131, South Africa.Voice: +27-11-882-3164; fax: +27-11-882-3741.
juppy@mweb.co.za

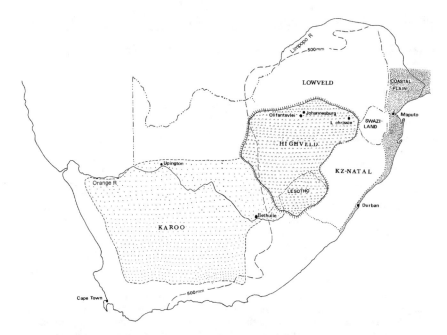

FIGURE 1. South Africa, showing the inland plateau (Karoo and Highveld) and the KwaZulu-Natal coastal plain. The 500 mm isohyet bisects the country into eastern moist and western arid parts.

arid semidesert with a mean rainfall of less than 500 mm, while the Highveld is cooler grassland with 500–700 mm of rainfall. The coastal plain of KwaZulu-Natal (KZN), the other region where studies were undertaken, is a lowland strip on the eastern seaboard with a moist subtropical climate except near the Mozambique border to the north where it becomes tropical.

Neutralizing antibodies to WNV are widely distributed in humans in South Africa and also in neighboring Mozambique, as well as along the northern borders of Namibia and Botswana. The virus was isolated at 11 localities on the inland plateau and at 2 localities on the KZN coast. Neutralizing antibodies were found in humans more frequently on the inland plateau (17.1% in the Karoo and 8% in the Highveld) than in the KZN coastal localities (2%).[1-5] This difference has correlated positively with mosquito infection rates, observed human illness, and avian infection and is believed to be due to the presence of the efficient vector *Culex univittatus* on the plateau, which is replaced by a much less efficient vector, *Culex neavei*, on the KZN coast.[6] From the various aspects of the ecology of WNV studied on the plateau, it became clear that a maintenance or enzootic cycle existed in which the virus was transmitted between various species of wild birds by the mosquito *Cx. univittatus*.[7,8]

Sporadic human cases of WNV—invariably a mild febrile illness with myalgia, arthralgia and a maculopapular rash—occur annually each summer on the Highveld.[9] On two occasions this usual pattern changed: there was an epidemic of WNV in the Karoo in 1974[10] and an unusual epizootic accompanied by more human cases than usual in the Highveld in 1984.[11]

TABLE 1. West Nile virus isolations from mosquitoes in South Africa, 1956–1980[a]

Region	Infected species	No. tested	No.isolations
Inland Plateau	Cx. univittatus	70,037	128
	Cx. theileri	82,995	6
	Cx. pipiens	128,967	1
	Ae. caballus sl	1809	1
KwaZulu-Natal	Cx. neavei	57,559	1
coastal lowlands	Cq. microannulata	254	1
	Ae. circumluteolus	201,427	1

[a]Isolations from the 1974 Karoo outbreak are not included; see TABLE 4.

TABLE 2. Results of quantitative vector competence tests with West Nile virus

	Culex univittatus			Culex neavei
Titer of infective feed $\log_{10}$ LD$_{50}$/mL	Infection rate[a]	50% Infection threshold $\log_{10}$ LD$_{50}$/mL[b]	Transmission rate[c]	50% infection threshold $\log_{10}$ LD$_{50}$/mL
5.8 –6.3	37/37		35/36 (97%)	
4.3	24/24		5/15 (33%)	
		2.1		4.4
2.7	21/25 (84%)			
1.9	12/29 (41%)			

[a]Numerator = No. mosquitoes infected; denominator = No. mosquitoes tested.
[b]This is calculated from infection rates and is titer of virus to infect 50% of mosquitoes.
[c]Numerator = No. mosquitoes transmitting virus; denominator = No. of infected mosquitoes feeding.

The *Alphavirus* Sindbis (SIN) has the same ecology as WNV and a very similar epidemiology. Hence, the two viruses have been studied simultaneously in South Africa and what has been said above applies to both. Observations on the SIN virus will sometimes be included in this paper where the comparison with WNV is considered important.

THE MOSQUITO VECTORS

TABLE 1 lists those mosquito species collected between 1956 and 1980 from which one or more isolates of WNV were made.[8,12,13] Multiple isolations were obtained from only two species, *Cx. univittatus* and *Cx. theileri,* and nearly all came from the former. Both these mosquitoes occur on the inland plateau; laboratory vector competence tests carried out with *Cx. univittatus* (TABLE 2) have shown that this species is highly susceptible to the virus with a low 50% infection threshold of 2.1 $\log_{10}$ LD$_{50}$/mL and that it has a high transmission rate (97%) after an infecting feed with

TABLE 3. Olifantsvlei birds and West Nile virus; highest viremias recorded after viral inoculation and percentage of certain species naturally infected (hemagglutination inhibition antibodies), 1962–1965

Species	Laboratory viremia $\log_{10}$ LD$_{50}$/mL	Natural infection: No. tested (% positive)
Bubulcus ibis (cattle egret)	6.1	39 (9)
Threskiornis aethiopicus (sacred ibis)	5.2	14 (14)
Anas undulata (yellow-bill duck)	5.4	104 (17)
Anas erythrorhyncha (red-bill teal)	4.2	56 (36)
Netta erythrophthalma (pochard)	3.9	NT
Fulica eristata (red-knobbed coot)	4.2	72 (22)
Columba livea (domestic pigeon)	4.7	NT
Streptopelia capicola (turtle dove)	5.1	NT
Streptopelia senegalensis (laughing dove)	6.7	39 (10)
Passer melanurus (Cape sparrow)[a]	4.4	NT
Ploceus velatus (masked weaver)	7.5	133 (9)
Quelea quelea (red-bill quelea)[a]	3.9	279 (11)
Euplectes orix (red bishop)	7.7	999 (11)
Acrocephalus gracilirostris (Cape reed warbler)	NT	32 (11)

NT = not tested.
[a]Bloods titrated after storage, hence actual titers possibly higher than values shown.

a titer of about 6.0 logs/mL.[14–16] This rate was still quite high (33%) following an infective feed on a viremic chick circulating 4.3 logs of virus.[16] As the maximum titers of virus reached in feral birds varies from about 4.0–7.7 logs/mL (TABLE 3) it is clear that Cx. univitattus would be able to infect a range of birds or become infected by feeding on such avian species when they were viremic. Although Cx. theileri has a low 50% infection threshold of 3.2 logs/mL, it has low transmission rates viz. 0% and 25% following an infective meal of 6.2 and 7.1 logs, respectively.[17] If Cx. theileri is almost as easily infected as Cx. univittatus in experiments, why are so few viral isolates made from wild populations? It is probably because of differences in feeding habits. Cx. univittatus is highly ornithophilic while Cx. theileri is only moderately so.[18,19] Furthermore there are differences between their host preferences among various avian species, Cx. theileri feeding largely at ground level while Cx. univitattus feeds both on the ground and in the canopy of trees.[19] Cx. theileri is thus regarded as only a minor vector. It is notewothy that no other mosquito species, particularly Aedes species, have been incriminated as vectors in South Africa.

As mentioned earlier, WNV activity is low on the KZN coastal plain as compared to the inland plateau. An explanation for this is the poorer susceptibility of Cx. neavei to the virus as compared to Cx. univittatus (TABLE 2).[6] Cx. univittatus is replaced by Cx. neavei in the coastal plain,[20] and only one virus isolation has been made from this species. Apparently, therefore, Cx. neavei is less readily infected after feeding on birds.

THE AVIAN HOST

Thirteen common avian species collected at our study site Olifantsvlei (near Johannesburg) have circulated the virus at significant titers after inoculation in the laboratory (TABLE 3).[21] Viremia lasted 3–4 days and no illness or mortality was attributed to the virus.

Fifty-seven of 62 birds (92%) had hemagglutination inhibition (HI) antibodies and 42 of 60 birds (70%) had neutralizing (N) antibodies on the 30th day. From 1962–1965 wild birds were trapped at Olifansvlei and tested for antibodies and infection by WNV.[22] Two hundred and fifty-two of 2022 birds (12.5%) were found to have HI antibodies to WNV in their plasmas. Twenty-seven species were among the positively reacting birds. TABLE 3 shows the percentage of reacting birds from among 10 of these species which are common on the plateau. No isolation of WNV was made from 1015 plasmas tested for virus by inoculation into infant mice.

Both fowls and pigeons have been used for surveillance of virus transmission in the field. Fowls were exposed in fowl-pen mosquito traps at Olifantsvlei and at another site on the plateau—Lake Chrissie—over three consecutive summers from 1962–1965.[7] They were bled periodically for HI antibody tests. Infections (antibody conversions) were recorded at both localities each summer, with a total of 38 infections at Olifantsvlei (53% of the fowls) and 13 at Lake Chrissie (54% of the fowls). Later, fowls were replaced by pigeons as sentinels. Pigeons were preferred since they were as susceptible to the virus as fowls but hardier, easier to handle, and less expensive to maintain. These were exposed at Olifansvlei from 1967–1971 and at Bethulie in the Karoo from 1968–1971.[23] At Olifansvlei a total of 20 infections were recorded during four of the five years and at Bethulie a total of 41 during three of the four years. Infections mainly occurred in the summer and but sometimes in the autumn. The higher infection rate in Bethulie compared to Olifansvlei was significantly different ($P < 0.025$). Insects collected in suction traps, which were sometimes suspended at the bottom of the sentinel cages, revealed the numerical prevalence of *Cx. univitattus*.[23] This type of trap proved to be the most efficient of the various methods used for sampling ornithophilic mosquitoes.

HUMAN INFECTION AND EPIDEMICS

Host preference studies in the Highveld region of the plateau showed that while *Cx. univitattus* is strongly ornithophilic it does feed on humans to a limited extent and even enters houses.[19] This limited anthropophily must be an important factor limiting the number of human cases of WNV and preventing the regular occurrence of epidemics. Human infections occur annually on the plateau, but in small numbers, and humans are incidental hosts to the virus. Because of low viremia in man, human infection is totally dependent spatially and temporally on avian infection and humans are "blind alleys" in the transmission cycle.

Since work started on WNV in South Africa, there has been only one large epidemic and one more localized epizootic accompanied by an increase in human infections. The epidemic occurred in the summer of 1973–1974 in the Karoo following exceptional summer rains. The mosquitoes collected at Upington in April 1974 are shown in TABLE 4. Thirty-three isolations were obtained from only 1325 *Cx. univit-*

TABLE 4. Number of mosquitoes collected in April 1974 at Upington during the Karoo epidemic and number of isolations of West Nile and Sindbis viruses made from them

Species	No. of mosquitoes tested	No. isolations		MIR^a (IR^b)	
		WN	SIN	WN	SIN
Cx. univittatus	1325	33	8	24.9	6.0
Cx. theileri	4889	4	4	(39.0)	(6.5)
Cx. pipiens	1200			0.8 (0.8)	0.8
5 other species	100				(0.8)

[a]Minimum infection rate = No. infected mosquitoes/1000.
[b]Statistical infection rate/1000 calculated by method of Chiang and Reeves (1962).

tatus and four isolations from 4889 *Cx. theileri*. This epidemic was accompanied by one of SIN virus, although the mosquito infection rates were much higher for WNV (TABLE 4). This event and the related studies have been fully reported by McIntosh et al.[10] Studies of the mosquitoes, birds and humans in the Upington area revealed that WNV was much more active than SIN virus. Further mosquito collections made at Upington during the first wet summer after the outbreak (1976), which also had unusually heavy rain, showed that *Cx. univittatus* was an important anthropophilic species there. This might have been due to a very high population density of *Cx. univittatus* or it could indicate that the local population of the mosquito is more anthropophilic than the Highveld population. All eight species of birds trapped and bled in the Karoo at Upington after the epidemic revealed a high positivity in antibody tests for WNV, and there was also a high percentage positive in the sera of some bird species for SIN virus (TABLE 5). A mean of 55% human sera were positive for WNV after the epidemic and 16% were positive to SIN virus. The outbreak covered 2500 km², from the Orange river in the north, Laingsburg to the south, Beaufort West to the east and the Atlantic seaboard to the west. It is thought that two key factors favoring the occurrence of this epidemic were the unusual rains, which led to a greatly increased *Cx. univittatus* population density, and the higher summer temperatures in the Karoo, which enhanced viral replication in the vector.

TABLE 5. Percentage of bird sera, collected from various species in Upington after the Karoo epidemic in 1974, reacting in hemagglutination inhibition and/or neutralization tests with West Nile virus

Species	No. sera tested	Percent sera positive
Turdus olivaceus (olive thrush)	24	92
Streptopelia senegalensis (laughing dove)	72	86
Streptopelia capicola (turtle dove)	2	100
Pycnostictus nigricans (red-eyed bulbul)	9	22
Passer domesticus (house sparrow)	48	50
Euplectes orix (red bishop)	153	40
Quela quela (red-billed quelea)	5	60
Ploceus velatus (masked weaver)	9	33
Total/Mean	322	53

TABLE 6. Isolations of Sindbis and West Nile viruses from *Culex univittatus* collected at four Witwatersrand (Gauteng) localities in February–March 1984

Locality	No. *Cx. univittatus* tested	No. pools	Sindbis No. isolations	Sindbis MIR (IR)	West Nile No. isolations	West Nile MIR (IR)
Germiston	1980	79	5	2.5 (2.5)	19	9.6 (10.9)
Rietfontein	817	33	2	2.4 (2.5)	3	3.7 (3.8)
Modderfontein	558	23	3	5.4 (5.6)	1	1.8 (1.6)
Florida/Rietfontein	22	1	—		1	—

The 1983–1984 epizootic of WN and SIN viruses occurred in the Witwatersrand-Pretoria (Gauteng) area of the Highveld.[11] The spring and early summer experienced unusually good rains (October to December). This was followed by higher than average temperatures in January to March, which again are thought to have increased the transmission of the virus by *Cx. univittatus*. The number of *Cx. univitattus* collected at four localities in the Witwatersrand, the number of isolations of both WN and SIN viruses, and the field mosquito infection rates are shown in TABLE 6. The infection rates of both WN and SIN viruses were higher than usual in the *Cx. univittatus* populations, indicating that an epizootic of both viruses had occurred. However, the number of human infections was much higher in the case of SIN virus, reaching epidemic level, while the increase in WNV cases over the previous season was only slight. It is unclear why the transfer from the feral cycle to humans occurred to such a limited extent with WNV.

There have only been four human cases of WNV in South Africa in which the usual mild illness has developed into a more serious condition. In two cases there has been renal failure associated with the virus. The first of these was a 55-year-old man who tested with an HI titer of 1:1280 and a positive IgM by ELISA.[24] The second was a 33-year-old man from whose serum the virus was isolated, but this patient had a three-year history of brucellosis.[25] The remaining two cases, also males, were a 60 year old who had meningoencephalitis, an HI titer of 1:1280 and positive IgM but who recovered[24] and a 28 year old who died from liver failure. WNV was isolated from a liver biopsy from the latter patient, who has been the only fatality in South Africa associated with the virus.[25]

INFECTION IN MAMMALS

Serological surveys undertaken on the inland plateau have shown the presence of neutralizing antibodies in cattle and to a lesser degree in sheep and horses.[3,4] These hosts are all considered to be incidental ones and the mammals concerned blind alleys in the transmission cycle. Experimental viremia studies have concurred with this view, since after inoculation with virus calves and goats had no detectable viremia.[5] However, if pregnant ewes are inoculated their lambs may have developmental abnormalities including hydranencephaly.[26] *Otomys* rodents showed no detectable viremia,[5] and of six other rodent species inoculated with the virus, only *Aethomys* circulated virus with a maximum titer of 3.2 $\log_{10}LD_{50}$/mL.[27] Blackburn *et al.* inoculated three dogs with WNV, and one developed a slight viremia with a maximum of 2.8 logs/mL.[28] At this level of viremia some of the *Cx. univittatus* mosquitoes could become infected, but the efficiency of their subsequent transmission to feral birds would be limited after such a low infecting dose. Hence dogs might be able to feed back a small amount of virus into the enzootic mosquito-avian cycle.

GENETIC RELATEDNESS OF WNV ISOLATES

The genetic relatedness of South African WNV isolates with isolates from other countries has been investigated by the comparison of nucleotide sequences determined for each isolate. This study showed two lineages as follows. The first comprises 17 isolates which originate from Europe (3), Israel (2), New York (1), India (1), North Africa (3), The Central African Republic (CAR) (2), Kenya (1), Senegal (1), Ivory Coast (1), and Australia (Kunjin virus). The second lineage comprises 35 isolates from South Africa (25), Mozambique (1), Botswana (1), Namibia (1), Madagascar (3), Uganda (1), Senegal (1), Kenya (1), and CAR (1). The sequence homology of the South African isolates was 86.3%–100%, which indicates that the virus is remarkably constant in this country. This in turn may indicate the infrequency with which new strains of the virus are being imported into the country in infected migrant birds. Furthermore this may have a bearing on the mechanism which is responsible for survival of the virus through the relatively mild winter period on the inland plateau. This mechanism is probably the continuation of transmission between endemic birds and *Cx. univittatus* at a very low level, perhaps at only certain foci on the plateau. A minimum of genetic variability would be expected in South Africa if the virus overwinters here and if the enzootic cycle does not depend upon annual reintroduction of the virus by migrant birds.

CONCLUSION

The studies indicated that WNV is widespread in South Africa, where it is the cause of one of the most common arbovirus infections in humans. Although most active on the inland plateau, where it uses a highly efficient mosquito vector, it has adapted to diverse climates and is active on the KZN coast as well as in other southern African countries. The virus uses a variety of avian species as vertebrate hosts, which presumably provide it with the means to move from locality to locality, perhaps even from region to region, although there has been no evidence to suggest that birds reintroduce the virus into South Africa each year onto the South African plateau. The remarkable genetic constancy of South African isolates of the virus supports this view. Humans, livestock, and other mammals are all blind alleys in the transmission cycle except perhaps dogs. There is no evidence of a real amplifying nonavian host that would promote human infection, nor is there a likelihood of an alternative more anthropophilic and equally efficient vector superseding *Cx. univittatus* on the plateau. Owing to these factors, the pattern of endemic human infection with intermittent epidemics is expected to continue.

REFERENCES

1. KOKERNOT, R.H., K.C. SMITHBURN & M.P. WEINBREN. 1956. Neutralizing antibodies to arthropod-borne viruses in human beings and animals in the Union of South Africa. J. Immunol. **77:** 313–323.
2. MCINTOSH, B.M., E.T. SERAFINI, et al. 1962. Antibodies against certain arbor viruses in sera from human beings resident in the coastal areas of southern Natal and eastern Cape Provinces of South Africa. S. Afr. J. Med. Sci. **27:** 77–86.
3. MCINTOSH, B.M., D.B. DICKINSON, et al. 1962. Antibodies against certain arbor viruses in sera from human beings and domestic animals from the South African Highveld. S. Afr. J. Med. Sci. **27:** 87–94.
4. DICKINSON, D.B., G.M. MCGILLIVRAY, et al. 1965. Antibodies against certain arboviruses in sera from human beings and domestic animals from the south-western and north-western regions of the Cape Province of South Africa. S. Afr. J. Med. Sci. **30:** 11–18.
5. ANONYMOUS. Arbovirus Research Unit, South African Institute for Medical Research and National Institute for Virology, Johannesburg. Unpublished data, 1963–1973.
6. JUPP, P.G., B.M MCINTOSH & N.K. BLACKBURN. 1986. Experimental assessment of the vector competence of Culex (Culex) neavei Theobald with West Nile and Sindbis viruses in South Africa. Trans. R. Soc. Trop. Med. Hyg. **80:** 226–230.
7. MCINTOSH, B.M., P.G. JUPP, et al. 1967. Ecological studies on Sindbis and West Nile viruses in South Africa. I. Viral activity as revealed by infection of mosquitoes and sentinel fowls. S. Afr. J. Med. Sci. **32:** 1–14.
8. MCINTOSH, B.M., P.G. JUPP & I. DOS SANTOS. 1978. Infection by Sindbis and West Nile viruses in wild populations of Culex (Culex) univittatus Theobald (Diptera: Culicidae) in South Africa. J. Entomol. Soc. Sth. Afr. **4:** 57–61.
9. MCINTOSH, B.M., G.M. MCGILLIVRAY & D.B. DICKINSON. 1964. Illness caused by Sindbis and West Nile viruses in South Africa. S. Afr. Med. J. **38:** 291–294.
10. MCINTOSH, B.M., P.G. JUPP, et al. 1976. Epidemics of West Nile and Sindbis viruses in South Africa with Culex (Culex) univittatus Theobald as vector. S. Afr. J. Sci. **72:** 295–300.
11. JUPP, P G., N.K. BLACKBURN, et al. 1986. Sindbis and West Nile virus infections in the Witwatersrand-Pretoria region. S. Afr. Med. J. **70:** 218–220.
12. BROOKE WORTH, C., H.E. PATERSON & BOTHA DE MEILLON. 1961. The incidence of arthropod-borne viruses in a population of culicine mosquitoes in Tongaland, Union of South Africa (January, 1956, through April, 1960). Am. J. Trop. Med. Hyg. **10:** 583–592.
13. MCINTOSH, B.M. & P.G. JUPP. 1982. Ecological studies on West Nile virus in southern Africa 1965–1980. In Arbovirus Research in Australia. T.D. St. George & B.H. Kay, Eds. Proceedings of the 3rd symposium of the Commonwealth Scientific and Research Organization and the Queensland Institute for Medical Research, 15–17 February, 1982, Brisbane, Australia.
14. JUPP, P.G. 1976. The susceptibility of four South African species of Culex to West Nile and Sindbis viruses by two different infecting methods. Mosq. News **36:** 166–173.
15. JUPP, P.G. & B.M. MCINTOSH. 1970. Quantitative experiments on the vector capability of Culex (Culex) univittatus Theobald with West Nile and Sindbis viruses. J. Med. Ent. **7:** 371–373.
16. JUPP, P.G. 1974. Laboratory studies on the transmission of West Nile virus by Culex (Culex) unitittatus Theobald; factors influencing the transmission rate. J. Med. Entomol. **11:** 455–458.
17. JUPP, P.G., B.M. MCINTOSH & D.B. DICKINSON. 1972. Quantitive experiments on the vector capability of Culex (Culex) theileri Theobald with West Nile and Sindbis viruses. J. Med. Entomol. **9:** 393–395.
18. JUPP, P.G., B.M. MCINTOSH & E.M. NEVILL. 1980. A survey of the mosquito and Culicoides faunas at two localities in the Karoo region of South Africa with some observations on bionomics. Onderstepoort J. Vet. Res. **47:** 1–6.
19. JUPP, P.G. 1973. Field studies on the feeding habits of mosquitoes in the Highveld region of South Africa. S. Afr. J. Med. Sci. **38:** 69–83.

20. JUPP, P.G. 1971. The taxonomic status of *Culex (Culex) univittatus* Theobald (Diptera: Culicidae) in South Africa. J. Entomol. Soc. Sth. Afr. **34:** 339–357.
21. MCINTOSH, B.M., D.B. DICKINSON & G.M. MCGILLIVRAY. Ecological studies on Sindbis and West Nile viruses in South Africa. V. The response of birds to inoculation of virus. S. Afr. J. Med. Sci. **34:** 77–82.
22. MCINTOSII, B.M., G.M. MCGILLIVRAY, *et ul.* 1968. Ecological studies on Sindbis and West Nile viruses in South Africa. IV. Infection in a wild avian population. S. Afr. J. Med. Sci. **33:** 105–112.
23. MCINTOSH, B.M. & P.G. JUPP. 1979. Infections in sentinel pigeons by Sindbis and West Nile viruses in South Africa, with observations on *Culex (Culex) univittatus* (Diptera: Culicidae) attracted to these birds. J. Med. Entomol. **16:** 234–239.
24. ANONYMOUS. South African virus laboratories surveillance bulletin. 1991, April, p. 3. The National Institute for Virology. Johannesburg, South Africa.
25. GROBBELAAR, A.A., F.J. BURT, *et al.* National Institute for Virology, unpublished data.
26. BARNARD, B.J.H & S.F. VOGES. 1986. Flaviviruses in South Africa: pathogenicity for sheep. Onderstepoort J. Vet. Res. **53:** 235–238.
27. MCINTOSH, B.M. 1961. Susceptibility of some African wild rodents to infection with various arthropod-borne viruses. Trans. Roy. Soc. Trop. Med. Hyg. **55:** 63–68.
28. BLACKBURN, N.K., F. REYERS, *et al.* 1989. Susceptibility of dogs to West Nile virus: A survey and pathogenicity trial. J. Comp. Pathol. **100:** 59–66.

Kunjin Virus

An Australian Variant of West Nile?

ROY A. HALL, JACQUELINE H. SCHERRET, AND JOHN S. MACKENZIE

*Department of Microbiology and Parasitology,
University of Queensland, Brisbane, Queensland 4072, Australia*

ABSTRACT: Kunjin (KUN) is a flavivirus in the Japanese encephalitis antigenic complex that was first isolated from *Culex annulirostris* mosquitoes captured in northern Australia in 1960. It is the etiological agent of a human disease characterized by febrile illness with rash or mild encephalitis and, occasionally, of a neurological disease in horses. KUN virus shares a similar epidemiology and ecology with the closely related Murray Valley encephalitis (MVE) virus, the major causative agent of arboviral encephalitis in Australia. Based on traditional antigenic methods, KUN was initially found to be similar to, but distinct from, reference strains of West Nile (WN) virus and designated as a new species. However, more recent phylogenic analyses have revealed that some strains of WN virus, including the isolates from New York, are more similar to KUN virus and form a separate lineage to other WN viruses. An unusual KUN isolate from Malaysia and the African virus Koutango appear to form additional lineages within the WN group of viruses. While these findings are in agreement with the Seventh Report of the International Committee for the Taxonomy of Viruses that designates KUN as a subtype of West Nile, they also suggest that the species should be further subdivided into additional subtypes.

KEYWORDS: Kunjin virus; West Nile virus; Japanese encephalitis; Murray Valley encephalitis; Australia

INTRODUCTION

Kunjin (KUN) virus is a member of the Japanese encephalitis (JE) antigenic complex in the *Flavivirus* genus. Kunjin takes its name from a local aboriginal tribe of Kowanyama in North Queensland, where the virus was first isolated in 1960 from captured mosquitoes.[1] KUN virus is endemic to the tropical north of Australia where virus activity is regularly detected by seroconversions in sentinel chickens, and isolations are made in most years from captured mosquitoes.[2,3] It is antigenically and genetically very similar to some strains of West Nile (WN) virus and produces a similar disease in humans.[4,5] Indeed, the International Committee for the Taxonomy of Viruses (ICTV) has recently designated KUN as a subtype of WN virus.[6] In this paper, we describe the epidemiology, ecology, and etiology of KUN virus in Australia and discuss recent molecular phylogenic studies that have helped to resolve its taxonomic position in relation to WN within the *Flavivirus* genus.

Address for correspondence: Roy A. Hall, Department of Microbiology and Parasitology, University of Queensland, Brisbane, Queensland 4072, Australia. Voice: 61-7-33654647; fax: 61-7-33654620.

royboy@biosci.uq.edu.au

THE VIRUS

Like all members of the *Flavivirus* genus, KUN is a spherical, enveloped, single-stranded RNA virus approximately 50 nm in diameter.[6] Upon infection of mammalian cells, the positive sense flavivirus genome is released into the cytoplasm and acts as messenger RNA to code for the structural proteins, core (C), premembrane (prM: precursor to M), and envelope (E), that make up the virion and the nonstructural proteins (NS1, NS2A, NS2B, NS3, NS4A, NS4B, and NS5) that are involved in RNA replication.[7] The virion E protein has been shown to induce a protective, neutralizing antibody response in the infected host.[8] The nonstructural protein NS1, which is expressed on the surface of and secreted from infected vertebrate cells, also induces a protective antibody response that is mediated via immune cytolysis.[9,10] The NS3 protein has been shown to induce virus-specific cytotoxic T cells.[11] Once the infection has been resolved by the immune system, the host has lifelong immunity to the homologous virus.

THE DISEASE

KUN virus occasionally causes disease in humans with clinical symptoms of mild fever, headache, photophobia, rash, arthralgia, myalgia, and lymphadenopathy.[12,13] On rare occasions, KUN has also been associated with severe encephalitis.[14,15] Importantly, the symptoms of the latter, which may include severe headache, neck stiffness, slurred speech, mental confusion, ataxia, cranial nerve palsies, and respiratory failure, are clinically indistinguishable from those of the encephalitis caused by infection with the antigenically related Australian flavivirus, Murray Valley encephalitis (MVE).[15] Since KUN and MVE have a similar distribution, the specific diagnosis of flavivirus encephalitis in Australia is often difficult. This is further compounded by the presence of a third member of the JE serogroup, Alfuy virus, in northern Australia.[16] Although Alfuy virus has not been clearly associated with human disease, serological surveys have established that it does infect humans, although probably as a subclinical infection.[17] The most recent cases of KUN virus disease occurred in central and Western Australia during the summer of 2000, concurrent with an outbreak of MVE virus activity.[18,19]

Like WN virus, KUN virus has also been associated with disease in horses. Badman *et al.*[20] reported the isolation of KUN virus from the cervical spinal cord of a horse suffering severe nervous signs including lateral recumbency, cutaneous anesthesia marked dullness, and convulsions. The pathology revealed severe nonsuppurative encephalomyelitis, with lesions in the thalamus, midbrain, pons, and medulla.

VECTORS AND VERTEBRATE HOSTS

Culex annulirostris mosquitoes have yielded the majority of isolates of KUN virus; however, isolates have also occasionally been recovered from *Ae. tremulus*, *Cx. australicus*, *Cx. squamous*, and *Cx. quinquefasciatus*.[3,21,22] Based on the high frequency of virus isolation and the results of vector competence studies, *Cx.*

annulirostris mosquitoes are thought to be the major vectors of KUN virus in Australia.[3,21]

As with WN, MVE, and JE viruses, birds also appear to play a key role in the ecology and epidemiology of KUN virus. Serological studies on avian sera collected from various areas of Australia have indicated that many species of birds, particularly ardeid waterbirds of the order Ciconiiformes, are involved in the natural cycles of KUN virus.[22,23] KUN virus has also been isolated from the blood and organs of wild caught birds,[16] while experimental infection studies revealed that inoculated herons and egrets were viremic for 3–5 days, confirming their potential as vertebrate hosts.[24]

DISTRIBUTION OF KUNJIN

KUN virus has been isolated from all mainland states of Australia; however, the vast majority of isolates have come from the tropical regions of northern Western Australia, the Northern Territory, and northern Queensland, where the virus appears to be endemic.[2,3] KUN virus activity, as detected by virus isolation from mosquitoes, by serologically confirmed clinical disease, or by seroconversions in sentinel chickens, has been less frequent in the temperate regions of central and southern Australia, although significantly more common than MVE. It is thought that the virus is introduced from the endemic foci in the north via migration of viremic waterbirds following flooding of the main watercourses in central and southeastern Australia.[2] A similar scenario has been hypothesized for MVE virus. Indeed, unusually heavy rainfall in regions of Western and central Australia during the summer of 1999/2000 was followed by the appearance of several cases of MVE and KUN disease during March to July 2000, predominantly in areas south of the endemic foci.[18,19] Further heavy rains in the summer of 2000/2001 have also resulted in further cases of MVE in central Australia, with seroconversions to MVE and KUN viruses detected in chicken flocks in southeastern Australia during February/March 2001 (A.K. Broom and J. Azoulas, personal communication). This latest seeding of MVE and KUN viruses into epidemic areas of central and southeastern Australia is a worrying scenario, particularly if these regions experience another wet summer.

Based on serological evidence, KUN is probably also active in Papua New Guinea and Irian Jaya[2] and possibly the islands of the Indonesian archipelago and other parts of Southeast Asia.[25] Indeed, isolation of three KUN-like viruses from *Cx. pseudovishnui* mosquitoes trapped in Sarawak, Malaysia, in 1966 and of a similar virus from Cambodia have also been reported.[26] However, in the context of KUN epidemiology, these isolations should be viewed with caution as one of the Malaysian isolates has since been shown to be quite distinct from the Australian KUN isolates and probably represents a separate genetic lineage within the KUN/WN group of viruses (see below for further discussion).

SURVEILLANCE OF KUN AND MVE VIRUSES

KUN and MVE viruses are primarily zoonotic and use birds as their major vertebrate hosts. To monitor flavivirus activity and the relative risk to public health, flocks of sentinel chickens are tested regularly to detect seroconversions to specific flavi-viruses.[27] The sentinel flocks are located strategically near small towns and villages, with at least 12 birds per flock. To specifically detect seroconversions to flaviviruses in sentinel chickens, competitive ELISAs, using monoclonal antibodies (Mabs) targeting immunodominant epitopes on flavivirus proteins, are used.[28] These assays target MVE-specific and KUN-specific epitopes on the nonstructural protein NS1 of these viruses. Using this assay, KUN infections can be reliably differentiated from MVE infections in sentinel chickens, as well as in laboratory rabbits and naturally infected humans. The assays were pivotal in the specific detection of MVE and KUN seroconversions in sentinel chicken flocks prior to the first human cases in 2000.[19]

Of note, the KUN virus–specific serological assay described above targets an epitope that is common to both KUN and WN viruses.[5,29] In the wake of the out-break of WN in North America, we decided to evaluate the assay for use in testing sentinel animal sera for seroconversion to WN virus infection. Indeed, seroconver-sions to WN were clearly detected in naturally infected chickens, while sera from SLE-infected chickens were unreactive (R.A. Hall, K. Pham, A. Glasser, and L. Stark, unpublished results). These results indicate that these reagents may be useful for serosurveillance of WN in sentinel chickens in North America. Further evalua-tion of the specificity and sensitivity of these assays with sera from WN-infected humans and horses and from a range of avian species is currently being undertaken.

THE PHYLOGENY OF KUN VIRUS

KUN virus was initially deemed to be a distinct virus within the group B arbo-viruses based on cross-neutralization and complement fixation assays using a panel of reference viruses and polyclonal antisera (M. Theiler, personal communication cited in Ref. 1). Further cross-neutralization studies also revealed that KUN shared a close antigenic relationship with WN virus.[30,31] This relationship was confirmed when the prototype strain of WN virus (Wengler) and an Australian isolate of KUN virus (MRM61C) were found to have 82% nucleotide sequence identity in the coding region of the viral genome and 93% identity in the deduced amino acid sequence of the viral translation products.[32] Additional similarities between KUN and WN were identified at the epitope level by examining the reaction patterns of Mabs produced to WN and KUN viruses in ELISA, IFA, and hemagglutinin inhibition.[33,34]

Further studies on a large panel of KUN virus isolates from various regions of Australia collected over a 25-year period revealed these viruses to be genetically and antigenically homogenous.[29,35,36] These findings are consistent with the belief that viremic waterbirds regularly disperse the virus from an endemic foci in northern Australia to other regions, thereby maintaining a single genotype throughout the continent.[37] However, a KUN isolate from Sarawak, Malaysia,[26] was found to be genetically and antigenically distinct from the Australian viruses and actually shared closer sequence homology to some WN viruses[29,38] (see TABLE 1 and FIG. 1).

In a similar study on the genetic relationship between the KUN prototype strain (MRM61C) and a large panel of WN viruses from Europe and Africa, Berthet et al.[39] compared the nucleotide sequence of a region of the E gene. They were able to sep-arate the WN isolates into two lineages (I and II), with isolates from lineage I show-

TABLE 1. Reaction of monoclonal antibodies to WN and KUN virus isolates in ELISA

Virus	Monoclonal antibody ID					
	10A1	H5.46	2B2	3.67G	3.91D	3.1112G
Australian KUN	+	−	+	+	+	+
Malaysian KUN	−	−	+	+	+	+
WN lineage I	−	+	+	+	+	+
WN lineage II	−	+	+	+	+	+
Indian WN	−	+	+	+	+	+
Sarafend WN	−	−	+	−	−	+
Koutango	−	−	+	+	+	−

NOTE: See Ref. 5 for details of virus isolates, monoclonal antibodies, and ELISA methods.

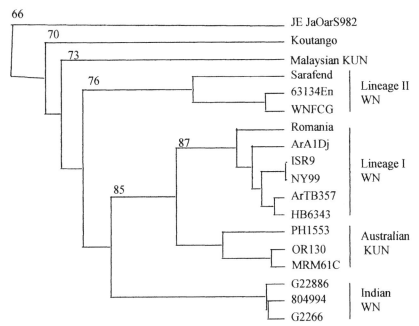

FIGURE 1. Phylogenic tree based on nucleotide sequences of a region of the E gene of KUN and WN isolates (see Ref. 5 for details of virus isolates and methods used for sequencing and phylogenic analysis). JE virus was used to outgroup the tree.

ing divergence of up to 29% from isolates in lineage II. However, KUN virus showed >80% nucleotide identity with WN isolates of lineage I and was designated as a subtype of this lineage. On the basis of these results, the authors proposed that KUN be designated as a subtype of WN virus, a change that has since been adopted by the ICTV. [6]

Additional analysis of recent isolates of WN from Romania, Israel, and New York revealed that these viruses all grouped with the viruses of lineage I and were more similar to the prototype Australian KUN virus (MRM61C) than to the WN viruses of lineage II.[40,41] However, sequence analysis of regions of the E gene and the NS5/3'UTR of a comprehensive panel of KUN- and WN-like viruses also revealed that the Malaysian KUN-like virus and the WN-like virus, Koutango virus, exist as separate lineages with <75% nucleotide identity to each other and the two main lineages.[5] This study also confirmed the relationship between KUN viruses and lineage I WN viruses; however, it also highlighted that KUN viruses were genetically distinct from the remaining viruses in the study. Similarly, the WN viruses from India were also shown to be a discrete genetic group, as a branch within lineage I viruses with relatively low bootstrap confidence levels.[5]

Further analysis of this panel of viruses with Mabs produced to KUN or WN viruses also showed the existence of several antigenic types[5] (TABLE 1). These Mab binding patterns identified the Australian KUN viruses, the Malaysian KUN virus, a Koutango virus isolate, and the Sarafend WN virus isolate as antigenically distinct subgroups. Failure to differentiate between lineage I, lineage II, and Indian WN viruses may have been due to the selection of the Mabs used in these studies. The significance of the unique reactions observed with the Sarafend isolate is uncertain. This isolate has served as the reference strain of WN virus in many Australian laboratories for several decades; however, its passage history prior to importation in the 1950s and its origins are unknown.

CONCLUSIONS AND FUTURE DIRECTIONS

The above studies have demonstrated that isolates of KUN, WN, and Koutango comprise a closely related group of viruses that can be subdivided into several distinct subgroups by antigenic and genetic means. The fact that some subgroups of WN are more closely related to Australian KUN viruses than to other WN subgroups seems to vindicate the decision of the ICTV to reclassify KUN as a subtype of WN. However, based on the findings summarized above, it could be argued that additional subgroups should be defined within this group of viruses (see TABLE 1). The geographical separation of many of these subgroups suggests that they represent a biological cline, evidence of the evolution of WN viruses. Indeed, genetic and antigenic analysis of additional WN-like viruses isolated from Southeast Asia may provide further clues. Future research should also be aimed at determining the biological properties of representatives of each subgroup, including virulence in mice and birds and the competence of mosquito vectors to transmit them.

REFERENCES

1. DOHERTY, R.L. *et al.* 1963. Studies of arthropod-borne virus infections in Queensland. III. Isolation and characterisation of virus strains from wild-caught mosquitoes in north Queensland. Aust. J. Exp. Biol. Med. Sci. **41:** 17–40.
2. MARSHALL, I.D. 1988. Murray Valley and Kunjin encephalitis. *In* The Arboviruses: Epidemiology and Ecology. Volume III, pp. 151–189. CRC Press. Boca Raton, FL.
3. MACKENZIE, J.S. *et al.* 1994. Arboviruses causing human disease in the Australasian zoogeographic region. Arch. Virol. **136:** 447–467.

4. HALL, R.A. 2000. The emergence of West Nile virus: the Australian connection. Viral Immunol. **13:** 447–461.
5. SCHERRET, J.H. *et al.* 2001. Studies on the relationships between West Nile and Kunjin viruses. Emerg. Infect. Dis. **7:** 697–705.
6. HEINZ, F.X. *et al.* 2000. Family *Flaviviridae*. *In* Virus Taxonomy: Seventh Report of the International Committee for the Taxonomy of Viruses, pp. 859–878. Academic Press. San Diego.
7. RICE, C.M. 1996. *Flaviviridae*: the viruses and their replication. *In* Fields Virology. Third edition, volume 1, pp. 931–959. Lippincott-Raven. Philadelphia.
8. MONATH, T.P. & F.X. HEINZ. 1996. Flaviviruses. *In* Fields Virology. Third edition, volume 1, pp. 961–1034. Lippincott-Raven. Philadelphia.
9. SCHLESINGER, J.J. *et al.* 1990. Cell surface expression of yellow fever virus non-structural glycoprotein NS1: consequences of interaction with antibody. J. Gen. Virol. **71:** 593–599.
10. TIMOFEEV, A.V. *et al.* 1998. Immunological basis for protection in a murine model of tick-borne encephalitis by a recombinant adenovirus carrying the gene encoding the NS1 non-structural protein. J. Gen. Virol. **79:** 689–695.
11. LOBIGS, M. *et al.* 1994. The flavivirus nonstructural protein NS3 is a dominant source of cytotoxic T cell peptide determinants. Virology **20:** 195–201.
12. PHILLIPS, D.A. *et al.* 1992. Isolation of Kunjin virus from a patient with a naturally acquired infection. Med. J. Aust. **157:** 190–191.
13. PHILLIPS, D.A. *et al.* 1992. Epidemiology of arbovirus infection in Queensland, 1989–1992. Arbovirus Res. Aust. **6:** 245–248.
14. MULLER, D. *et al.* 1986. Kunjin virus encephalomyelitis. Med. J. Aust. **144:** 41–42.
15. MACKENZIE, J.S. *et al.* 1993. Australian encephalitis in Western Australia, 1978–1991. Med. J. Aust. **158:** 591–595.
16. WHITEHEAD, R.H. *et al.* 1968. Studies of the epidemiology of arthropod-borne virus infections at Mitchell River Mission, Cape York Peninsula, north Queensland. III. Virus studies in wild birds, 1964–1976. Trans. R. Soc. Trop. Med. Hyg. **62:** 439–445.
17. HAWKES, R.A. *et al.* 1985. Arbovirus infections of humans in New South Wales. Med. J. Aust. **143:** 555–561.
18. CORDOVA, S.P. *et al.* 2000. Murray Valley encephalitis in Western Australia in 2000, with evidence of southerly spread. Comm. Dis. Intell. (Aust). **24:** 368–372.
19. BROOM, A.K. *et al.* 2001. An outbreak of Australian encephalitis in Western Australia and central Australia (Northern Territory and South Australia) during the 2000 wet season. Arbovirus Res. Aust. **8:** 37–42.
20. BADMAN, R.T., J. CAMPBELL & J. ALDRED. 1984. Arbovirus infection in horses—Victoria. Comm. Dis. Intell. (Aust.) **17:** 5–6.
21. RUSSELL, R.C. 1995. Arboviruses and their vectors in Australia: an update on the ecology and epidemiology of some mosquito-borne arboviruses. Rev. Med. Vet. Entomol. **83:** 141–158.
22. DOHERTY, R.L. *et al.* 1964. Studies of arthropod-borne virus infections in Queensland. IV. Further serological investigations of antibodies to group B arboviruses in man and animals. Aust. J. Exp. Biol. Med. Sci. **42:** 149–164.
23. MARSHALL, I.D. *et al.* 1982. Variation in arbovirus infection rates in species of birds sampled in a serological survey during an encephalitis epidemic in the Murray Valley of south-eastern Australia, February 1974. Aust. J. Exp. Biol. Med. Sci. **60:** 471.
24. BOYLE, D.B., R.W. DICKERMAN & I.D. MARSHALL. 1983. Primary viraemia responses of herons to experimental infection with Murray Valley encephalitis, Kunjin, and Japanese encephalitis viruses. Aust. J. Exp. Biol. Med. Sci. **61:** 655–664.
25. KANAMITSU, M. *et al.* 1979. Geographic distribution of arbovirus antibodies in indigenous human populations in the Indo-Australian archipelago. Am. J. Trop. Med. Hyg. **28:** 351–363.
26. BOWEN, E.T.W. *et al.* 1970. Arbovirus infections in Sarawak: the isolation of Kunjin virus from mosquitoes of the *Culex pseudovishnui* group. Ann. Trop. Med. Parasitol. **64:** 263–268.
27. MACKENZIE, J.S. *et al.* 1994. Surveillance of mosquito-borne viral diseases: a brief overview and experiences in Western Australia. *In* Rapid Methods and Automation in Microbiology and Immunology, pp. 191–202. Intercept Limited. Andover.

28. HALL, R.A., A.K. BROOM, A.C. HARTNETT *et al.* 1995. Immunodominant epitopes on the NS1 protein of MVE and KUN viruses serve as targets for a blocking ELISA to detect virus-specific antibodies in sentinel animal serum. J. Virol. Methods **51:** 201–210.
29. ADAMS, S.C. *et al.* 1995. Glycosylation and antigenic variation among Kunjin virus isolates. Virology **206:** 49–56.
30. DE MADRID, A.T. & J.S. PORTERFIELD. 1974. The flaviviruses (group B arboviruses): a cross-neutralization study. J. Gen. Virol. **23:** 91–96.
31. CALISHER, C.H. *et al.* 1989. Antigenic relationships between flaviviruses as determined by cross-neutralization tests with polyclonal antisera. J. Gen. Virol. **70:** 37–43.
32. COIA, G. *et al.* 1988. Nucleotide and complete amino acid sequence of Kunjin virus: definitive gene order and characteristics of the virus-specified proteins. J. Gen. Virol. **69:** 1–21.
33. BESSELAAR, T.G. & N.K. BLACKBURN. 1988. Antigenic analysis of West Nile virus strains using monoclonal antibodies. Arch. Virol. **99:** 75–88.
34. HALL, R.A. *et al.* 1991. Monoclonal antibodies to Kunjin and Kokobera viruses. Immunol. Cell Biol. **69:** 47–49.
35. LOBIGS, M., R.C. WEIR & L. DALGARNO. 1986. Genetic analysis of Kunjin virus isolates using HaeIII and TaqI restriction digests of single-stranded cDNA to virion RNA. Aust. J. Exp. Biol. Med. Sci. **64:** 185–196.
36. FLYNN, L.M., R.J. COELEN & J.S. MACKENZIE. 1989. Kunjin virus isolates of Australia are genetically homogenous. J. Gen. Virol. **70:** 2819–2824.
37. MACKENZIE, J.S. *et al.* 2000. Molecular epidemiology and phylogeny of Australian arboviruses. *In* The Molecular Epidemiology of Infectious Diseases, pp. 297–315. Arnold. London.
38. POIDINGER, M., R.A. HALL & J.S. MACKENZIE. 1996. Molecular characterisation of the Japanese encephalitis serocomplex of the flavivirus genus. Virology **218:** 417–421.
39. BERTHET, F.X. *et al.* 1997. Extensive nucleotide changes and deletions within the envelope glycoprotein gene of Euro-African West Nile viruses. J. Gen. Virol. **78:** 2293–2297.
40. LANCIOTTI, R.S. *et al.* 1999. Origin of the West Nile virus responsible for an outbreak of encephalitis in the northeastern United States. Science **286:** 2333–2337.
41. JIA, X.Y. *et al.* 1999. Genetic analysis of West Nile New York 1999 encephalitis virus. Lancet **354:** 1971–1972.

The West Nile Virus Encephalitis Outbreak in the United States (1999–2000)

From Flushing, New York, to Beyond Its Borders

DEBORAH S. ASNIS, RICK CONETTA, GLENN WALDMAN, AND ALEX A. TEIXEIRA

Department of Internal Medicine, Flushing Hospital Medical Center, Flushing, New York 11355, USA

ABSTRACT: Viruses cause most forms of encephalitis. The two main types responsible for epidemic encephalitis are enteroviruses and arboviruses. The City of New York reports about 10 cases of encephalitis yearly. Establishing a diagnosis is often difficult. In August 1999, a cluster of five patients with fever, confusion, and weakness were admitted to a community hospital in Flushing, New York. Flaccid paralysis developed in four of the five patients, and they required ventilatory support. Three, less severe, cases presented later in the same month. An investigation was conducted by the New York City (NYC) and New York State (NYS) health departments and the national Centers for Disease Control and Prevention (CDC). The West Nile virus (WNV) was identified as the etiologic agent. WNV is an arthropod-borne flavivirus, with a geographic distribution in Africa, the Middle East, and southwestern Asia. It has also been isolated in Australia and sporadically in Europe but never in the Americas. The majority of people infected have no symptoms. Fever, severe myalgias, headache, conjunctivitis, lymphadenopathy, and a roseolar rash can occur. Rarely, encephalitis or meningitis is seen. The NYC outbreak resulted in the first cases of WNV infection in the Western Hemisphere and the first arboviral infection in NYC since yellow fever in the nineteenth century. The WNV is now a public health concern in the United States.

KEYWORDS: West Nile Virus, encephalitis; arbovirus

BACKGROUND

Encephalitis is an inflammation of the brain parenchyma. Infectious agents can invade the brain either directly or indirectly. There are a variety of pathways that organisms can use to establish their presence in the central nervous system; the most common is via the blood. This is how the majority of viruses, rickettsia, bacteria, and fungi initiate infection. Some pathogens can enter and replicate in the respiratory tract (measles, mumps, varicella-zoster), the gastrointestinal tract (poliovirus, echovirus, Listeria monocytogenes), the genital tract (herpes simplex virus), or subcutaneous tissue (arthropod-borne viruses, rickettsia, trypanosomes). Others may enter

Address for correspondence: Deborah S. Asnis, M.D., Flushing Hospital Medical Center, 4500 Parsons Boulevard, Flushing, New York 11355. 718-670-3012; fax 718-670-4510. IDDOC@erols.com

through peripheral nerves (rabies, poliomyelitis). Rarely, entry can occur through the olfactory nerve via the nasal mucosa (free-living amebas). Other, less common noninfectious causes of encephalitis include drug reactions, carcinoma, and vasculitis.[1] Once the agent enters the nervous system, only selected cells become infected. Cortical neuronal infection may cause encephalopathy with focal or diffuse seizures, oligodendroglial disease can cause demyelination, and brain stem infection may change a person's level of consciousness. Most people present with altered consciousness ranging from lethargy and confusion to stupor and coma.[1]

Most encephalitis is not diagnosed accurately. Enteroviruses and arboviruses cause the majority of encephalitis. Enteroviruses have the greatest activity during the summer, affecting those younger than 16 years of age or persons in contact with swimming pools. Arboviruses are also most active during the summer. In a two-year period (1996–1997), health departments in 19 states reported to the CDC 286 cases of arboviral encephalitis: 252 cases of La Crosse encephalitis, 15 cases of St. Louis encephalitis, and 19 cases of Eastern equine encephalitis.[2] Sporadic cases are due to herpes simplex virus and can present with bizarre behavior, hallucinations, focal seizures, and temporal lobe localization on an electroencephalogram (EEG). This is the only viral encephalitis that is treatable with acyclovir.

More than 75% of encephalitis cases do not have a known etiology. According to the New York City Department of Health (NYCDOH), there were approximately ten cases of encephalitis and 172 cases of aseptic meningitis reported by passive surveillance annually from 1989 to 1998. After active surveillance was initiated in 1999, the NYCDOH found more than 650 suspected cases of meningitis/encephalitis in 1999 without a specific etiology. There were over 2000 specimens sent for WNV testing to the CDC's Division of Vector-Borne Infectious Disease laboratory in Fort Collins, Colorado.[3] These data underscore the importance of identifying cases of encephalitis and our inability to isolate the exact cause of illness in these people. The CDC has initiated an unexplained death project that will use innovative techniques to test human samples in deaths in previously healthy people, recognizing the limitations that exist in identification of specific organisms as causes of death. It is easy to appreciate the difficulty in establishing a diagnosis in the initial cluster at Flushing Hospital. Arboviruses had not been reported in NYC since yellow fever during the 1800s, and there was no parallel enterovirus outbreak in the community to raise this suspicion.

THE OUTBREAK

The initial cluster of WNV infection in the United States (1999) was previously reported.[4] The first five patients were adults between the ages of 57 and 87 years old who lived within a two square mile radius of one another in northern Queens, a borough of NYC. All of them had been spending a significant amount of time outdoors. As they became acutely ill with fever, headache, and encephalopathy, they were admitted to the same hospital. All went to the intensive care unit (ICU). Three, less severe, cases presented shortly thereafter. The cerebrospinal fluid (CSF) and CT head findings are summarized in TABLE 1. Patients one through six had encephalitis, and the latter two patients had meningitis. All the patients had a CSF pleocytosis except for patient two. There was a lymphocytic predominance in the CSF except in patient

TABLE 1. Cerebrospinal fluid and CT head findings[a,4]

Cases	Days after onset	CSF WBC cells/ mm³	CSF %P/%L	CSF RBC cells/mm³	CSF protein (<45 mg/ dL)	CSF glucose (50–80 mg/dL)	CT scan head
1	8	35	0/90	0	69	83	Central atrophy
2	8	0	0	47	62	89	Mild atrophy
3	0	93	96/4	1346	117	133	Mild atrophy
4	10	14	6/84	8	51	91	N/A
5	3	100	2/78	800	129	96	Old right basal ganglia Infarct
6	3	10	10/56	195	78	76	Normal
7[b]	8	85	4/94	15	81	66	Normal
8[b]	3	37	22/62	4	66	58	NA

ABBREVIATIONS: %P: % polymorphonuclear cells; %L: % lymphocytes cells; NA: not available.
[a]Patients 1–5 were in the ICU cluster.
[b]Patients with meningitis only.

three who presented earlier in his illness than the other patients. A repeat lumbar puncture (LP) in this patient showed a shift to lymphocytes. All patients had an elevated protein and none had a depressed glucose value.

Four of the first five patients developed severe muscle weakness and required ventilatory assistance. Two appeared to have a Guillain-Barré type syndrome and were treated with plasmapheresis. Paresis/paralysis has been reported rarely in WNV.[5-7] Severe muscle weakness was a unique feature, and this abnormality was studied on electromyogram (EMG)/nerve conduction velocities (NCV). In the patients who were alert enough to examine motor strength, diffuse weakness of both proximal and distal muscles was noted, which was well out of proportion to their level of consciousness. No sensory disturbances were found and reflexes were preserved. Four patients had EMG/NCV studies in the ICU setting performed between nine and twenty-one days after onset of symptoms. Slowing of NCV was not demonstrated in any of the cases. Only one of the surviving encephalitis patients underwent serial electrophysiological studies while he was hospitalized. These studies demonstrated improvement in low amplitude sensory and motor responses and appeared to parallel clinical recovery. Needle electromyography in some of the patients demonstrated active denervation. Muscle weakness, especially flaccid paralysis, is not a typical feature of encephalitis and seemed to carry with it a poorer prognosis in our patients.

Relative lymphocytopenia was present in all of our cases and has been reported previously.[7] Relative lymphocytopenia is defined in our hospital laboratory as <20% lymphocytes on the peripheral smear. The relative lymphocyte differential counts on admission for the eight patients ranged from 4–14% (see TABLE 2). The absolute lymphocyte counts ranged from 400 to 2200 cells/mm³ (normal value 1100–2800 cells/mm³). The duration of lymphocytopenia can be prolonged and last up to fifty-

TABLE 2. Admission WBC and percent lymphocytes

Patient	WBC $4.2–11.4/mm^3$	Percent lymphocytes $(20–40\%)$	Absolute number of lymphocytes; $1.1–2.8 \ k/mm^3$
1	17.9	7.0	1.3
2	9.5	4.2	0.4
3	4.3	13.2	0.6
4	12.5	4.9	0.6
5	15.5	14.2	2.2
6	9.1	7.4	0.7
7	12.3	7.2	0.9
8	13.0	14.0	1.8

TABLE 3. T lymphocyte subsets

Patient	Days after onset	$CD4/mm^3$ 490–1740	$CD8/mm^3$ 180–1170	CD4/CD8 0.86–5.00
1	16	314	550	0.59
1	40	340	522	0.65
1	180	708	1386	0.51
2	22	245	492	0.50
3	17	190	62	3.12
4		ND	ND	ND
5	6	909	189	4.64

NOTE: ND: not done.

two days.[7] Four of the five initial ICU cluster had lymphocyte subsets performed as well. All had CD4 lymphopenia except one; this patient was not weak. One patient had sequential lymphocyte testing that improved with time (see TABLE 3). In a previous study from Romania, both humoral and cellular immunity were tested in 27 patients aged 15 to 77 years with the diagnosis of acute encephalitis or acute meningitis. The IgA, IgM, and IgG values were normal. The CD4 value was $49–648/mm^3$ (average $300/mm^3$) and the CD8 value $13–275/mm^3$ (average $119/ mm^3$), which was way below the control group with CD4 and CD8 mean values of $1030/mm^3$ and $553/ mm^3$, respectively.[8]

When it was suspected that a communicable outbreak could be taking place, public health officials were notified, and an investigation was launched. Preliminary serologic testing was positive for St. Louis encephalitis. Subsequent tests demonstrated that the true agent was the WNV. The viral DNA was more than 99.8% identical to a WNV strain from an Israeli goose's brain in 1998 where there was no concurrent human outbreak.[9] Prior to this, there were no known cases of WNV in the Western Hemisphere.

TABLE 4. Profile of symptoms in patients with WNV meningitis/encephalitis[4]

Symptoms	Case 1	Case 2	Case 3	Case 4	Case 5	Case 6	Case 7[a]	Case 8[a]
Fever > 39.0°C	+	+	+	−	+	+	+	+
Headaches	−	+	−	+	−	−	+	+
Stiff neck	−	−	+/−	−	−	−	+	−
Change in mental status	+	+	+	+	+	+	−	−
Skin rash	−	−	−	−	−	−	+	+/−
Gastrointestinal complaints	+	+	−	+	+	+	+	+
Severe muscle weakness	+	+	+	+	−	−	−	−

[a]Patients with meningitis only.

During the summer of 1999, most WNV cases were in people over age fifty, with three in children younger than 16 years. Clinical presentations are summarized as follows: encephalitis with muscle weakness (39%, median age 75 years), encephalitis without muscle weakness (22%, median age 71 years), aseptic meningitis (32%, median age 60 years), and fever and headache syndrome (7%, median age 64.5 years). There was an increased severity of illness in the older patients. Fever (90%), headache (46%), altered mental status (44%), and rash (22%) were a few of the signs and symptoms.[10] In the initial group of eight patients, the majority had temperatures above 39°C, gastrointestinal complaints (nausea, vomiting, and diarrhea), and muscle weakness (see TABLE 4).

Three of our patients expired and five survived. Three had neurologic sequelae, including difficulty concentrating and muscle weakness. One of the most severely ill still has minimal neurological impairment 18 months later.

DISCUSSION

The West Nile virus (WNV) is a member of the family Flaviviridae. It belongs to the Japanese encephalitis complex along with Japanese encephalitis, St. Louis encephalitis, Murray Valley encephalitis, Kunjin, and others. It was initially isolated in 1937 from the blood of a febrile Ugandan woman.[11] Ecology of the disease was first described in Egypt in the 1950s. Epidemics have been reported in Israel (1951–1954), followed by the largest outbreak in South Africa (1974) affecting about 3000 people and in India (1980). More recently, WNV outbreaks have been reported in Algeria (1994), Romania (1996–1967), the Czech Republic (1997), the Democratic Republic of the Congo (1998), Russia (1999), the United States (1999–2000), and Israel (2000). WNV is found throughout Africa, the Middle East, parts of Europe, Russia, India, and Indonesia. It is transmitted principally by the *Culex* species of mosquitoes but is also found in *Aedes* and *Anopheles* species as well. In total, the virus has been isolated in over 43 mosquito species.[12] WNV has been isolated in wild ixodid and argasid ticks, but their role is unclear.[13] Birds are the natural hosts. Humans, horses, and domestic animals are usually incidental hosts.[14]

The incubation period of West Nile fever is five to fifteen days.[15] If infected, approximately 1 in 140–300 people will become clinically ill. The clinical presentation is characterized by a flu-like illness with fever, headache, backache, and myalgia lasting three to six days. Pharyngitis, conjunctivitis, nausea, vomiting, diarrhea, and abdominal pain are also reported. About one-half develop a nonpruritic, roseolar, or maculopapular rash on the chest, back, and arms that lasts seven days. Diffuse lymphadenopathy is also common.[14] Rarely, neurological infection ranging from aseptic meningitis, meningoencephalitis, myelitis, optic neuritis, or polyradiculitis can occur. The most severe neurologic disease is seen in the elderly and, less commonly, in children. Extraneurologic inflammation can include myocarditis, pancreatitis, and hepatitis. Common laboratory findings include leukocytosis,[12] leukopenia,[14] and, in neurological infections, CSF pleocytosis with elevated protein.[14] Virus can be recovered from the blood in an immunocompetent febrile patient for up to ten days. In the immunocompromised patient, viral isolation can be prolonged up to 22 to 28 days after infection.[12] Viremia peaks between four to eight days,[12] but the concentration is usually low at 10^3/mL.[13] Standard precautions should be followed with handling specimens. Virus is not found in feces, urine, or throat washings.[16]

The diagnosis is made by serology, PCR, or viral isolation. Serum IgM detection by antibody-capture enzyme immunosorbent assay (EIA) is one of the best methods for identification. The presence of IgM in CSF reflects intrathecal production. Cross-reactions with other flaviviruses may occur, therefore the plaque reduction neutralization test (PRNT) antibody to WNV is used to exclude other endemic viruses.[13] This cross-reaction was the main reason that the US outbreak was first mistaken for St. Louis encephalitis virus, one of the common North American arboviruses. Serial rising antibody titers can be demonstrated by EIA, complement fixation, neutralization, or hemagglutination inhibition (HI) tests.[13] In patients with meningoencephalitis, virus can be isolated from blood, CSF, and autopsied brains. Although PCR is specific for WNV, the immunohistochemical (IHC) stain will detect flaviviral antigens in the Japanese encephalitis complex. IHC staining can be performed on a formalin- fixed biopsy or necropsy material. The virus may be grown in the laboratory by intracranial inoculation into suckling mice or on continuous cell lines of mosquito or mammalian origin.[13] WNV is classified as a biosafety level-three agent.[17] On one occasion, a laboratory-acquired infection was transmitted through the aerosolized route.[18]

For public health purposes a case is confirmed if a patient with encephalitis or aseptic meningitis has one of the following: (1) isolation of WNV from (or WNV antigen or genomic sequences in) tissue, blood, CSF, or other body fluid; (2) demonstration of IgM antibody to WNV in CSF by IgM-capture EIA; (3) a four-fold serial rise in PRNT antibody titer to WNV in paired, timed serum or CSF samples; or (4) demonstration of both WNV-specific IgM by EIA and IgG (screened by EIA or HI and confirmed by PRNT antibody in a single serum specimen).[19] A study done by the NYCDOH and CDC, on 22 case patients tested for IgM antibody six months after their onset of illness, showed that about 55% had detectable antibody. IgM positivity lasted longer in the younger patients (70% in those <65 years old versus 45% among persons >65 years).[20] Persistence of IgM antibody beyond two months was reported in 50% of patients tested in Romania.[21] This explains why any patient in whom the diagnosis rests on IgM antibody in sera alone (or borderline positive findings in CSF) be confirmed with a greater than four-fold rise in WNV neutralizing antibody in paired acute and convalescent sera two to three weeks apart. This applies especially to the areas of northern Queens, the South Bronx, and, now, Staten Island.

Autopsy findings on four of the seven deaths in the 1999 outbreak revealed two cases of encephalitis and two cases of meningoencephalitis. All four had scattered microglial nodules comprised of lymphocytes and histiocytes in the grey and white matter, with a predilection for the brain stem. The thalamus, cortex, and cerebellum were less involved. There was a mononuclear perivascular inflammatory infiltrate in the same areas of the brain. Leptomeningitis was seen in two cases and a mononuclear inflammation was seen around cranial nerve roots in two cases. The spinal cords and peripheral nerves were not examined. Pancreatitis was found as well,[4,22] which has been reported before.[23] WNV has also been isolated in the spleen, lymph nodes, liver, and lungs in postmortem tissues.[16]

The source of this outbreak is unknown, but it could have been from an infected bird (either migrated or imported), infected mosquitoes, or a viremic individual. WNV normally does not cause birds to become ill, but in the NYC outbreak, thousands of crows and other bird species died. An avian die-off was never previously recorded with WNV and misled scientists in the beginning to think that the bird and human outbreaks were not connected.[15] In the past, epizootics occurred in horses with encephalitis in Egypt, France, Portugal, Morocco, and Italy, but this is not common.[13,24] In 1999, there were approximately twenty-five horses that became sick on the North Fork of Long Island due to the WNV of which nine died and sixteen recovered. One cat died of WNV in New Jersey, and both cats and dogs seroconverted in NYC. During the 2000 WNV outbreak in the US, there were 65 horses that contracted WNV from 7 states, and 26 animals, including bats, squirrels, raccoons, cats, skunks, and chipmunks, that developed WNV. In 1999 bird and mosquito surveillance demonstrated WNV activity in New York, New Jersey, Connecticut, and Maryland (the latter had only a bird). In 2000, WNV spread beyond the NYC borders to encompass 12 states (Connecticut, Delaware, Maryland, Massachusetts, New Hampshire, New Jersey, New York, North Carolina, Pennsylvania, Rhode Island, Vermont, and Virginia) and the District of Columbia.[25]

WNV was actually in the US prior to 1999 as part of a study inoculating volunteers with neoplastic disease refractory to therapy in an attempt to achieve pyrexia. The theory was based on observations that certain viruses had an antineoplastic effect on experimental animals. Eighty-nine percent of the patients had no clinical illness except fever. Eleven percent had signs of diffuse encephalitis with twitching and mental confusion, and one of the patients had flaccid paralysis of the extremities. The neurological signs were transient, and all recovered completely.[16]

During the Romanian epidemic of 1996, WNV presented with mainly neurologic infections and presented similarly to the NYC outbreak in 1999. There were 393 patients who had confirmed or probable WNV infection; 352 had acute central nervous system infections: meningitis (40%), meningoencephalitis (44%), and encephalitis (16%). Typical findings were fever (91%), headache (77%), stiff neck (57%), and confusion (34%). Disorientation and generalized weakness was common. Abnormal reflexes, hypotonia, ataxia, and extrapyramidal signs were described less frequently. Coma developed in 17%. There were seventeen deaths, all above fifty years old with a case fatality ratio (CFR) of 4.3%. Age-specific CFR increased with age, from zero in those under 50 years old to 14.7% in people over 70 years. WNV was isolated from the *Culex pipiens* mosquito, and antibodies were found in 41% of domestic fowl. The clinical to subclinical infection ratio was 1 to 140-320. Serosurveys estimated a seroprevalence of 4.1%, with over 90,000 people who were infected.[26]

The presentation of a Guillain-Barré–like syndrome was unusual for WNV. Guillain-Barré syndrome (GBS) presents with subjective paresthesias or weakness, or both, which can progress over four weeks. GBS typically follows a respiratory or gastrointestinal illness, immunization, trauma, or metabolic insult. *Campylobacter jejuni* is most frequently associated, but other pathogens include cytomegalovirus, Epstein-Barr virus, HIV, *Mycoplasma pneumoniae,* and Lyme disease.[1,27] Japanese encephalitis virus[28] and dengue virus[29] have also caused GBS. In GBS, the CSF usually is acellular and has an elevated protein (albuminocytologic dissociation). Ten percent may have between 10 to 50 cells/mm^3. On EMG/NCV, there are decreased amplitudes in the motor action potential and slowed conduction velocity or conduction block.[27]

There was a single case report of an elderly patient from an endemic area with classical GBS. He had a rapidly progressive areflexic quadriparesis associated with the characteristic CSF abnormalities and EMG/NCV findings. His serum and CSF were positive for IgM capture ELISA for WNV, and the CSF PCR was positive as well.[30] The profound weakness common to all our patients made GBS a strong early consideration. None of our patients developed the characteristic areflexia, CSF, or electrophysiological finding necessary to make the diagnosis of GBS. The EMG data from our ICU indicated both an axonal and demyelinating lesion. One of the patients had a follow-up EMG/NCV at one year. His mental status had returned to baseline. Focal weakness persisted in the proximal left upper extremity and the distal right lower extremity. A four-limb EMG study was performed in October 2000 that demonstrated normal sensory and motor distal latencies, late responses, and conduction velocities. Low amplitude motor responses were noted in the lower extremities. The needle exam revealed both active and chronic denervation in all muscles tested, both symptomatic and asymptomatic, indicating a diffuse motor axonopathy or neuronopathy. Based on the currently available EMG data from a small number of patients, no definite conclusions can be made. WNV infection can present acutely with classical signs, symptoms, and laboratory findings consistent with GBS. In our experience, the cases presented with encephalopathy, with weakness out of proportion to the level of consciousness. None presented with clinical signs or laboratory data supportive of GBS. The early EMGs suggested both a demyelinating and axonal peripheral lesion, and one patient continues to have a motor axonopathy or neuronopathy at one year.

Treatment of WNV encephalopathy is largely supportive. *In vitro*, ribavirin has been shown to reduce WNV RNA levels and cause a cytopathic effect in neural cells.[31] Recovery is complete but slower in adults than children. Myalgias and weakness can persist for a long time, but permanent sequelae have not been recorded.[12]

The 1999 outbreak affected 62 people in NYC and one Canadian tourist who had just visited Queens. There were seven deaths with a case fatality rate of 12%. The seroprevalence was 2.6%, with up to 1900 people exposed.[6] Scientists demonstrated that the WNV was able to overwinter in hibernating mosquitoes.[32] During 2000, there were 21 infections, 14 in NYC, 6 in New Jersey and 1 in Connecticut. The epicenter moved to Staten Island (71% of the NYC cases) from Flushing. There were two deaths. A serosurvey done reflecting the 2000 season centered on three locations: Suffolk County (Babylon area), Staten Island in NYC, and Fairfield County, Connecticut. Based on data from nearly 2500 randomly tested individuals, about

1700 people (1574 from Staten Island, 120 in Babylon, and none in Connecticut) were likely to have been infected with WNV during 2000 in all three areas.[33] These three locations were selected because of the intense bird and mosquito activity. The exposure rate of 0.5% in Staten Island was substantially lower than the 2.6% in northern Queens the previous year. Possible explanations for this difference include the following: (1) the 1999 epizootic in Queens was more intense than in Staten Island, exemplified by WNV neutralizing antibody titers found in house sparrows that were six times higher in northern Queens than in Staten Island; (2) the 1999 Queens sampling site was 3 square miles instead of the more evenly dispersed 56 square miles of Staten Island; (3) the prevention measures implemented by the DOH perhaps had an effect (public health message campaign, mosquito larviciding prior to the transmission season, reduction of mosquito breeding sites, intensive insecticide spraying to control adult mosquitoes);[33] or (4) perhaps just the sporadic nature of WNV outbreaks was the explanation.[11] Why the outbreak in 2000 was smaller than in 1999 is not exactly known, but some explanations include (1) a greater public awareness about personal protection against mosquitoes and increased precautions around home property; (2) mosquito and bird surveillance with directed mosquito control, both larva and adult mosquitoes; and (3) a difference in the weather conditions. (In 1999, the winter was warm, followed by a very hot summer with heavy rains at the end of the season, favoring mosquito overpopulation; in 2000, the summer was colder and wetter).

Since 1999, the important lessons learned include strengthening relationships among the community physicians, health departments, veterinarians, and entomologists, reestablishing a solid mosquito and avian surveillance system and improving local and state public health laboratory capacity to diagnose unusual microbial pathogens. These mechanisms will benefit recognition of both natural and unnatural (bioterrorism) emerging infections.

ACKNOWLEDGMENTS

We wish to thank Drs. M. Layton and A. Fine and the NYCDOH, along with Drs. L. Grady and S. Wong and the NYSDOH. We also thank Drs. S. Yee (EMG/NCV), G. Campbell, J. Roehrig (serology), R. Lanciotti (PCR), S. Zaki (IHC), D. Gubler, and the CDC Arbovirus Diseases Branch, Division of Vector-Borne Infectious Diseases who assisted us with the specimens.

REFERENCES

1. GRIFFIN, D.E. 2000. Encephalitis, myelitis, and neuritis. *In* Principles and Practice of Infectious Diseases. G. Mandel, J. Bennett & R. Dolin, Eds: 1009–1016. Churchill Livingstone. Philadelphia, PA.
2. ARBOVIRAL INFECTIONS OF THE CENTRAL NERVOUS SYSTEM—UNITED STATES, 1996–1997. 1998. Morb. Mortal. Wkly. Rep. 47(25): 517–522.
3. FINE, A. & M. LAYTON. 2001. Lessons from the West Nile viral encephalitis outbreak in New York City, 1999. Implications for bioterrorism preparedness. Clin. Infect. Dis. **32:** 277–282.

4. ASNIS, D.S. *et al.* 2000. The West Nile virus outbreak of 1999 in New York: The Flushing Hospital experience. Clin. Infect. Dis. **30:** 413–418.
5. GADOTH, N., S. WELTZMAN & E.E. LEHMANN. 1979. Acute anterior myelitis complicating West Nile fever. Arch Neurol. **36:** 172–173.
6. LEPORT, C. *et al.* 1984. Meningo-myelo-encephalite a virus West Nile-Interet des dosages d'interferon dans les encephalitis primitives. Ann. Med. Interne **135:** 460–463 (in French with English abstract).
7. CUNHA, B.A. *et al.* 2000. Profound and prolonged lymphocytopenia with West Nile encephalitis. Clin. Infect. Dis. **31:** 1116–1117.
8. CEAUSU, E.M. *et al.* 1997. Clinical manifestations in the West Nile virus outbreak. Rom. J. Virol. **48**(1–4): 3–11.
9. LANCIOTTI, R.S. *et al.* 1999. Origin of the West Nile virus responsible for an outbreak of encephalitis in the northeastern United States. Science **286:** 2333–2337.
10. THE NEW YORK CITY DEPARTMENT OF HEALTH. West Nile virus: a briefing. 2000. City Health Information **19**(1): 1–5.
11. SMITHBURN, K.C. *et al.* 1940. A neurotropic virus isolated from the blood of a native of Uganda. Am. J. Trop. Med. **20:** 471–492.
12. HUBALEK, A. & J. HALOUZKA. 1999. West Nile Fever—a reemerging mosquito-borne viral disease in Europe. Emerg. Infect. Dis. **5**(5): 643–650.
13. PEIRIS, J.S.M. & F.P. AMERASINGHE. 1994. West Nile fever. *In* Handbook of Zoonoses Section B:Viral. G.W. Beran & J.H. Steele, Eds.: 139–148. CRC Press. Boca Raton, FL.
14. MONATH, T.P. & T.F. TSAI. 1997. Flaviviruses. *In* Clinical Virology. D.D. Richman, R.J. Whitley & F.G. Hayden, Eds.: 1133–1185. Churchill Livingston. New York.
15. CDC. Outbreak of West Nile-like viral encephalitis—New York, 1999. 1999. Morb. Mortal. Wkly. Rep. **48:** 845–849.
16. SOUTHAM, C.M. & A.E. MOORE. 1954. Induced virus infections in man by the Egypt isolates of West Nile virus. Am. J. Trop. Med. Hyg. **3:** 19–50.
17. CDC. 2000. Guidelines for surveillance, prevention, and control of West Nile virus infection—United States. Morb. Mortal. Wkly. Rep. **49**(2): 25–28.
18. NIR, Y.D. 1959. Airborne West Nile virus infection. Am. J. Trop. Med. Hyg. **8:** 537–539.
19. CDC. 1997. Case definitions for infectious conditions under public health surveillance. Morb. Mortal. Wkly. Rep. **46:** 12–13.
20. CDC. 2000. Update: West Nile virus activity-northeastern United States, January-August 7, 2000. Morb. Mortal. Wkly. Rep. **49**(31): 714–717.
21. TARDEL, G. *et al.* 2000. Evaluation of immunoglobulin M (IgM) and IgG enzyme immunoassays in serologic diagnosis of West Nile virus infection. J. Clin. Microbiol. **38**(6): 2232–2239.
22. SAMPSON, B.A. *et al.* The pathology of human West Nile virus infection. Hum. Pathol. **31**(5): 527–531.
23. PERELMAN, A. & J. STERN. 1974. Acute pancreatitis in West Nile fever. Am. J. Trop. Med. Hyg. **23**(6): 1150–1152.
24. SCHMIDT, J.R. & H.K. EL MANSOURY. 1963. Natural and experimental infection of Egyptian equines with East Nile virus. Ann. Trop. Med. Parasitol. **57:** 415–427.
25. THE NEW YORK CITY DEPARTMENT OF HEALTH. West Nile Virus Final Update for the 2000 Season, November 24, 2000: 1–4.
26. TSAI, T.F. *et al.* 1998. West Nile encephalitis epidemic in southeastern Romania. Lancet **352:** 767–771.
27. ADAMS, R.D., M. VICTOR & A.H. ROPPER. 1997. Diseases of the peripheral nerves. *In* Principles of Neurology. R.D. Adams, M. Victor & A.H. Ropper, Eds.: 1302–1369. McGraw-Hill. New York.
28. RAVI, V. *et al.* 1994. Association of Japanese encephalitis virus infection with Guillain-Barre syndrome in endemic areas of south India. Acta Neurol. Scand. **90**(1): 67–72.
29. ESACK, A., S. TEELUCKSINGH & N. SINGH. 1999. The Guillain-Barre syndrome following dengue fever. West Indian Med. J. **48**(1): 36–37.

30. AHMED, S. *et al.* 2000. Guillain-Barre syndrome: an unusual presentation of West Nile virus infection. Neurology **55:** 144–146.
31. JORDAN, I. *et al.* 2000. Ribavirin inhibits West Nile replication and cytopathic effect in neural cells. J. Infect. Dis. **182:** 1214–1217.
32. CDC. Update: Surveillance for West Nile virus in overwintering mosquitoes—New York. 2000. Morb. Mortal. Wkly. Rep. **49**(9):1789.
33. CDC. Serosurveys for West Nile virus infection—New York and Connecticut counties, 2000. 2001. Morb. Mortal. Wkly. Rep. **50**(03): 37–39.

West Nile Encephalitis

The Neuropathology of Four Fatalities

BARBARA A. SAMPSON AND VERNON ARMBRUSTMACHER

Office of Chief Medical Examiner of the City of New York,
520 First Avenue, New York, New York 10016, USA

ABSTRACT: West Nile virus was identified by immunohistochemistry (IHC) and polymerase chain reaction (PCR) as the etiologic agent in four encephalitis fatalities in New York City in the late summer of 1999. Fever and profound muscle weakness were the predominant symptoms. Autopsy disclosed encephalitis in two instances and meningoencephalitis in the remaining two. The inflammation was mostly mononuclear and formed microglial nodules and perivascular clusters in the white and gray matter. The brain stem, particularly the medulla, was involved most extensively. In two brains, cranial nerve roots had endoneural mononuclear inflammtion. In addition, one person had acute pancreatitis. On the basis of our experience, we offer recommendations for the autopsy evaluation of suspected WNV fatalities.

KEYWORDS: West Nile virus; encephalitis; pathology; autopsy

INTRODUCTION

West Nile virus, a member of the Flaviviridae family, was first isolated from the blood of a febrile Ugandan woman in 1937.[1] It is a single-stranded RNA virus, usually transmitted by *Culex* species mosquitoes, with wild birds as hosts. Humans and domestic animals are incidental hosts.[2] Although it is found throughout Africa, the Middle East, and parts of Europe and Western Asia, little is known about the pathological changes caused by this virus in humans. In endemic areas, such as Egypt, a seroprevalence of 40% has been reported in adults.[3]

The incubation period is 5–15 days. Infections are usually asymptomatic or may cause mild, nonspecific symptoms.[2] In more serious cases, pancreatitis,[4] myocarditis,[5] and hepatitis[6] have been reported. Treatment is currently nonspecific and supportive. Fatalities generally occur in older people, although child fatalities have been documented.[7,8]

We report the autopsy results of four fatalities from West Nile virus infection that occurred during an outbreak in New York City in the late summer of 1999. This is the first West Nile virus outbreak reported on this continent.[9] On the basis of our experience, we offer recommendations for autopsy procedures to best evaluate and study cases of suspected West Nile virus infection.

Address for correspondence: Barbara A. Sampson, M.D., Ph.D., Office of Chief Medical Examiner of the City of New York, 520 First Ave., New York, NY 10016. Voice: 212-447-2335; fax: 212-447-2716.

basampson@yahoo.com

MATERIAL AND METHODS

Case Selection

The Office of Chief Medical Examiner of the City of New York accepted under our jurisdiction all suspected cases of West Nile virus infection because of the obvious public health implications. Four decedents were confirmed to be positive for West Nile virus by immunohistochemistry (IHC) and polymerase chain reaction (PCR) of brain tissue by the Centers for Disease Control. Two of the four decedents had limited autopsies due to religious objection, which are empowered by law in New York State. The limited autopsies included gross inspections of all organs, but only the most necessary tissue samples were taken for routine histology, IHC, and PCR. The other two decedents had full autopsies, with all organs examined grossly and by routine histology; tissue also was obtained for IHC and PCR.

Protocol for Tissue Collection

Tissue for IHC and PCR was collected following guidelines provided by the New York City Department of Health and by the Centers for Disease Control. Two tubes of CSF and one container with sections of fresh brain were submitted on dry ice. Two purple-top tubes of blood and formalin-fixed tissues were submitted in a separate container without dry ice. We recommend submission of pancreas, liver, heart, lung, spleen, and kidney for routine histologic exam and special studies. Brain sections should include several from the brain stem, particularly from the medulla and the spinal cord, including dorsal and ventral roots.

Immunohistochemistry

Sections of formalin-fixed, paraffin-embedded tissue were cut onto positively charged glass slides and stained using a modified avidin-biotin immunoperoxidase technique [10] and an automated staining system (Ventana, Tucson, AZ). Briefly, sections were dewaxed in xylene and hydrated through graded alcohols to deionized water. Pretreatment of slides for optimum antigen retrieval was performed as follows: for CD20 (L26), slides were microwave heated on medium-low power for 10 minutes in citrate buffer, pH 6.0; for CD4, slides were boiled in 0.01M EDTA, pH 8.0 for 20 minutes; for CD8, the slides were microwave heated on medium-low power in citrate buffer, pH 8.0 for 20 minutes. Following inhibition of endogenous peroxidase, primary antibodies CD20 (mouse monoclonal, Dako, Carpinteria, CA) and CD4 (mouse monoclonal, Novacastra Laboratories, Ltd., United Kingdom) were applied at a 1:250 dilution, and CD8 (mouse monoclonal, Dako, Carpinteria, CA) was used at 1:50 dilution. The reaction was visualized using a commercially prepared detection system (Basic DAB Detection Kit, Ventana, Tucson, AZ) using biotinylated secondary antibody and the standard avidin-biotin-complex technique with copper-enhanced 3,3' diaminobenzidine (DAB) and hematoxylin counterstain. Slides were dehydrated in ascending grades of alcohol, fixed in xylene, and mounted.

RESULTS

The average age of the four decedents was 81.5 years. They each had coexistent medical problems. Their clinical course has been described elsewhere.[11] General autopsy showed no myocarditis or hepatitis. One patient had an acute, hemorrhagic pancreatitis.

Histology

The neuropathological examination of each West Nile encephalitis–related fatality revealed a grossly normal brain. Histologically all showed microglial nodules composed mainly of lymphocytes and histiocytes. Some nodules included degenerating neurons. These were present predominantly in the grey matter but also in the white matter (FIG. 1A). Variable mononuclear perivascular inflammation was present (FIG. 1B). The medulla and thalamus were involved most consistently, but similar pathological changes were also present in the frontal lobe, temporal lobe, parietal lobe, hippocampus, and cerebellum in some instances. Scattered mononuclear inflammatory infiltrate was present in the leptomeninges in two of the four cases (FIG. 1C). Two autopsies revealed encephalitis with involvement of cranial nerve roots. Focal mononuclear inflammation was present in cranial nerve roots of the medulla (FIG. 1D).

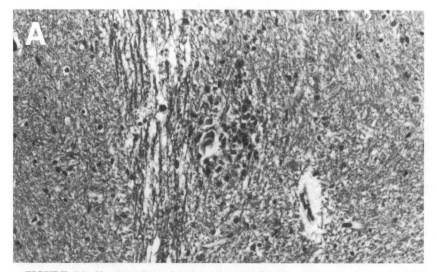

FIGURE 1A. Hematoxylin and eosin–stained section of medulla, showing a microglial nodule composed of histiocytes and occasional lymphocytes (70× magnification). (From Sampson et al.[18] Reproduced by permission.)

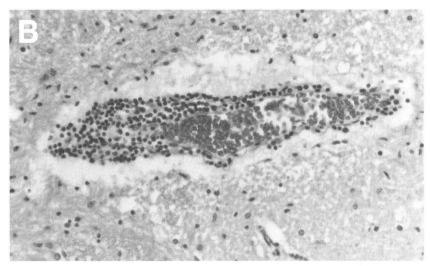

FIGURE 1B. Hematoxylin and eosin–stained section of medulla, showing a perivascular collection of lymphocytes (50× magnification). (From Sampson et al.[18] Reproduced by permission.)

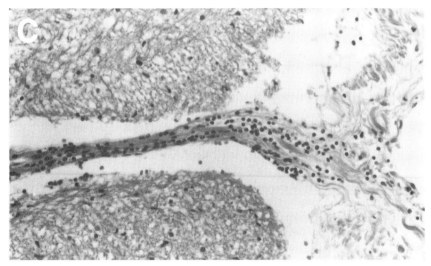

FIGURE 1C. Hematoxylin and eosin–stained section of medulla, showing extension of the perivascular inflammation into the leptomeninges (50× magnification). (From Sampson et al.[18] Reproduced by permission.)

Immunohistochemistry

Immunohistochemistry was performed to analyze the populations of lymphocytes prominent in this infection. CD8+ T cells were numerous and were present within the microglial nodules, in the perivascular infiltrates, in the meninges, and in the cranial nerve roots.

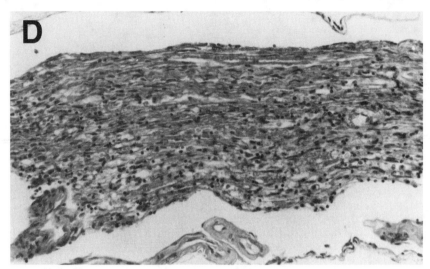

FIGURE 1D. Hematoxylin and eosin–stained section, showing a cranial nerve as it exits from the medulla with endoneural lymphocytic inflammation (50× magnification). (From Sampson et al.[18] Reproduced by permission.)

CD4+ T cells also were present in these areas but were far fewer. In the most heavily involved areas of the medulla, CD8+ T cells were found scattered throughout the parenchyma. CD20+ B cells were scattered and most prominent around the blood vessels.

CONCLUSIONS

These are the first fatalities due to complications of West Nile virus encephalitis in North America. A detailed description of the clinical course of three of these patients, as well as that of five people who survived WNV infection has recently been published.[11] WNV also caused the deaths of many New York City birds, particularly crows, and several exotic birds at the Bronx Zoo. Necropsies of the birds revealed meningoencephalitis, which was much more pronounced than in humans, and marked myocarditis.[12]

In 1954 a study using West Nile virus for the treatment of advanced cancer was published.[13] Eleven percent of their patients developed encephalitis.[14] The neuropathology of the 1999 New York City fatalities was significant for scattered microglial nodules composed of lymphocytes and histiocytes and mononuclear perivascular inflammatory infiltrate. These findings were most common in the brain stem but were also found in the thalamus, cerebellum, and cerebral cortex. Leptomeningitis was present in two instances, and mononuclear inflammation was seen around cranial nerve roots in two instances. The predominant T cell was CD8+.

These pathological changes are quite different from the more fulminant arbovirus encephalitides, such as Eastern and Western equine encephalitis. In West Nile virus encephalitis the inflammatory infiltrate is focal and slight. There is no vasculitis. This difference probably results from the less fulminant course of this infection with prolonged survival with maximal medical support after infection. In St. Louis encephalitis the distribution of lesions is predominantly cerebral, while with West Nile virus the brain stem is involved most consistently.

The most striking clinical manifestation of West Nile virus encephalitis present in over half of the confirmed WNV encephalitis cases (including nonfatal and fatal cases) in this outbreak is profound muscle weakness, often with axonal neuropathy and requiring mechanical ventilation. Clinically Guillain-Barré syndrome was considered a possible diagnosis. Instances have been described with chronic neurologic sequelae, in particular persistent muscle weakness (M. Layton, personal communication). Our examinations revealed a mononuclear cranial nerve root infiltrate in two brains with a nerve root included incidentally in the examination of the medulla. The spinal cord was not examined in any of the four fatalities. Examination of the entire spinal cord and nerve roots in a confirmed death due to WNV infection might help explain the clinical presentation and emphasizes the need for autopsies in all deaths suspected or confirmed to be due to West Nile virus. Although an instance of acute anterior myelitis complicating WNV encephalitis has been reported,[15] the type of severe axonal neuropathy observed in our study population usually is not associated with the epidemic encephalitides and has not been documented pathologically.

It appears that West Nile virus is now endemic in the New York area. West Nile virus RNA was detected in overwintering mosquitoes.[16] Moreover, in 2000, 21 cases of West Nile virus associated illness were reported in New York, New Jersey, and Connecticut.[17] One fatality in New York City in 2000 has been attributed to West Nile virus. No autopsy was performed.

The threshold for suspecting WNV infection should be low, because the symptoms are common and nonspecific. Also, the scope of the possible manifestations of this infection are not yet clearly established. The New York City Department of Heath requested that any patients be reported to them with fever $>38.0°$, altered mental status, CSF pleocytosis with predominant lymphocytes and/or elevated protein, and muscle weakness (especially flaccid paralysis) confirmed by neurologic exam or EMG. Also to be reported are any patients with a presumed diagnosis of viral encephalitis or with focal CNS findings and fever, any patients with fever and presumed Guillain-Barré syndrome or acute flaccid paralysis, or any patients with aseptic meningitis. At autopsy, particular attention should be paid to complete neuropathologic examination, including the spinal cord and nerve roots. If autopsy is limited for any reason, the brain stem, particularly the medulla, should be sampled. We recommend submission of pancreas, liver, heart, lung, spleen, and kidney for routine histologic exam and special studies.

ACKNOWLEDGMENTS

We would like to thank Drs. R. Lanciotti (PCR) and S. Zaki (IHC). In addition we thank Drs. M. Layton and D. Asnis for many thought-provoking discussions.

REFERENCES

1. SMITHBURN, K.C., T.P. HUGHES, A.W. BURKE, *et al.* 1940. A neurotropic virus isolated from the blood of a native of Uganda. Am. J. Trop. Med. **20:** 471–492.
2. MONATH, T. & F.X. HEINZ. 1996. Flaviviruses. *In* Virology. B.N. Fields, D.M. Knipe & P.M. Howley, Eds.: 1004–1006. Raven Press. New York.
3. CORWIN, A., M. HABIB, D. WATTS, *et al.* 1993. Community-based prevalence profile of arboviral, rickettsial and Hantaan-like viral antibody in the Nile River delta of Egypt. Am. J. Trop. Med. Hyg. **48:** 776–783.
4. PERELMAN, A. & J. STERN. 1974. Acute pancreatitis in West Nile fever. Am. J. Trop. Med. Hyg. 23(6): 1150–1152.
5. ALBAGALIC, C.R. 1959. A case of West Nile myocarditis. J. Med. Assoc. Isr. **57:** 274–275.
6. GEORGES, A.J., J.L. LESBORDES, M.C. GEORGES-COURBOT, *et al.* 1987. Fatal hepatitis from West Nile virus. Ann. Inst. Pasteur/Virol. **138:** 237–244.
7. GEORGE, S., M. GOURIE-DEVI, J.A. RAO, *et al.* 1984. Isolation of West Nile virus from the brains of children who died of encephalitis. Bull. W.H.O. 62(6): 879–882.
8. LE GUENNO, B., A. BOUGERMOUH, T. AZZAM & R. BOUAKAZ. 1996. West Nile: a deadly virus? Lancet **348:** 1315.
9. CENTERS FOR DISEASE CONTROL. 1999. Outbreak of West Nile-like viral encephalitis— New York. Morb. Mortal. Wkly. Rep. **48:** 845–849.
10. HSU, S-M., L. RAINE & H. FANGER. 1981. Use of avidin-biotin-peroxidase complex (ABC) in immunoperoxidase technique: a comparison between ABC and unlabeled antibody (PAP) procedures. J. Histochem. Cytochem. **29:** 577-580.
11. ASNIS, D.S., R. CONETTA, A.A. TEIXEIRA, *et al.* 2000. The West Nile virus outbreak of 1999: The Flushing Hospital Experience. Clin. Infect. Dis. **30:** 413–418.
12. STEELE, K.E., M.J. LINN, R.J. SCHOEPP, *et al.* 2001. Pathology of Fatal West Nile virus infections in native and exotic birds during the 1999 outbreak in New York City, New York. Vet. Pathol. **37:** 208–224.
13. NEWMAN, W. & C.M. SOUTHAM. 1954. Virus treatment in advanced cancer: a pathological study of fifty-seven cases. Cancer **7:** 106–118.
14. SOUTHAM, C.M. & E. MOORE. 1954. Induced virus infections in man by the Egypt isolates of West Nile virus. Am. J. Trop. Med. **3:** 19–50.
15. GADOTH, N., S. WEITZMAN & E. LEHMANN. 1979. Acute anterior myelitis complicating West Nile fever. Arch. Neurol. **36:** 172–173.
16. CENTERS FOR DISEASE CONTROL. 2000. Update surveillance for West Nile virus in overwintering mosquitoes—New York, 2000. Morb. Mortal. Wkly. Rep. **49:** 178–179.7
17. CENTERS FOR DISEASE CONTROL. 2001. Serosurveys for West Nile virus infection— New York and Connecticut counties, 2000. Morb. Mortal. Wkly. Rep. **50:** 37–39.
18. Sampson, B.A., C. Ambrosi, A. Charlot, *et al.* 2000. The pathology of human West Nile virus infection. Hum. Pathol. **31:** 527–531.

Laboratory Testing for West Nile Virus
Panel Discussion

GRANT L. CAMPBELL, *Moderator*
Division of Vector-Borne Infectious Diseases,
Centers for Disease Control and Prevention, Fort Collins, Colorado 80522, USA

LEO J. GRADY, *Moderator*
Division of Infectious Diseases, Griffin Laboratory, Wadsworth Center,
New York State Department of Health, Slingerlands, New York 12159, USA

CINNIA HUANG
Griffin Laboratory, Wadsworth Center,
New York State Department of Health, Slingerlands, New York 12159, USA

ROBERT LANCIOTTI
Arbovirus Diseases Branch, Centers for Disease Control and Prevention,
Fort Collins, Colorado 80521, USA

LAURA KRAMER
Griffin Laboratory, Wadsworth Center,
New York State Department of Health, Slingerlands, New York 12203, USA

JOHN T. ROEHRIG
Arbovirus Diseases Branch, Division of Vector-Borne Infectious Diseases, Centers for
Disease Control and Prevention, Fort Collins, Colorado 80522, USA

ROBERT E. SHOPE
Department of Pathology, University of Texas Medical Branch,
Galveston, Texas 77555-0609, USA

GRANT L. CAMPBELL: This panel session is entitled Laboratory Testing for West Nile Virus. We have five excellent panelists with us today. My co-moderator, Dr. Leo Grady is from the New York State Department of Health. My name is Roy [Grant] Campbell from CDC in Fort Collins, Colorado.

LEO J. GRADY: Good morning. Sitting directly to my right is Dr. Cinnia Huang from the New York State Department of Health; to her right is Dr. Laura Kramer, also from the New York State Department of Health. Dr. Rob Lanciotti from the CDC, Fort Collins, is next, and then comes Dr. John Roehrig, also from the CDC. At the end is Dr. Bob Shope from the University of Texas Medical Branch in Galveston, Texas. Each of the panelists will make a few brief comments about their involvement in laboratory testing, and then we will open the floor for discussion. Dr. Huang begins this session.

CINNIA HUANG: Our lab is involved in human testing. The new state experiments with RT-PCR for West Nile virus are similar to what has been done at Fort Collins. The only difference we find is that a two-step regular RT-PCR is as sensitive as Taq-Man. The two-step RT-PCR is the protein protocol used now for the encephalitis PCR panel. Our panel includes different viruses, and West Nile is one of them. Based on our data, there are cases other than West Nile virus, such as enterovirus and the herpes virus, and the enterovirus season overlaps with West Nile virus. For this reason, our lab will continue to perform tests using PCR batteries.

ROBERT LANCIOTTI: I want to run through the most commonly used diagnostic tests, both for serology and for virus detection. For human diagnostics, our gold standards are the IgM and IgG ELISAs, and we confirm those by plaque-reduction neutralization testing. The molecular amplification tests, such as RT-PCR and TaqMan have limited usefulness in human diagnostics, and I think it's important to emphasize that. There are some people with a misconception that those could be front-line tests for human diagnostics. We have data showing—and it's limited data from the 1999 epidemic—that a positive PCR certainly is diagnostic but a negative doesn't mean a whole lot. There are a lot of other reasons. We have serologically confirmed cases, where you can't detect viral RNA, and I think that has a lot to do with the duration and level of viremia. Many times we're looking for virus pretty far out beyond the febrile phase, so the molecular tests have been most useful in the fatal cases, less useful in CSF, and even less in serum. Again, the ELISA serological tests are really our gold standard for human diagnostic testing. Virus isolation also should be attempted, but in many cases, the virus samples that we're getting to test and isolate are, in the diagnostic lab, beyond the viremic stage in many cases. But I think they're still important tests and ought to be attempted. For the surveillance of mosquito pools and birds, this is an application where the molecular tests are very useful—the RT-PCR and TaqMan. NASBA is another amplification technology that works very well. Those are the most commonly used tests, not only in our lab, but also in other state health departments. There's also immunofluorescence and immunohistochemistry, and there was a poster here describing antigen capture ELISA for West Nile detection as well. I think Dr. Kramer is going to talk about the importance of having a confirmatory algorithm in the lab. I think for any one of these tests, whether serological or virological, there needs to be a way of confirming positives. The other issue that I'll just mention is the importance of standardization. You may be aware that the CDC has done a lot of training in the last few months. We've trained, at this point, representatives from almost every state health department in the country, and we are now initiating a huge proficiency panel program where we're sending out both molecular and serology samples to every state health department that chooses to participate. This will be a large undertaking, but we think it's very important for states that anticipate testing to participate in the standardization proficiency panel.

LAURA KRAMER: To follow up on Dr. Lanciotti's comment, I think proficiency testing is crucial, especially with all the new labs coming online now doing surveillance testing. I also think that there's got to be quality control to make sure that what is positive is really positive. Because PCR is such a powerful and sensitive tool, it's a double-edged sword, and it's very easy to pick up contaminating RNA, either by aerosol or on your glove when you open up a tube. It's just so sensitive. We know that it detects less than one plaque-forming unit. We diluted avian tissues out 10^{-6}, and we still detect a positive. So, it's very easy to think that you have a positive tissue and not really have it because your RNA is contaminated. I think some water blanks need to be included in all the assays, particularly with the bird tissues, where there's such a high load of viral RNA. The water blank needs to be in there from the very beginning. Where you're homogenizing the tissue, an aerosol is being created; it's closed, the system is closed, but when that tube gets opened it's very easy to carry over some viral material and think that you have a host of new positives. So if your water blank comes up positive, whether it's from the beginning or whether it's from the RNA extraction stage, you need to go back to the tissue and reextract and repeat the process to confirm that that tissue is truly positive. And as part of this, when labs are setting up new TaqMan or PCR assay rooms, they have to be fully knowledgeable about how the flow needs to go. There are many books on it, but if you're doing standard PCR and writing gels, you never take those pipe headers from that room after you clean your area, which is your pre-PCR area. For a confirmatory assay, just to reiterate what Dr. Lanciotti said, there needs to be an independent confirmatory assay. One set of primers may be more sensitive than the other, but we don't know what you're detecting if you keep on repeating that set of primers and saying, "Well we did two assays," when, in fact, it's really one assay repeated. It needs to be two totally independent assays. So, either two sets of primers or an RT-PCR and an IFA or a NASBA—some other totally separate assay. I think that while RT-PCR is wonderful and it's rapid and you can get the results out there, I don't think we should stop trying to isolate virus and cell culture. First of all, you can pick up viruses that the PCR is not specific for. PCR is a very specific assay because of the primers, and with the TaqMan probe, it's even more specific. But, it's important for research to understand the virus and for confirmation that this is an infectious virus to inoculate cell cultures. What does a PCR positive mean? I think we need to try to sort out what's happening with the mosquito pools and the bird tissues as well, where we do see RT-PCR-positive tissues that we cannot get out in cell culture. And I think we need to determine how we're going to interpret these.

CAMPBELL: John?

JOHN T. ROEHRIG: I have a few comments. It's come to our attention that some of you are setting up BSL-3 laboratories in which you want to do plaque assays for serology and also virus isolation. That can be a dangerous approach to take if you're trying to do isolation in the same place that's using standardized West Nile for plaque assays because you're liable to get cross-contamination. Last year when we talked in Fort Collins about the best approaches for RT-PCR, one of the suggestions that we had was that for the plaque assay it may be useful to use a prototype strain like Egypt 101. In our hands it looks as though the New York 1999 strain and the Egypt 101 strain are pretty interchangeable. If you were to use a strain like Egypt 101 in your plaque-reduction neutralization test and happen to get that cross-contaminated into a tissue that you were trying to do isolation from, you could actually tell those viruses apart by sequencing the amplimers by RT-PCR. Unfortunately, at the time, everybody demanded New York 1999, but now that we're a year and a half out, you may want to reconsider how you're doing that plaque assay and go over to something that's actually distinguishable from what you might get from isolates from the environment. My history in arbovirology has been less on nucleic acid and more on proteins and protein structure and function. I just want to remind you that there's another component to viruses besides nucleic acid and it's actually protein that can be used as a confirmatory test. Laura's laboratory uses IFAs on tissues and isolates. There are plenty of monoclonal antibodies available to you that will allow you to identify West Nile and other arboviruses that you may be isolating or seeing. Yesterday, there was a poster on an antigen detection assay that's been developed for West Nile that's as sensitive as the SLE assay. It's been out for a number of years and can be used in tandem either with mosquito pools, or, in this case, it was also shown in tissues of birds, where luckily the virus titers are even higher than in mosquitoes and a relatively good assay. It could be used either as a front-line assay or as a confirmatory assay for other tests. So, be aware that that's out there and should be available to you if that's what you desire to use as well. Later on today or tomorrow, Denise Martin will talk about some of the work she's done looking at the cross-reactivity of IgMs between SLE and West Nile. I'd like to remind you that there are other things out there besides PCR, although PCR is quite good. But, there are other things out there besides ELISAs that you can use to identify antibody reactivities in other species. But you have to be careful when you do things like hemagglutination inhibition assays on birds. The extraction protocols for the sera are a little different than what you may be used to as far as the other nonspecific inhibitors that may be in bird sera that are not removed by the standard sucrose acetone extraction. Bear in mind that there's a lot of literature out there and, you know, one of the implications that's come out of this meeting is that there's a lot of new information that's coming out that people haven't thought about. I think lots of people have thought about these issues for a long time before we've even thought about them. Nothing substitutes for going back and looking at what's been done in the past and seeing how you can apply it to the present and the future.

CAMPBELL: Bob?

ROBERT E. SHOPE: Let me first agree completely about the use of Egypt 101 as a strain for neutralization tests for the reason that you're giving but also because I think you'll find that it produces much nicer plaques than the New York strain does. I don't know why, but that's a practical reason to use it. I'd like to make some comments about cross-reactions among flaviviruses. I first learned about the cross-reactions from Jordy Casals, who incidentally just lives down the road here in northern Manhattan, but he described the cross-reactions and flaviviruses using the hemagglutination inhibition test and later using the neutralization test. What happens is that in a primary infection the serological reaction is relatively specific during the first week or ten days postinfection, but then it broadens out and you can use any one of the serological tests against any one of the flaviviruses to show that the person has had a flavivirus infection. As in 1999, it was discovered, even with the capture IgM test, which is relatively specific, that you can misdiagnose closely related flaviviruses. What was called St. Louis encephalitis was really West Nile, and this isn't surprising. This is what one would have expected. I don't have the benefit of working with very many West Nile human sera, and I look forward to hearing the talk tomorrow, but in our animal models—we have an animal model of West Nile—Bob Tesh has developed a model in a hamster that, as far as the clinical syndromes go, is very close to the human picture. About 40% of these animals die following an interperitoneal inoculation. These animals develop a muscle weakness prior to death, and they also develop serological reactions by day six after inoculation; they have relatively specific antibodies in the hemagglutination inhibition test, and they also start to get IgM. The IgM is gone by day 60, which I think is probably very close to the picture in humans. Is that right?

ROEHRIG: I should have mentioned that. Actually, it goes a little bit longer than that.

SHOPE: OK. But it certainly decreases rapidly just before that time. Regarding the secondary infections, if you inoculate a hamster with yellow fever or Japanese encephalitis virus, follow it and a month later or so inoculate with West Nile virus you get a very brisk anamnestic reaction, which is broadly cross-reacting in all of the tests that we use, so that you need to be careful how you interpret results. Bob Tesh and and his colleagues have been testing human serum in a study collaborating with the Department of Defense using recruit sera from the postal codes zones of the epicenter of the 1999 epidemic. There are no identifiers on these sera. Other than the fact that they're probably eighteen, nineteen, or twenty year olds, we don't know much about them. But we do know where they were recruited from. They're using an HI test, a hemagglutination inhibition test, and many of these sera have positives. Many of the reaction patterns when you test with multiple flavivirus antigens look either like dengue or like multiple reaction sera. These people were bled before they were vaccinated with yellow fever, but some of them may have had prior vaccinations also. So the message here is to be very careful about interpreting serological reactions. A positive with West Nile does not necessarily mean that that person has been infected with West Nile virus. This stimulated us to look at some of our dengue sera. We have four prototype sera that were supplied through Jim LaDuke from dengue patients. There's one from Malaysia, one from the Philippines, one from India, and I forget where the fourth one was from, but we went back and did both West Nile IgM ELISAs on those sera and they're positive, in addition to being positive for dengue. And Bob Tesh also went back and did neutralization tests. Three out of the four sera are positive in the West Nile neutralization test. He uses a 90% plaque reduction, so it's a very stringent test. So, the message is to be careful. In the hamster experiments, we've done a vaccination challenge. The vaccine that Bob Tesh used was the live attenuated Japanese encephalitis vaccine, the vaccine that has been given to millions of horses in China. Those hamsters did not get sick from the vaccination. They were challenged a month later with West Nile virus, and in the controls there was about 40% mortality. There was no mortality in the vaccination challenge test with West Nile virus. So here's an example of a vaccination challenge test that also shows more cross-reaction. There are other implications in the vaccination challenge experiment. I mean it must be obvious to you that the vaccine for horses used in China probably would be a good vaccine to use for horses in the United States.

CAMPBELL: Thank you, Bob.

MIKE L. BUNNING (*Centers for Disease Control and Prevention, Fort Collins, CO*): Can I ask John to follow up on the IgM persistence?

ROEHRIG: Sorry, I didn't get that written down on my list. We've been collaborating with the New York City Health Department doing follow-up studies on the longevity of the IgM from some of the patients from the 1999 outbreak, and it's been pretty revealing, although not totally surprising about the longevity of the IgM in some of these patients. Clearly what Dr. Shope said is true: if you look at the IgM response early in infection, and some of these were pretty early infections in 1999, there's a clear spike of IgM activity. This is serum now we're talking about, not CSF. In the early serum infection after 30 to 60 days, it will drop down to lower levels. However, many of these patients carried IgM and continued to carry IgM in their serum specimens above the cutoff level for the IgM ELISA. Not many at this point. I think the last lead was around 500 days postinfection, and at this point the study has been terminated. But it was a very valuable study. What we were interested in looking at and why this was so important from a public health perspective was whether or not IgM could persist from one transmission season to the next at a level that if you happened to have an individual from outside the United States come in with encephalitis the following season, and you did an IgM on them, or something was suspicious of encephalitis, and the IgM was positive but at a lower level, is this truly a recent infection of West Nile or a past infection of West Nile? I think our conclusions are that you actually can be confused by that. That's why earlier on this season, we were recommending acute and convalescent specimens that could be tested as paired sera to actually sort out whether it's an active immune response or if it was a stable older immune response. So it's clear that some patients can carry IgM from one transmission season to the next. Up to this point I think that six months was about as long as this had been investigated, although never with West Nile. With Japanese encephalitis it had been looked at, and actually I guess with West Nile with some of the Romanian patients, Dr. Tsai looked at six-month specimens. So bear that in mind. As people who do serology will tell you, it's clearly always better to have acute and convalescent specimens that you can actually titer. This especially becomes important when West Nile travels into regions where there is more activity from St. Louis encephalitis and you may actually be looking at an SLE infection versus a West Nile infection.

CAMPBELL: So we know now that, at least in a few patients, that IgM would persist for up to a year, and that might have a couple of implications. It goes back to something that Dr. Shope and others have said and that's to be careful because you'd have to imagine a scenario. First of all, a couple of things: the seroprevalence rates in Queens and in Staten Island after the epidemic were quite low. Queens was higher at 2.6% and in Staten Island, less than 1%. So you'd have to imagine a scenario where a person was, say, subclinically infected in the year 2000 in Staten Island and in the next year was unlucky enough to get encephalitis from some other cause and then you test them for West Nile antibody and find IgM antibody. Well, we would not expect that outcome; that would be a very rare event. Second of all, we would not expect that the IgM would persist in the cerebrospinal fluid. Nobody's going to do those studies because they'd be unethical. But at that point when that patient comes into your laboratory like that this summer, you're going to test CSF for one thing and that will help you, but also acute and convalescent serum for development of IgG. So, you've got to look at the whole serological picture in that case. There should be no serious problem in sorting that kind of case out clinically. I think where it has more application or it causes more confusion is in seroprevalence studies where you might have only 1% of people who were infected the year before, and a smaller percentage of those are going to still have antibody later. So, I think it's more of a theoretical concern than a practical impediment. Bob?

SHOPE: From what I've heard this morning, I think there might be a possibility that IgM in the spinal fluid might persist. I have no basis other than seeing some of those pathology pictures.

CAMPBELL: Well, I guess it's theoretically possible, but from what I've heard, persistence of IgM and the CSF would imply that there is active plasma cell production due to ongoing infection of the cerebrospinal fluid. So, from what you saying—from everything we've been able to find in the literature, and Tony Marfin has done a lot of the literature review in this—there's not that much information available. But in the human IgM and CSF it's cleared very quickly, and unless you have active plasma cell production—unless there's a plasma cell that's being stimulated in that sequestered space—the IgM is cleared very quickly. So, that would imply persistent infection to most infectious disease physicians, I think. Maybe you're right. But we'll have to see. I don't know how we're ever going to figure that out, though, because nobody's going to do serial lumbar punctures on patients.

SHOPE: Changing the subject a little bit, I meant to mention that Dr. Hall is here from Australia, and he's developed a test for use in sentinel chickens, which might be more broadly applicable—I don't know. But it might be worth hearing comments from him as to what we really need is a specific serological test, and his approach might be something that's helpful.

CAMPBELL: At this point, we'd invite questions or comments from the audience.

LANCIOTTI: I want to make a quick comment about neutralization, and this is to build on what others, especially Dr. Shope, have had to say. In our lab, when I mention confirmation of the ELISA test by neutralization, that doesn't mean we do neutralization just with West Nile. It's important to do the whole panel of the flaviviruses that occur in North America. So last year we routinely did dengue, because of potential for travel, West Nile, SLE, and Powassan. In most cases when we can demonstrate specific sera conversion to West Nile, the titers to West Nile may have been 1:512 or greater. There was an accompanying dengue and SLE neutralizing antibody titer much less—1:20 or 1:40—but I would say in most cases we do see a cross-reactivity, and so I think it's very important when you do the neutralization tests to include the other flaviviruses.

SHOPE: I think it may be important also to test dengue patients, especially the other way around using that same panel against convalescent sera from a dengue patient. And you may find that some of these crosses are more one-way.

DALE L. MORSE (*New York State Department of Health, Albany, NY*): A number of panel members have mentioned the need for caution in interpreting human serological tests and the need for quality control in confirmatory testing. It wasn't well publicized, but a small number of the laboratories in New York State, New York City, and the CDC last year that had experience with this had some anxious moments as we followed up on screening tests on the serologic IgM that were low level titer or intermediate and as we tracked back to find out whether these really were going to be cases or not. Now as more laboratories are going to come on board, private and commercial, the potential testing that we'll presumably be doing will probably be just a screening test because they don't have BSL-3 or don't have the capability to do neutralization tests. There's a potential for a much larger concern and for following up all these tests or potential reporting of a potential case without confirmatory testing. New York has fairly strong regulations so we can try to have some quality control for those labs coming on, but a number of states don't have that ability to regulate, so I have three questions in this regard. What are the capabilities nationally for quality control of commercial labs that might come on during testing in the coming year? Number two: What is the capability for confirmatory testing for those labs that are going to start showing some potential positive tests on the screening test? And third: Should there be a requirement for a two-step testing before labs can be certified to test for West Nile?

LANCIOTTI: We strongly recommend confirmation by neutralization. Last year, there were a handful of specimens that we couldn't confirm by neutralization. And we're following up on some of those to see what they could have been. But clearly, you need to have a confirmatory test. We would caution any state from reporting a result without confirmation. Now, if they don't have the ability to do that, that is one of the things that CDC certainly is offering. Many states made use of this where they got a positive IgM, ELISA result, and forwarded the specimens to us for confirmation. If you can't do that in your lab, I think you'd want to have the neutralization tests.

CAMPBELL: I want to ask when MRL [Materials Research Laboratory] may be going to release their test kit for general commercial use.

QUESTION: Well, in theory, they can't because it's not FDA approved, so they could only use a home brew at MRL. So they can't even pass it off as specialty.

LANCIOTTI: We are trying to establish a relationship with MRL so that when they receive specimens—and they have done this—they'll contact us for confirmatory testing. There's also a need for improved communication that's being set up between MRL and the states where the samples came from, because in some cases state health departments are bypassed, where samples are sent directly to MRL and the state epidemiologist is not even aware of it. So, we are trying as best we can to set up all that communication, but certainly MRL is aware, and we have received samples from them for confirmatory testing.

GRADY: I believe New York State also is going to require any laboratory that is permitted to do West Nile testing for New York residents to provide material for confirmation, either at the state laboratory or at CDC, Fort Collins.

ROEHRIG: I think that's a good point. I mean, I think it's kind of a double-edged sword here. It's not necessarily bad to have commercial testing for West Nile because you're casting a broader net to try to find these cases, but somehow the link has to be made for those laboratories to get confirmatory testing. I'm not sure the two-tier testing requirement is going to be the answer because if you do that, it's going to just close out those laboratories that will never do neutralization. The important part is to get the confirmatory testing done somewhere and to make the link back to the state or back to us at the CDC. We can probably do the confirmatory testing. I don't think that's an issue.

DUANE J. GUBLER (*Centers for Disease Control and Prevention, Fort Collins, CO*): New York is probably one of the few states around that has a system in place where they do actual proficiency testing of local laboratories before they can be certified. And, in fact, do we have a representative here from APHL [Association of Public Health Laboratories]? APHL is really the key to the answer. We went through this with Lyme disease testing, and CDC has no regulatory authority to enforce this kind of proficiency testing. It's really at the state level. We need to bring APHL into this discussion and develop a proficiency-testing scheme probably modeled after the New York program that certifies local laboratories that were testing. And, I agree with John that commercial tests are a good thing as long as they're controlled reasonably well so that there is some quality control. Another solution is to use regional laboratories to do the confirmatory testing. The CDC can't do it all, and New York can't do it all, so we really need to work with APHL to set up regional laboratories to do the quality control confirmatory testing.

THOMAS P. MONATH (*Acambis Inc., Cambridge, MA*): The requirement to use BL-3 for West Nile and St. Louis and other viruses you'd like to use in performing neutralization tests is an issue for many labs. I'd like to gauge the interest of this group, in particular, on the question of interest in the way of converting these viruses to BL-2 agents so that one could use them safely for neutralization virtually in a large number of labs. Now, the approach that we suggested is to use our chimeric yellow fever technology, which is being applied for attenuated vaccines, so that one would wind up with a family of BL-2 viruses, or basically yellow fever 17D vaccine. But the envelope genes of West Nile, St. Louis, Japanese encephalitis could be used then because they're specifically neutralized only by antibody against each of the respective flaviviruses. They could be used in the neutralization tests to distinguish sera that neutralized a specific virus of interest. So one could actually perform confirmatory neutralization tests in any BL-2 lab with a series of these chimeric flaviviruses that were specific for each of the virus types. Now we already have Japanese encephalitis and West Nile available, and St. Louis needs to be made, and we're willing to undertake that. We're actually working with Dr. Gubler's group now. But it would be useful to know whether this, in fact—if we're going the right direction with this— would be useful. Would it broaden the capability of labs to do confirmatory diagnosis? It might be very useful in the situation of surveillance of birds and other animals as well. It would be interesting to hear some comment from the panel or anybody else in the room to get a sense of how hard to push this, because it would take quite a bit of work to actually validate the technology.

ROEHRIG: For example, with Japanese encephalitis chimera, when you have it approved for human use as a vaccine, clearly at that point that chimera can be classified as a BSL-2 agent. How much characterization do you need to have as far as pathogenesis or virulence in humans before it really will go from a BSL-3 to a BSL-2?

MONATH: Well, we had classified the Japanese encephalitis construct to BL-2 long before human trials.

ROEHRIG: Yes, but that was a vaccine, vaccine chimera.

MONATH: Right.

ROEHRIG: But for West Nile, you're talking about taking a wild type and trying to attenuate.

MONATH: Well, we have mutants now too. They're even more attenuated than the wild-type construct. But, I think the answer is we need data, and there are very good animal models, both mouse and monkey, that can be used. The critical question: Is the chimera less neurovirulent than yellow fever 17D, which is a BL-2 human vaccine? We're testing the appropriate animal system. I think in the case of West Nile, we'll have those data, including monkey data, within a few months. And so at that point what we would do is currently BL-3; we would ask our biosafety, institutional biosafety committee and other collaborators to reevaluate this at BL-2. We might ask the subcommittee, Arbovirus Laboratory Safety, ACAB, to look at this question independently—or the CDC for that matter. But I think it's just a matter of providing the data.

ROEHRIG: So you think preclinical data in monkeys and mice will be enough to downgrade it?

MONATH: Yes.

SHOPE: With Japanese encephalitis virus, is it necessary to use the chimera? The parent of the chimera has been tested in literally millions of humans in China.

MONATH: Right. You could use a vaccine strain.

SHOPE: Yes, the SA14-14-2 strain.

MONATH: We don't have one for West Nile though. There are attenuated strains of St. Louis and you can make the same argument. But I think that the ideal thing is that the yellow fever backbone allows you then to use the yellow fever vaccine for comparison in assessing relative virulence. And so you have a very convincing story about attenuation. So I think for St. Louis and West Nile, that's going to be essential.

SHOPE: I think you make a good case, yes.

ROY A. HALL (*University of Queensland, Brisbane, Queensland, Australia*): I want to respond to Bob Shope's mention of the competitive assay that I briefly alluded to in my talk yesterday. Basically we designed it for animal surveillance that works quite well for primary infections. We have a batch of sera that CDC had sent to us from New York, and in the initial trial, samples came out positive in the ELISA—not all, but some. And we've yet to compare the data with neutralization tests, and Ann Hunt said she's got the data and we're going to compare them. But at this stage it's still a bit early. It's certainly worthwhile to evaluate it with West Nile.

NANCY HALPERN (*New Jersey Department of Agriculture, Trenton, NJ*): I have a question for Dr. Shope. You mentioned, I believe, a Japanese encephalitis vaccine for horses. I was wondering if you or anyone in the room might know the mechanism to allow its use while we're waiting for the vaccine's development in this country.

SHOPE: I don't know the proper mechanism, but a great deal is known about the vaccine itself.

HALPERN: I know. I know it's in use for horses, right.

SHOPE: It's also been tested for its ability to infect mosquitoes. Dr. Barry Beatty and Dr. Tenbo Chong did those experiments; they're published. It does not readily infect mosquitoes; since it's alive, the attenuated strains are one of the things you'd be worried about. Maybe someone else knows how veterinary vaccines are licensed.

ALEXANDER E. PLATONOV (*Central Research Institute of Epidemiology, Moscow, Russia*): What use are the specific ligands for West Nile, for example—not like a physical concentration, but a specific concentration of a sample.

LANCIOTTI: I'm not aware of anyone who has done that with West Nile. So you're saying concentration before one of the nucleic acid tests?

PLATONOV: Yes, for example, or before RT-PCR, before application of any diagnostic tools.

LANCIOTTI: Again, I'm not aware of anyone who has attempted that. I will say that when we use PCR or NASBA or any of those assays looking for West Nile in bird tissues, there is such a large amount of virus that in most cases it's not really a sensitivity issue. There are always going to be a handful of cases where you would like to concentrate before, and mosquito pools are pretty much the same. There's a large amount of virus, so that there are not too many ambiguous samples. It's really in human diagnostics that we run into, I think, an issue either of sensitivity of the test or as likely the timing of the specimen. We're looking at CSF or serum beyond the febrile phase. So there may not be any virus there at all, because we also didn't detect virus by isolation as well.

GUBLER: I want to come back to your point about persistence of IgM antibody in the cerebrospinal fluid, Roy. I know I've read this in Kuno's review of persistence on page nine—I just looked it up. On page nine he says—this is a reference paper published in 1983—monkeys inoculated with West Nile virus presented an asymptomatic infection, but the virus persisted in the brain for up to 5.5 months without viremia. So, in other words, they isolated virus five and a half months after, and so this would explain the persistence of the IgM if this is occurring in humans.

CAMPBELL: I don't remember.

GUBLER: We need to keep an open mind.

CAMPBELL: Did they test cerebral spinal fluid for IgM?

GUBLER: Yes, well they didn't test CSF, or at least he doesn't cover it in here, but it was brain. But indicating that there's virus in the brain meant it may be intrathecal production of antibodies.

ROEHRIG: Well, Duane, I don't think that's a problem, but I think that you're comparing apples to oranges even though monkeys are closer to humans than mice.

GUBLER: I think the point is that we should keep an open mind.

ROEHRIG: Well, I think we should keep an open mind about everything. I don't think that that's an issue. But the point of having cerebrospinal fluid taps, to actually answer the question, is going to be hard to get for humans.

DENISE MARTIN (*Centers for Disease Control and Prevention, Fort Collins, CO*): I'd like to bring up another point that hasn't been really driven home yet about confirmatory testing. There was a fair amount of concern last year about the length of time it takes to do a confirmatory test in several capacities. There was a lot—especially in states that were looking at the possibility of the first case in their state—of push for doing a neutralization on a very acute specimen last year. And a lot of these extremely acute specimens have not allowed for time for neutralizing antibody to be formed. I think we need to make the point that you can detect IgM by an ELISA test before you can detect IgM in a neutralization test. So, it's extremely important to do a classical neutralization test and see a rise and fall in antibody to get that convalescent specimen. In the push to identify West Nile in each new state, often it doesn't seem to be acceptable to wait for that convalescent specimen, and yet ruling out West Nile on a very acute specimen might be erroneous in the long run.

SHOPE: I think that one could make a case for having a diagnosis that's called a presumptive diagnosis: that's what you do I think. I guess I would be even more conservative, and even after you've done the neutralization test and confirmed the positive reaction that you still call it a presumptive diagnosis, unless you've actually identified the virus either by isolation or by sequencing, because of the cross-reactions that can occur in flaviviruses. I don't know, is anybody else with me on that wavelength? Probably not.

ROEHRIG: I think I missed that.

SHOPE: I don't think we ever have a definitive diagnosis on the basis of serology, and we should keep that in the back of our minds. I understand that the patient and the press demand that you tell them what they have, but we should always, as scientists, keep a little bit of doubt when we're basing our diagnosis solely on serology. That's a personal feeling.

ROEHRIG: So you would say if you had a patient that had presented with clinical encephalitis with muscle weakness, had a huge IgM response in the CSF, and in acute and convalescent specimens showed an 8- to 16-fold titer rise against West Nile encephalitis, and stable or no antibody against the rest of the cross-test as flaviviruses—this isn't a dead person, so you don't have autopsy specimens, and you can't get PCR or isolation positive—that you wouldn't be comfortable that that was a West Nile case?

SHOPE: I would be comfortable on a presumptive basis (*general laughter*). I think one of the keys to your statement is that you've tested it against all of the other flaviviruses. We continue to find new flaviviruses. In fact, New York City is a case in point; one did find a new flavivirus.

ROEHRIG: Yes, and as we did the neutralization tests, it became clear that it wasn't St. Louis (*general laughter*).

CAMPBELL: I want to say one thing: Earlier, Rob Lanciotti used the term "gold standard" in terms of serology, and I think, just to go back to basic principles, most of us would agree that if you're really a purist that the gold standard for the diagnosis of West Nile virus infection is isolation of the virus from the patient, and that's rarely possible. So we all realize that serology is not the same as viral isolation.

GRADY: I should throw in too that we had one case in New York that, based on the capture IgM, was suspect for West Nile, and it turned out to be dengue when the PCR was done on serum. When the folks followed it up, it turned out that it was a travel history; the patient had actually become ill while in Haiti, but didn't bother to seek medical attention until back in New York.

PATRICIA REPIK (*Charles River Tektagen, Malvern, PA*): This question is for Rob. Are you recommending a virus isolation by any standardized method, say, looking at it for over a period of however many days and doing subpasses, like one subpass or two subpasses? Or is it just plaque isolation? Are you allowing replication to proceed?

LANCIOTTI: There are two ways we do it. For the mosquito testing, we actually just do it with an overlay and look for plaques. But in the human, trying to isolate virus from the human cases, we went the extra mile and did multiple tests and liquid culture and multiple cell lines, and mice, as well. So, we tried everything that we had available to us besides direct mosquito inoculation. I don't think we ever tried that. So, for humans I think that's what we would recommend just because we try everything that is available, not just mammalain cells, but C6-36 cells as well.

ROEHRIG: There's a practical side to this. I mean, we can do that as a reference laboratory, but in the heat of trying to diagnose outbreak at a state laboratory, a local laboratory gets to be a bit tedious when you have a thousand other samples coming in and trying to deal with them. Duane, didn't Bruce do mosquito inoculation with some of those West Nile specimens?

GUBLER: No, unfortunately we didn't do mosquito inoculation, but I think Bruce did show that the fluid culture of Vero cells was probably the most sensitive of the systems. They were all fairly close. Laura and I were just talking about this yesterday. We should do mosquito inoculation in some of these samples. We haven't done them.

HELENE PAXTON: (*PanBio InDx, Inc., Baltimore, MD*): Rob, at the ASTMH meeting when we had our first West Nile meeting and Duane was chairing it, you talked a lot about using IFA and using slides that had all of the relevant viruses in the United States or outside the United States on your slides so that you could do cross-reactivity studies. In the last two meetings, there's been very little said about the usefulness of indirect IFA. As a commercial company, we constantly get barraged with whether you're going to do an IFA titer. Is there any strength in doing, say, a 1:40 screen and a 1:320 screen for each of the viruses that might be circulating in the United States? Can you define any true seropositivity? From what Bob said it sounds like you probably can't, but we do get asked that question an awful lot. The other issue is whether or not, in animal models, if you're doing chickens or horses or some of the other mammals, whether or not the IFA would hold up better. Because most labs—and I'm getting ten or twelve phone calls a day—can't do the more sophisticated techniques, and they want to have a way of screening to see whether or not there's a possibility that West Nile is in the differential diagnosis.

KRAMER: I can answer for use of IFA for bird serology. Susan Wong can answer for the human serology, but we do indirect IFAs on all our ELISA-positive bird sera as the second test, and then if that still is positive we go on and do a plaque-reduction neutralization assay. And it's been very useful in cutting back the number of neutralization tests we need to do, so it's one more refined step after the ELISA. We also use an indirect IFA to confirm positivity in tissues and in cell culture after the cells are inoculated. If cytopathology is seen we spot slides with the infected cells and do IFA on that, and not just for West Nile but for other viruses that are active in New York State.

PAXTON: That's direct FA though, right?

KRAMER: No. Indirect.

PAXTON: You're doing an indirect on the tissues?

KRAMER: Yes. Those were the slides that I showed yesterday and that were in Alan Dupuis' poster.

PAXTON: So you're using positive sera against a substrain as your antigen that could possibly be infected?

KRAMER: We're using the antibody to make sure that what we're seeing is the virus.

PAXTON: I have one other comment. Duane knows this well: the issue of getting FDA clearance. I talked to Woody DuBois at length about this in the microbiology branch, and he is very aware that there is a tremendous need to get these tests cleared. You can't purchase IFA slides as analyte-specific reagents from various manufacturers, and the analyte-specific reagents statute requires that you make a disclaimer in your patient reports saying that this has not been cleared by the FDA. Whole kits have not been cleared and are more problematic, and so you may have a situation where you'll find components floating around where their "label" is ASR. That's really not the intent of the law. But Woody has strongly suggested that if you could get dengue cleared, then West Nile could be treated as a predicate against dengue. If the major problem of West Nile is getting enough samples to be able to do an FDA submission that would hold up, then let's keep that in the back of our minds as we're collecting samples, because a commercial company totally has their hands tied behind their back in trying to get a clearance for an assay without having the proper samples.

ROEHRIG: I think that's a good point. I forget these things, but positive control specimens are really difficult to come by, and luckily over the last couple of years we've had cooperative physicians and cooperative patients, like Dr. Asnis pointed out in her talk, that have been able to donate serum specimens for use as positive control. So for the physicians around, keep this in mind, because this'll be an ongoing need, and you'd be surprised how quickly you go through it. This doesn't include the needs of a commercial company where they need large amounts of these specimens banked.

SHOPE: Let me make a comment. We found that dengue convalescent sera worked beautifully in the capture IgM ELISA for West Nile, and you can get large quantities of that. I don't know whether that would be permitted as a positive control by the FDA, but they work.

PAXTON: That's the problem, that the dengue is so cross-reactive.

SHOPE: You need to market the test as specific; your test could give you a flavivirus diagnosis, and that would be very useful I would think.

CAMPBELL: Dr. Bresnitz?

EDDY BRESNITZ (*New Jersey Department of Health and Senior Services, Trenton, NJ*): In the clinical setting where you have a patient who has the right clinical syndrome for encephalitis, and treatable infection has essentially been eliminated, nailing down the diagnosis, when you feel where it's no longer suspect or probable, really has no either clinical or public health practicality to it, to be honest with you. From a clinical perspective, once you nail down the diagnosis it really doesn't make a difference by then. And certainly from the control of mosquitoes it makes no difference either because it takes so many weeks. And I would argue that, in fact, it's what we will do in New Jersey as well: it's letting the mosquito control people know when you have an individual you suspect might have West Nile virus encephalitis—particularly if you're coming from an area where activity has been demonstrated in birds or mosquitoes or horses. That waiting for diagnosis, final diagnosis, or even a probable diagnosis is too late for enhancing mosquito control. So it's a nice theoretical discussion. From a practical perspective it really doesn't make a difference.

LANCIOTTI: We would agree that waiting is probably better, but I can't tell you how many times this year we've gotten calls that said we want you to confirm our ELISA result, and we have a press conference tonight at six. So, that's not uncommon.

SCOTT P. HENNIGAN (*Massachusetts State Laboratories, Boston, MA*): Is anybody looking into using the Western blot? We use the Western blot for HIV infection; we use it for Lyme in a two-tier method. Is it something that could be used as a quick three-hour—I don't like saying confirmation—but that type test. Instead of waiting for a couple of days for the neutralization, you can actually run a Western blot; you could probably do an IgM or IgG on it also.

ROEHRIG: I come from a laboratory that, before West Nile, dealt with Lyme disease. Where the Lyme disease test is, the Western blot is used as a confirmatory test for Lyme disease, which is, of course, a bacterial pathogen that has multiple antigens. Part of the differential for the Lyme disease Western blot is how many of these antigens are positive, how many are negative, and how many bands are seen. Flaviviruses are fairly simple organisms. There are really three proteins that you can see on a gel, one of which is the M protein, which is a very small membrane-bound protein that is immunogenic, but not overly immunogenic, so you're really looking at two bands on the blot that may actually elicit antibody responses. The nucleocapsid protein, for all viruses and including flaviviruses, is relatively conserved, and so you would get very little serospecificity out of a reactivity with a nucleocapsid. That also needs to be factored in with the nucleocapsid because it interacts with the nucleic acid. It's a highly charged protein and typically gives a very high background in a Western blot. So really you're talking about the envelope glycoprotein as being the most important antigen, and since you're really talking about one band, you can't separate out five or six bands' reactivity patterns. When you talk about the glycoprotein you're talking about other problems with the glycoprotein, which is the confirmational stability of epitopes, whether you run Western blots with mercaptomethanol sulphides or whether you leave it native. The problem is that the protein really isn't big enough to do a lot of differentiation from, let's say, a dengue serum from a West Nile serum from an SLE serum. So I don't think that the Western blot is going to help improve the specificity of the test. We've run a lot of Western blots over the years in my laboratory, and basically this is what you see. I could be wrong, and I want you to keep an open mind, but my best guess would be that a Western blot would not be specific for West Nile infection. A caveat could be that there are also nonstructural proteins that are synthesized by these viruses. A number of years ago, even before I came to CDC, Fort Collins, Dr. Dennis Trent and Ateef Qureshi looked at the immune response as five proteins, and their preliminary evidence was that this was a far more specific protein than the E glycoprotein. The problem with the NS5 protein is that not everybody makes antibody to NS5 to high enough levels that you can detect it on a Western blot. So if you did that sort of thing, you couldn't use virion E (protein); you'd probably have to use infected cells where you'd be looking at the nonstructural or structural proteins. I think that it's a thing that could be used, but we would have to do a lot more work with the specific virus to try to determine whether or not it would be useful. My initial take on it would be that it's probably not going to add much over what we already have.

MONATH: I think the future is going to be very interesting with respect to diagnosis, because, fortunately, so far, West Nile has invaded an area of the United States where other flaviviruses are not so active. But as and if it moves west, West Nile will infect people who previously have seen St. Louis encephalitis. In fact, in the Midwest, there were big epidemics in the mid-1970s. This is the elderly population now that is going to get sick, so the complexity of flavivirus serology, serological diagnosis, is really highest where you have multiple flaviviruses circulating and affecting human population. And the complexities of the patterns of antibodies with respect to cross-reactivity are going to *really* be problems when this virus appears in the St. Louis country. So I think—if you want to look into the future and prepare yourself for it—that's how that is going to affect our ability to make a specific serological diagnosis. It would be a worthwhile model. We really don't understand very well what happens in these sequential infections to see what happens in the St. Louis–infected animal that's later infected with West Nile. It's going to be a real headache when that happens.

ROEHRIG: Well, at least, Tom, from a public health perspective, if we diagnose it as a flaviviral encephalitis, they can use control and, we hope, try to get it under containment. But yes, actually trying to define exactly what the agent is could be problematic. It will be problematic.

CAMPBELL: It reminds me of something that Dr. Bill Reeves from the University of California-Berkeley reminded Duane and me of recently. Tom, you may know this, but there was some early work—and again, going back to John's point about looking at the early work and trying to appreciate what was already done and not re-inventing the wheel; there was some laboratory work done by some scientists years ago, including Dr. Hammon, who is a pioneer in arbovirology—looking at cross-protection of dengue antibodies against West Nile virus in laboratory animals. And there is some cross-protectivity there, and I wonder what we know. I'm not familiar with any similar studies with SLE, but I would suspect there is some cross-protection at least.

SHOPE: There's a large literature on this. Dr. Winston Price did a whole series of experiments in primates. And, yes, there is cross-protection as Tom says.

CAMPBELL: It could be that those people that were infected in Chicago in 1975 are going to be the least likely to get West Nile encephalitis now that they're old.

GRADY: Before we end our panel, I'd like to throw out something else for your consideration: Although West Nile is new, it hasn't replaced the usual causes of viral encephalitis that one sees, particularly enteroviruses and herpes group viruses. And you've got to keep in mind that that has to be part of the differential diagnosis. We have data suggesting that in the same time period in the greater metropolitan and surrounding counties, that there were probably, at a minimum, as many cases due to other viruses as there were due to West Nile. And I say at a minimum because enteroviruses can be recovered by culture, and there are a substantial number of laboratories that have that capability. We don't know what their results were, and likewise more and more labs are coming on line able to do PCR for herpes group viruses. Again, we don't know what their results are. We only know the results of specimens that were tested in our laboratory. Before we leave, I'd like you to remind you to keep that in mind. The outbreak doesn't replace other viruses; it merely is superimposed on what is normally going on.

KRAMER: I wanted to add to that—Dr. Monath reminded me. I mentioned that we do cell culture because we don't want to miss other viruses that are there. And I think it's very important that as this virus moves into Florida, where there's St. Louis, and as it moves toward the West Coast where there's St. Louis, that if people use PCR to look for West Nile in mosquito pools, they might be missing St. Louis. So it's very important to do assays so that you don't miss the other viruses that are there on the mosquitoes as well, because you may not see human cases that will tell you there's another virus there, except that they may be spotty. We don't want to narrow down our focus on West Nile alone, even in the mosquitoes.

CAMPBELL: OK, it's time to wrap it up. Thank you very much to our excellent panel.

Variations in Biological Features of West Nile Viruses

V. DEUBEL,[a] L. FIETTE,[b] P. GOUNON,[b] M. T. DROUET,[b] H. KHUN,[b] M. HUERRE,[b] C. BANET,[c] M. MALKINSON,[c] AND P. DESPRÈS[b]

[a]Institut Pasteur, Lyon, France

[b]Institut Pasteur, Paris, France

[c]Kimron Veterinary Institute, Beit Dagan, Israel

ABSTRACT: Pathological findings in humans, horses, and birds with West Nile (WN) encephalitis show neuronal degeneration and necrosis in the central nervous system (CNS), with diffuse inflammation. The mechanisms of WN viral penetration of the CNS and pathophysiology of the encephalitis remain largely unknown. Since 1996, several epizootics involving hundreds of humans, horses, and thousands of wild and domestic bird cases of encephalitis and mortality have been reported in Europe, North Africa, the Middle East, Russia, and the USA (see specific chapters in this issue). However, biological and molecular markers of virus virulence should be characterized to assess whether novel strains with increased virulence are responsible for this recent proliferation of outbreaks.

KEYWORDS: West Nile virus; central nervous system; flavivirus infection

INTRODUCTION

West Nile (WN) virus belongs to the genus *Flavivirus* of the family Flaviviridae. The genus comprises 70 viruses classified on the basis of their serological and genetic relatedness.[1,2] WN virus is a member of the Japanese encephalitis (JE) complex that includes St. Louis encephalitis (SLE), Murray Valley encephalitis (MVE), and the Kunjin (KUN) viruses (TABLE 1). KUN virus is closely related genetically to, but distinct antigenically from, WN virus.[3–5] These studies also demonstrated that WN viruses are clustered into two genetic lineages that differ epidemiologically. Whether viruses are introduced in epidemic areas by migrating birds and are then maintained in endemic states remains unknown.[3,6] The primary transmission cycle of WN virus involves birds and mosquitoes, mainly of the *Culex* species. Humans and some wild and domestic vertebrates are usually dead-end hosts that have low-level viremias, thereby diminishing their importance of their role in transmission cycles. Although all viruses in the JE complex have the potential to infect migratory birds, only SLE in South and North America and WN virus have been isolated from wide areas of the world (TABLE 1).

Address for correspondence: V. Deubel, Institut Pasteur, Unité de Biologie des Infections Virales Emergentes, 21 Avenue Tony Garnier, 69365 Lyon cedex 7, France.Voice: +33-437-282-442; fax: +33–437–282–441.

vdeubel@cervi-lyon.inserm.fr

TABLE 1. Japanese encephalitis complex and geographic repartition[a]

Africa	America	Asia	Australia	Europe
West Nile	West Nile	West Nile/Kunjin	Kunjin	West Nile
Koutango[a]	St-Louis encephalitis	Japanese encephalitis	Japanese encephalitis	
Usutu	Ilheus		Murray Valley encephalitis	
Yaounde[a]	Rocio		Alfuy	
	Cacipacore			

[a]There is no natural avian host known for these viruses.

In humans, WN virus causes an essentially mild infection with only rare signs of encephalitis.[7] In severe infections, clinical signs and symptoms include headache, acute onset of fever, encephalitis, and hemorrhages, according to virus virulence and age susceptibility. In this chapter, we review biological features of flaviviral and WN virus-induced encephalitis in natural and experimental infections with flaviviruses of the JE serocomplex.

STRUCTURE, REPLICATION, AND MORPHOGENESIS OF FLAVIVIRUSES

WN viruses are spherical particles 50 nm in diameter, with a unit-membrane envelope and dense core. The nucleocapsid contains a single-stranded RNA genome of positive sense packaged within the core protein C (FIG. 1). Protein C determinants that participate in RNA and protein interactions during nucleocapsid assembly have not been defined. The viral envelope protein is composed of the envelope E and membrane M proteins embedded in a lipid bilayer by their hydrophobic C-terminus spanning domains.[8] The M protein has a short ectodomain of 41 amino acids. Virions may contain variable amounts of the prM glycoprotein, the intracellular precursor of the virion-associated M protein, which reduces the infectivity of the virion.[9] The flavivirus E protein, as exemplified by the tick-borne encephalitis virus protein E[10], is a head-to-tail curved, elongated rod-shaped, dimer laying on the surface of the envelope, conferring a smooth appearance (no surface projections visible by electron microscopy). The ectodomain (470 aa) of the E protein is divided into three domains: central domain I that includes an antigenic domain composed of the 50 N-terminal amino acids and a segment that carries the N-glycosylation site; domain II is structured in two loops involved in dimer contacts that contain the highly conserved sequence from aa residues 98 to 111, and possibly a fusion sequence; and domain III, resembling an immunoglobulin constant domain, proposed to contain sequences that bind to cell receptor(s). The E protein has important biological roles, including virion assembly, cell receptor recognition, fusion with cell endosomal membranes, agglutination of red blood cells, and induction of B and T cell responses associated with protective immunity. Some of the WN/KUN virus E proteins are N-glycosylated.[3,11] The role of glycosylation in E function is still unclear,[11,12] although an association with neuroinvasiveness in the rodent model has been suggested.[13,14]

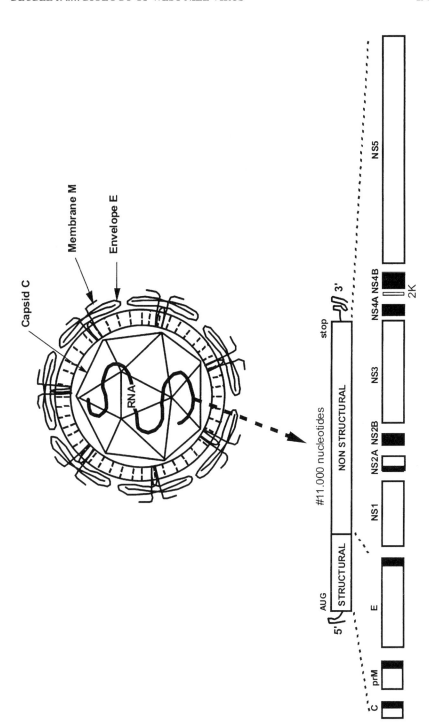

FIGURE 1. Structure of flavivirus virion and of the positive strand RNA genome.

WN virus RNA genome is approximately 11 kb long.[15,16] The genomic RNA carries a type 1 cap at the 5' end[15] but does not contain a polyadenylate tract at the 3' end.[17] The genome has a single open reading frame encoding for one polyprotein that is cleaved cotranslationally and posttranslationally at specific sites by host and viral proteases to produce the virion and replicase components (FIG. 1). The 5' end of the genome encodes the three structural proteins of the virus C-prM(M)-E, while the remaining 3' portion encodes at least seven nonstructural proteins NS1-NS2A-NS2B-NS3-NS4A-NS4B-NS5.[8] The 5' noncoding regions (NCR) of JE-complex viruses are 97 nucleotides long, but the 3' NCR have variable lengths.[8] Potential stem-loop secondary structures have been predicted at the 5' and 3' ends of the flaviviral genome, while conserved RNA sequences in both untranslated regions may be important for regulating translation, replication, and packaging.[18]

Flaviviruses replicate in a variety of cells of insect, mammal, or avian origin. Cell receptors specific for flaviviruses have not been identified, but it is believed that virus binding to the cell may be promoted through the initial interaction of E protein with highly sulfated heparan sulfate (HSHS) residues present on the surface of a wide variety of cells.[19] Recently, it has been suggested that a short segment of E protein (amino acids 306-314) present in a hydrophilic sequence in domain III of dengue E protein may be critical for virus infectivity.[20] This sequence as well as amino acid 306 of JE virus were shown to be associated with protein binding to cell surface glycoaminoaglycans.[21] Entry of WN/KUN viruses into host cells is believed to occur via receptor-mediated endocytosis in coated pit vesicles.[22,23] The fusion segment that is not apparent at the surface of the dimeric form of E protein may become active after reorganization of the E protein into a trimeric form on exposure to acid pH in the endosome.[24] Therefore, it can be assumed that neutralization of virus infectivity by anti-E antibodies could occur either by blocking virus binding to HSHS and to specific receptor(s) or by interfering with the structural rearrangements that occur at acid pH. This is consistent with the finding that potential neutralization sites defined by amino acid substitution present in monoclonal antibody escape mutants are located on the three domains of the upper side of E protein. However, subneutralizing concentrations of antibody or cross-reactive nonneutralizing antibodies acquired from a previous flaviviral infection may mediate the attachment and uptake of virus through Fc receptors.[25] This antibody-dependent enhancement of virus infection has been shown for WN and dengue viruses *in vitro* but is less evident *in vivo*.[26]

Flavivirus replication occurs in the perinuclear region of the endoplasmic reticulum (ER) of cells that become vacuolated and hypertrophic.[27,28] Translation of the polyprotein occurs in association with the rough ER, and proteins prM, E, and NS1 then translocate into the lumen of the ER. prM and E proteins heterodimerize[29] and are included in the immature virion formed in close association with the ER membranes. Electron microscopy shows virions associated with the ER.[30–33] The immature virions accumulate within membrane-bound vesicles and may form pseudocrystal structures (FIG. 2A). Virions are transported through the secretory pathway to the cell membrane. prM protein cleavage by furin occurs at the final stage of exocytosis, leading to production of mature virus[34] (FIGS. 2B and 2C). Alternative release of virions by budding from infected cells has also been observed with dengue 2 virus in mosquito cells and with the Sarafend strain of WN virus in Vero cells.[30,35]

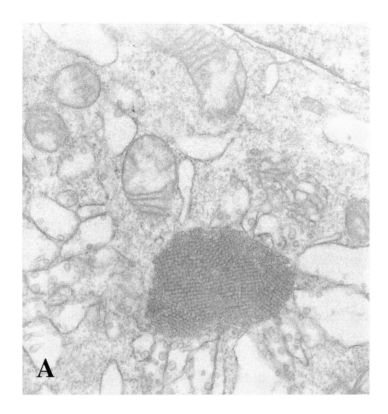

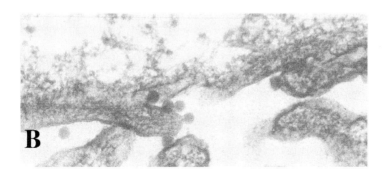

FIGURE 2. Electron miscroscopy of Aedes pseudoscutellaris AP61 cells infected at a multiplicity of infection of 10 with WN viruses isolated in Israel (stork, 1998). Infected cells were fixed with glutaraldehyde 1% 2 days postinfection. A: × 20,000; B and C: × 100,000.

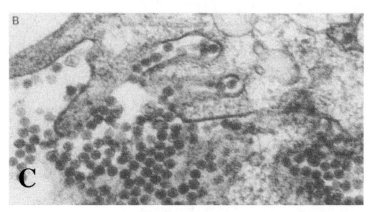

FIGURE 2C.

Exit of virus particles from infected cells may be associated with the glycosylation status of the envelope protein.[35]

    Flavivirus replication may be lytic for host cells, lead to syncytium formation, or may induce persistent noncytopathic infection.[36] Persistent infection has been observed in neuroblastoma cell lines infected with JE virus.[37] Production of defective interfering viruses appears to be an important mechanism in the expression of *Flavivirus* persistence.[37–39] Persistent infection also occurs in WN virus–infected hamsters with virus isolated from the brain up to 53 days after initial infection.[40] Persistent chronic JE virus infection has been observed in the CNS of a patient 117 days after the onset of clinical symptoms in the presence of specific IgM antibodies in the cerebrospinal fluid.[41]

PATHOGENESIS OF WN VIRUS

    In human and animals hosts, the outcome of flavivirus infection is influenced by several factors, including virus strain, dose and route of inoculation, and the age, genetic susceptibility, and immune status of the host.[36,42] The pathophysiology of invasiveness of the CNS and neuron damage, however, is largely unknown.

    In mice, WN virus, like others flaviviruses, is neurotropic and intracerebral inoculation is usually lethal. Experimental lesions are similar to those reported in natural infections of humans and horses. In the brain of mice infected with an Israeli strain of WN virus,[6] perivascular cuffing of macrophages and lymphocytes are found around small vessels (FIG. 3A). Neuronal degeneration and necrosis, neuronophagia,

---

FIGURE 3. Neuropathogenesis of 6-week-old mice infected intradermally with WN virus isolated in Israel (Stork/98). A: Hematoxylin-eosin staining of cortex (× 40); **B:** immunostaining of viral antigen in neurons of the cortex and (**C**) hippocampus (× 40); **D:** immunostaining of neurons in the cortex (× 100).

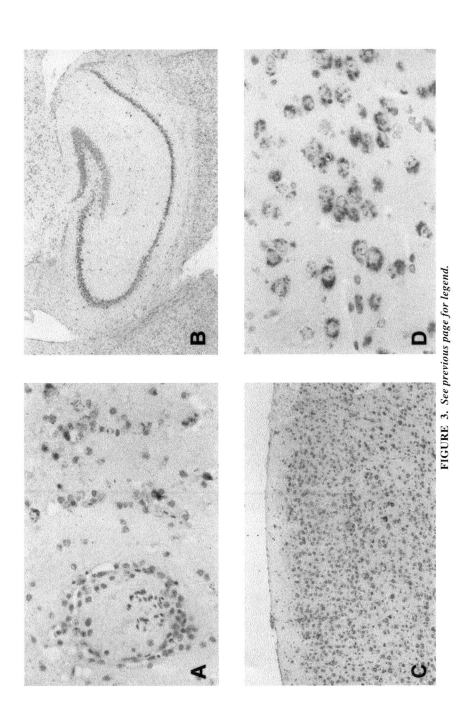

FIGURE 3. See previous page for legend.

spongy degeneration, and focal hemorrhages are observed.[43,44] Hippocampus and cortex areas are the main locations of the virus in the mouse (FIGS. 3B and 3C),[45] whereas preferential sites of infected cells are thalamus, cerebrum, cerebellum, medulla oblongata, and cervical spinal cord in humans, monkeys, horses, and birds.[46–50] Neurons (FIG. 3D) and glial cells are target cells of WN virus infection, and Purkinje cells of the cerebellum have been shown infected in dead birds.[48,51,52] Virus isolation from spleen, lymph nodes, liver, heart, kidney, lung, and pancreas has also been described in humans and birds.[46,48,53]

Pathways of entry and diffusion of WN virus in the CNS are not fully understood. Important variations in WN virus load may be observed in CNS of human and horses by the time of death. Viremia in these hosts is generally low, and processes of CNS invasion remain unknown. WN virus is often absent from the brain, whereas virus isolation is still possible from the lumbar part of the spinal cord.[49,54] The fact that scattered spotty necroses are observed in the cerebrum and cerebellum of horses at autopsy, whereas viable WN virus is often recovered in lower parts of the CNS only suggests that virus has migrated from the brain along the spinal cord (M. Huerre, L. Fiette, and V. Deubel, unpublished observations). Therefore, neuroinvasion of virulent WN virus with centripetal virus spray by peripheral nerves seems unlikely.

We have studied the influence of the route of inoculation in six-week-old Swiss mice using an Israeli WN virus strain isolated from a stork in 1998.[6] The intranasal route of infection requires about 100 times more virus than the intradermal and intraperitoneal routes to kill 50% of mice (data not shown). It allows delivery of virus to olfactory neurons and to the brain via the olfactory lobes. This route may introduce the virus to the CNS via olfactory epithelium by either passive diffusion across brain capillary endothelial cells or via virus replication in the endothelial cells and shedding into the brain parenchyma.[55] Neuroinvasive virions inoculated by intraperitoneal and intradermal routes may also cross the blood brain barrier by processes of extraneural replication, high viremia, and cytokine-induced damage to the capillary endothelial cells. Entry of WN virus into the CNS has been studied using mouse brain endothelium.[56] WN virus was detected in cells of small blood vessels of WN virus–infected mice. In vitro, WN virus was also able to replicate to a moderate level in mouse brain endothelial cells without cytopathic effect. However, release of viral particles was not polarized. Human umbilical vein endothelial cells (HUVEC) can be infected with WN virus.[57] WN virus infection increased the expression of E-selectin, VCAM-I, and ICAM-I within 30 min to 3 h after infection. Infected endothelial cells also produce nitric oxide that may potentiate monocyte adhesion. Recently, Wen et al.[58] showed an increase of nitrite secretion and a rearrangement of zonula occludens-1 (ZO-1) and β-catenin in HUVEC infected with WN virus. Thus, WN virus may modulate its entry into the CNS by altering cellular junctions of endothelial cells and leukocyte diapedesis across the endothelial cells.

Apoptosis has been shown to be a major pathway of death in mouse neuronal cells infected with dengue virus.[59] By contrast, it seems that neurons of mice infected with MVE virus do not show evidence of apoptosis, and the severity of the disease may be more linked to neutrophil infiltration and inducible nitric oxide synthetase activity in the CNS.[60] WN virus is neuroinvasive for adult mice at low doses.

Variation exists in neurovirulence and neuroinvasion for mice among JE virus strains.[61] We have assessed whether differences could be related to virus strain and dose of inoculation by causing WN encephalitis in six-week-old Swiss mice. Two WN virus strains have been compared: one that caused an outbreak in storks and geese in 1998 in Israel (shown to be similar to the strain isolated in New York[4,6]), and another one that was isolated from *Aedes aegypti* mosquitoes in Senegal in 1990. Thus the two strains differed epidemiologically and belonged to different lineages, as established on genetic criteria by Berthet *et al.*[3] Various doses of the two WN viruses were injected intradermally, and the percentages of mouse death were compared (data not shown). Hundreds of times more virus of the Senegalese strain (*Aedes*/90) than from the Israeli isolate (Stork/98) are required to kill mice. This result suggests that epidemic WN virus is more pathogenic than enzootic virus. However, we have not tested the amount of virus in the brains of mice that succumbed to infection with either virus dependent on the virus or the route of inoculation.

CONCLUSION

In conclusion, the extent of flavivirus infection and neuroinvasion depends on viral factors such as virus origin, attenuation by serial passages, and dose.[13,14] They may also depend on host factors, such as the age, genetic background, and immune status of susceptible hosts.[44] The degree of inflammatory changes in the CNS of natural hosts, birds, humans, and horses, and of experimental animals, mice, and monkeys infected with JE complex–related viruses may vary depending on the host and the virus strain. In a mouse model we have examined, intranasal and intraperitoneal or intradermal inoculations reveal variability in neuroinvasiveness of WN virus according to the virus strain and to the route of inoculation. The intranasal route of inoculation was less effective for WN virus neuroinvasion than the intradermal or intraperitoneal routes, despite direct infection of olfactory neurons. The mouse model of WN virus infection may help to determine the route of virus spread into the human CNS. Differences were observed in neuroinvasiveness between two wild strains of WN viruses isolated in different epidemiological conditions. These strains are genetically different and show about 20% amino acid divergence in the E protein gene. Moreover, the less virulent strain shows a deletion of four amino acids at the glycosylation site of the protein. Recombinant technology recently developed to produce infectious clones for WN and KUN viruses[62,63] may provide molecular tools to identify genetic markers of virus virulence.

ACKNOWLEDGMENTS

We are grateful to Dr. Charles Calisher for his critical and thoughtful review of the manuscript.

REFERENCES

1. CALISHER, C.H., N. KARABATSOS, J.M. DALRYMPLE, *et al.* 1989. Antigenic relationships among flaviviruses as determined by cross-neutralization tests with polyclonal antisera. J. Gen. Virol. **70:** 37–43.

2. HEINZ, F.X., M.S. COLLETT, R.H. PURCELL, et al. 2000. Family Flaviviridae. In Virus Taxonomy. Classification and Nomenclature of Viruses. 7th report of the International Committee for the Taxonomy of Viruses. M.H.V. van Reggenmortel, C.M. Fauquet, D.H.L. Bishop, et al., Eds.: 859–878. Academic Press. San Diego, CA.

3. BERTHET, F.X., H. ZELLER, M.T. DROUET, et al. 1997. Extensive nucleotide changes and deletions within the envelope glycoprotein gene of Euro African West Nile viruses. J. Gen. Virol. 78: 2293–2297.

4. LANCIOTTI, R.S., J.T. ROEHRIG, V. DEUBEL, et al. 1999. Origin of the West Nile virus responsible for an outbreak of encephalitis in the northeastern US. Science 286: 2333–2337.

5. SCHERRET, J.H., J.S. MACKENZIE, A.A. KHROMYKH & R.A. HALL. 2001. Biological significance of glycosylation of the envelope protein of Kunjin virus. Ann. N.Y. Acad. Sci. 951. This volume.

6. MALKINSON, M., C. BANET, Y. WEISMAN, et al. 2001. West Nile virus infection in white storks migrating into Israel. Emerg. Infect. Dis. In press.

7. SOUTHAM, C.M. & A.E. MOORE. 1954. Induced virus infections in man by the Egypt isolates of West Nile virus. Am. J. Trop. Med. Hyg. 3: 19–50.

8. RICE, C.M. 1996. Flaviviridae: the viruses and their replication. In Virology. N.D. Fields, D.M. Knipe, P.M. Kowley, et al., Eds.: 931–959. Lippincott-Raven. Philadelphia, PA.

9. WENGLER, G. & G. WENGLER. 1989. Cell-associated West Nile flavivirus is covered with E + Pre-M protein heterodimers which are destroyed and reorganized by proteolytic cleavage during virus release. J. Virol. 63: 2521–2526.

10. REY, F., F.X. HEINZ, C. MANDL, et al. 1995. The envelope glycoprotein E from tick-borne encephalitis virus at 2A resolution. Nature 375: 291–298.

11. ADAMS, S.C., A.K. BROOM, L.M. SAMMELS, et al. 1995. Glycosylation and antigenic variation among Kunjin virus isolates. Virology 206: 49–56.

12. WINKLER, G., F.X. HEINZ & C. KUNZ. 1987. Studies on the glycosylation of flavivirus E proteins and the role of carbohydronate in antigenic structure. Virology 159: 237–243.

13. HALEVY, M., Y. AKOV, D. BEN NATHAN, et al. 1994. Loss of active neuroinvasiveness in attenuated strains of West Nile virus: pathogenicity in immunocompetent and SCID mice. Arch. Virol. 137: 355–370.

14. CHAMBERS, T.J., M. HALEVY & A. NESTOROWICZ. 1998. West Nile virus envelope proteins: nucleotide sequence analysis of strains differing in mouse neuroinvasiveness. J. Gen. Virol. 79: 2375–2380.

15. CASTLE, E. & G. WENGLER. 1987. Nucleotide sequence of the 5′ terminal untranslated part of the genome of the flavivirus West Nile virus. Arch. Virol. 92: 309–313.

16. WENGLER, G., G. WENGLER & H.J. GROSS. 1978. Studies on virus-specific nucleic acids synthesized in vertebrate and mosquito cells infected with flaviviruses. Virology 89: 423–437.

17. WENGLER, G. & G. WENGLER. 1981. Terminal sequences of the genome and replicative-form RNA of the flavivirus West Nile virus: absence of poly (A) and possible role in RNA replication. Virology 113: 544–555.

18. CHEN, C., M. KUO, L. CHIEN, et al. 1997. RNA protein interactions. Involvement of NS3, NS5, and 3′ noncoding regions of Japanese encephalitis virus genomic RNA. J. Virol. 71: 3466–3473.

19. HILGARD, P. & R. STOCKERT. 2000. Heparan sulfate proteoglycans initiate dengue virus infection of hepatocytes. Hepatology 32: 1069–1077.

20. THULLIER, P., C. DEMANGEL, H. BEDOUELLE, et al. 2001. Mapping of a dengue virus neutralizing epitope critical for the infectivity of all serotypes: insight into the neutralization mechanism. J. Gen. Virol. 82: 1885–1892.

21. LEE, E. & M. LOBIGS. 2001. Mechanism of virulence attenuations of glycosaminoglycan-binding variants of encephalitic flaviviruses [Abstract]. International Symposium on Positive Strand RNA Viruses. no. P1-19. Paris, France.

22. GOLLINS, S.W. & J.S. PORTERFIELD. 1985. Flavivirus infection enhancement in macrophages: an electron microscopic study of viral cellular entry. J. Gen. Virol. 66: 1969–1982.

23. NG, M.L. & L.C.L. LAU. 1988. Possible involvement of receptors in the entry of Kunjin virus into Vero cells. Arch. Virol. **100:** 199–211.
24. ALLISON, S.L., J. SCHALICH, K. STIASNY, *et al.* 1995. Oligomeric rearrangement of tickborne encephalitis virus envelope proteins induced by acidic pH. J. Virol. **69:** 695–700.
25. GOLLINS, S.W. & J.S. PORTERFIELD. 1984. Flavivirus infection enhancement in macrophages: radioactive and biological studies on the effect of antibody on viral fate. J. Gen. Virol. **65:** 1261–1272.
26. KREIL, T.R. & M.M. EIBL. 1997. Pre- and post-exposure protection by passive immunoglobulin but no enhancement of infection with a flavivirus in a mouse model. J. Virol. **71:** 2921–2927.
27. MURPHY, F.A. 1980. Morphology and morphogenesis. *In* St. Louis Encephalitis. T.P. Monath, Ed.: 65–104. DC Apha. Washington.
28. WESTAWAY, E.G., J.M. MACKENZIE, M.T. KENNEY, *et al.* 1997. Ultrastructure of Kunjin virus infected cells: colocalization of NS1 and NS3 with double-stranded RNA and of NS2B with NS3, in virus-induced membrane structures. J. Virol. **71:** 6650–6661.
29. DESPRÈS, P., M.P. FRENKIEL & V. DEUBEL. 1993. Differences between cell membrane fusion activities of two dengue type-1 isolates reflect modifications of viral structure. Virology **196:** 209–219.
30. HASE, T., P. SUMMERS, K. ECKELS, *et al.* 1987. An electron and immunoelectron microscopic study of dengue-2 virus infection of cultured mosquito cells: maturation events. Arch. Virol. **92:** 273–291.
31. HASE, T.P., L. SUMMERS & D.R. DUBOIS. 1990. Ultrastructural changes of mouse brain neurons infected with Japanese encephalitis. Int. J. Exp. Pathol. **71:** 493–505.
32. DEUBEL, V., J.P. DIGOUTTE, X. MATTEI, *et al.* 1981. Morphogenesis of yellow fever virus in *Aedes aegypti* cultured cells. II. An ultrastructural study. Am. J. Trop. Med. Hyg. **30:** 1071–1077.
33. BARTH, O.M. 1999. Ultrastructural aspects of the dengue virus (flavivirus) particle morphogenesis. J. Submicrosc. Cytol. Pathol. **31:** 404–412.
34. STADLER, K., S.L. ALLISON, J. SCHALICH, *et al.* 1997. Proteolytic activation of tickborne encephalitis virus by furin. J. Virol. **71:** 8475–8481.
35. NG, M.L., J. HOWE, V. CREENIVASAN, *et al.* 1994(a). Flavivirus West Nile (Sarafend) egress at the plasma membrane. Arch. Virol. **137:** 303–313.
36. MONATH, T.P. & F.X. HEINZ. 1996. Flavivirus. *In* Virology. N.D. Fields, D.M. Knippe, P.M. Howley, *et al.*, Eds.: 961–1034. Lippincott-Raven. Philadelphia, PA.
37. SCHMALJOHN, C. & C.D. BLAIR. 1997. Persistent infection of cultured mammalian cells by Japanese encephalitis virus. J. Virol. **24:** 580–589.
38. BRINTON, M.A. 1982. Characterization of West Nile virus persistent infections in genetically resistant and susceptible mouse cells I. Generation of defective nonplaquing virus particles. Virology **116:** 84–98.
39. POIDINGER, M., R.J. COELEN & J.S. MACKENZIE. 1991. Persistent infection of Vero cells by the flavivirus Murray Valley encephalitis virus. J. Gen. Virol. **72:** 573–578.
40. XIAO, S.Y., H. GUZMAN, H. ZHANG, *et al.* 2001. West Nile virus infection in the golden hamster (*Mesocricetus auratus*): a model for West Nile encephalitis. Emerg. Infect. Dis. **7:** 714–721.
41. RAVI, V., A.S. DESAI, P.K. SHENOY, *et al.* 1993. Persistence of Japanese encephalitis virus in the human nervous system. J. Med. Virol. **40:** 326–329.
42. ELDADAH, A.H., N. NATHASON & R. SARSITIS. 1967. Pathogenesis of West Nile virus encephalitis in mice and rats. I: Influence of age and species on mortality and infection. Am. J. Epidemiol. **86:** 765–775.
43. HASE, T., R.R. DUBOIS & P.L. SUMMERS. 1990. Comparative study of mouse brains infected with Japanese encephalitis virus by intracerebral or intraperitoneal inoculation. Int. J. Exp. Pathol. **71:** 857–869.
44. SHIEH, W.J., J. GUARNER, M. LAYTON, *et al.* 2000. The role of pathology in an investigation of an outbreak of West Nile encephalitis in New York, 1999. Emerg. Infect. Dis. **6:** 370–372.
45. ELDADAH, A.H. & N. NATHASON. 1967. Pathogenesis of West Nile virus encephalitis in mice and rats. II. Virus multiplication, evolution of immunofluorescence, and development of histological lesions in the brain. Am. J. Epidemiol. **86:** 776–790.

46. SOUTHAM, C.M. & A.E. MOORE. 1954. Induced virus infections in man by the Egypt isolates of West Nile virus. Am. J. Trop. Med. Hyg. **3:** 19–50.
47. POGODINA, V.V., M.P. FROLOBA, G.V. MALENKO, *et al.* 1983. Study on West Nile virus persistence in monkeys. Arch. Virol. **75:** 71–86.
48. STEELE, K.E., M.J. LINN, R.P. SCHOEPP, *et al.* 2000. Pathology of fatal West Nile virus infections in native and exotic birds during the 1999 outbreak in New York City, New York. Vet. Pathol. **37:** 208–224.
49. CANTILE, C., G. DI GUARDO, C. ELENI, *et al.* 2000. Clinical and neuropathological features of West Nile virus equine encephalomyelitis in Italy. Equine Vet. J. **32:** 31–35.
50. SAMPSON, B.A., G. AMBROSI, A. CHARLOT, *et al.* 2000. The pathology of human West Nile virus infection. Hum Pathol. **31:** 527–531.
51. NIR, Y., A. BEEMER & R.A. GOLDWASSER. 1965. West Nile virus infection in mice following exposure to a viral aerosol. Br. J. Exp. Pathol. **46:** 443–449.
52. KOMAR, N. 2000. West Nile viral encephalitis. Rev. Sci. Tech. **19:** 166–176.
53. GEORGES, A.J., J.L. LESBORDES, M.C. GEORGES-COURBOT, *et al.* 1988. Fatal hepatitis from West Nile virus. Ann. Inst. Pasteur Virol. **138:** 237–244.
54. GUILLON, J.C., J. OUDAR, L. JOUBERT, *et al.* 1967. Lésions histologiques du système nerveux dans l'infection à virus West Nile chez le cheval. Ann. Inst. Pasteur **114:** 539–550.
55. MCMINN, P.C. 1997. The molecular basis of virulence of the encephalitogenic flaviviruses. J. Gen. Virol. **78:** 2711–2722.
56. DROPULIC, B. & C.L. MASTERS. 1990. Entry of neurotropic arboviruses into the central nervous system: an *in vitro* study using mouse brain endothelium. J. Infect. Dis. **161:** 685–691.
57. SHEN, *et al.* 1997. Early E-selectin, VCAM-1, ICAM-1 and a late major histocompatibility complex antigen induction on human endothelial cells by flavivirus and comodulation of adhesion molecule expression by immune cytokines. J. Virol. **71:** 9323–9332.
58. WEN, L., J. WONG, P.L. PENFOLD, *et al.* 2001. Changes in transcellular resistance in retinal pigment epithelium and endothelium after flavivirus infection correlate with changes in distribution of ZO-1 and β-catenin [Abstract]. Sixth International Symposium on Positive Strand RNA Viruses. Paris, France
59. DESPRÈS, P., M. FLAMAND, P.E. CECCALDI, *et al.* 1996. Human isolates of dengue type 1 induce apoptosis in mouse neuroblastoma cells. J. Virol. **70:** 4096–4090.
60. ANDREWS, D.M., V.B. MATTHEWS, L.M. SAMMELS, *et al.* 1999. The severity of Murray Valley encephalitis in mice is linked to neutrophil infiltration and inducible nitric oxide synthetase activity in the central nervous system. J. Virol. **73:** 8781–8790.
61. HUANG, C.H. & C. WONG. 1963. Relation of the peripheral multiplication of Japanese B encephalitis virus to the pathogenesis of the infection in mice. Acta Virol. **7:** 322–330.
62. YAMSCHIKOV, V.F., G. WENGLER, A.A. PERELYGIN, *et al.* 2001. An infectious clone of the West Nile flavivirus. Virology **281:** 294–304.
63. KHROMYKH, A.A., A. VARNAVSKI, P.L. SEDLAK, *et al.* 2001. Coupling between replication and packaging of flavivirus RNA [Abstract]. Sixth International Symposium on Positive Strand RNA Virus. Paris, France.

Host Factors Involved in West Nile Virus Replication

MARGO A. BRINTON

Biology Department, Georgia State University, Atlanta, Georgia 30303, USA

ABSTRACT: Viruses use cell proteins during many stages of their replication cycles, including attachment, entry, translation, transcription/replication, and assembly. Mutations in the cell proteins involved can cause disruptions of these critical host–virus interactions, which in turn can affect the efficiency of virus replication. These host–virus interactions also represent novel targets for the development of new antiviral agents. The different alleles of the murine *Flv* gene confer resistance or susceptibility to flavivirus-induced disease and provide a natural mutant system for the study of a host protein that can alter the outcome of a flavivirus infection. Since flaviviruses, such as West Nile virus, replicate in mosquitoes, mammals, and birds during their natural transmission cycles, it is expected that the critical cell proteins used by these viruses will be ones that are highly conserved between divergent host species. Our laboratory has focused on the identification and characterization of the flavivirus resistance gene product and of cell proteins that interact with the 3′ terminal regions of the West Nile virus genomic and antigenomic RNAs. The 3′ terminal regions of the viral RNAs function as promotors for viral RNA replication. Cell proteins that bind to the viral 3′ RNAs were detected by gel shift and UV-induced cross-linking assays. Individual proteins were then purified and partially sequenced. Mutation of a mapped, protein-binding site within the 3′ terminal region of the viral RNA in an infectious West Nile virus clone was used to demonstrate the functional importance of one of the cell proteins for efficient West Nile virus replication. Data from additional studies suggested possible roles for this viral RNA–cell protein interaction during the flavivirus replication cycle.

KEYWORDS: West Nile virus; host factors; genetic resistance; *Flv* gene; flavivirus replication; flavivirus translation

INTRODUCTION

Many studies have shown that viruses use cell proteins for multiple purposes during their intracellular replication cycles. For instance, viruses interact with cell proteins to facilitate their attachment to cells, entry into cells, the initiation and regulation of transcription and replication of their nucleic acids, the enhancement and regulation of the translation of their mRNAs, the transport of their proteins and nucleic acids within the infected cell, and the assembly of progeny virions. Viruses

Address for correspondence: Margo A. Brinton, Ph.D., Biology Department, Georgia State University, Kell Hall, Room 402, 24 Peachtree Center Avenue, Atlanta, GA 30303. Voice: 404-651-3113; fax: 404-651-2509.

biomab@panther.gsu.edu

also interact with cell proteins to alter the intracellular environment and/or cell architecture so that it is more favorable for virus replication and to inactivate intracellular defense mechanisms, such as apoptosis and interferon pathways. Since many aspects of the replication cycles of different types of viruses are unique, the cell proteins used by different types of viruses also differ.

Because flaviviruses, such as West Nile virus (WNV), cycle between vertebrate host species and insect vectors in nature, it is predicted that the critical cell proteins used by these viruses will be ones that are highly conserved among divergent host species. Identification of the cell proteins that flaviviruses depend upon during their replication cycles and analysis of the functions that these proteins provide for the virus are critical to furthering our understanding of virus–host interactions at the intracellular molecular level. These studies will also reveal additional targets for the development of novel antiviral therapies. It can be postulated that a spontaneous mutation in a cell protein required by a virus during its replication cycle could provide a selective advantage for host survival.

VARIATION IN THE HOST RESPONSE TO FLAVIVIRUS INFECTION

Individual variation in virus-induced disease susceptibility has been repeatedly observed after the exposure of populations of plants or animals to viral pathogens. The differences in the responses of individual hosts are often subsequently shown to be inherited. Studies with inbred mice have identified a number of unique genes that confer resistance to diseases induced by DNA or RNA viruses.[1] In some cases, resistance is controlled by a single locus, while in other cases two or more genes are involved. These genes map to different chromosomes, and only a few of them map within the major histocompatibility locus. The resistance phenotype is sometimes inherited as a dominant allele and sometimes inherited as a recessive allele. In a few cases, resistance and susceptibility are co-dominant. Additional host factors, such as age, nutritional state, hormone levels, and immune status can modulate the effect of the genetic background. The virulence, dose, and route of infection of the virus can also affect the outcome of an infection. For flaviviruses, it has been shown that younger mice (newborn to three weeks) develop higher levels of viremia and are more susceptible than adult mice.[2,3] This is due both to an immature immune system and to the higher susceptibility of immature neurons.

Variation in the response of mice to flavivirus infection was first observed in the 1920s, when individual mice in wild populations were shown to differ in their susceptibility to flavivirus-induced disease.[4] Breeding studies demonstrated that the alleles of a single gene, designated *Flv*, were responsible for this variation and that resistance segregated as a Mendelian dominant trait.[5,6] The majority of the inbred mouse strains currently in use were derived from a small number of progenitors and are susceptibile to flavivirus-induced disease[7] (TABLE 1). Only the BRVR, BSVR, Det, and PRI mouse strains are resistant.[1] The resistant PRI strain was used to create the resistant C3H/RV strain, which is congenic to the susceptible C3H/He strain.[8] Studies with wild *Mus musculus domesticus* (house mouse) from the United States[7] and Australia[9] showed that the resistant *Flv* allele continues to segregate in wild mouse populations. Studies with other taxonomic groups within the house mouse complex, such as *M. m. musculus, M. spretus, M. spicilegus, M. m. molossinius*, and

TABLE 1. The susceptibility of inbred strains of mice and of wild *Mus musculus* to yellow fever virus (YFV), strain 17D

Mouse strain[a]	No., sex	1	2	3	4	5	6	7	8	9	10	11	12	13	14	Percent susceptible[b]
DBA2	5F	—	—	—	—	—	—	—	—	—	2[c]	3	—	—	—	100
A	10F	1[d]	—	—	—	—	—	2	—	3	—	3	1	—	—	100
BALB/c	10M	—	—	—	—	—	—	—	2	6	2	—	—	—	—	100
C57Bl/6	5M, 4F	—	—	—	—	—	—	1	—	2	1	3	2	—	—	100
C57Bl/10	5F	—	—	—	—	—	—	—	2	3	—	—	—	—	—	100
AKR	8M	—	—	—	—	—	—	2	1	1	—	3	—	—	—	88
Swiss	5F	—	—	—	—	—	—	—	—	1	3	1	—	—	—	100
SJL	10F	—	—	—	—	—	—	—	1	3	—	4	1	—	—	90
SWR	10M	—	—	—	—	—	—	—	2	4	3	—	—	—	—	90
BIOD2 (old strain)	5M, 11F	—	—	—	—	—	—	—	1	7	5	3	—	—	—	100
BIOD2 (new strain)	5M, 5F	1	—	—	—	—	—	2	2	—	—	5	—	—	—	100
Wild[e] (Maryland)	4M, 6F	—	—	—	—	—	—	—	—	—	1	1	—	—	—	20
Wild (Soledad, Calif)[f]	5M	—	—	—	—	—	—	—	—	—	—	—	—	—	—	0
Wild (LaPuenta, Calif.)	5F	—	—	—	—	—	—	—	—	—	—	—	—	—	—	0
Wild (Devonshire, Calif.)	5F	—	—	—	—	—	—	—	—	—	—	—	—	—	—	0
C3H/RV	22M, 12F	1	—	—	—	—	—	—	—	—	—	13	4	2	—	0
C3H/HE	24M, 14F	—	—	—	—	—	—	—	2	9	7	13	4	2	1	100

[a]Mice were given an intracerebral injection of 0.03 mL of undiluted 17D-YFV. [b]% = number of animals killed by YFV/number of animals injected. [c]Day of death; some animals showed signs of sickness and paralysis one to two days prior to death. [d]Deaths occurring before the sixth day after infection were due to the trauma of the injection. [e]Third and fourth generation randomly bred wild mice. [f]Canyon where mice were trapped.

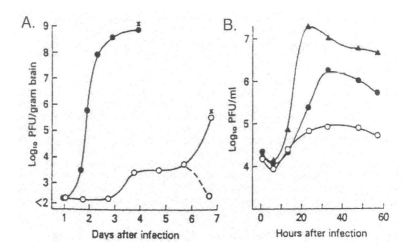

FIGURE 1. Replication of West Nile virus, Eg101, in congenic resistant (C3H/RV) and susceptible (C3H/He) mice and embryofibroblast cultures. A: Adult mice were injected intracerebrally with $10^{5.5}$ PFU. Brain titers for C3H/He (*closed circles*) and C3H/RV (*open circles*) are shown. All of the C3H/He mice died by day 5 postinfection, but less than half of the C3H/RV mice died by day 8. (*x*, signifies moribund state). Virus titers in the brains of moribund C3H/RV mice increased somewhat (day 7) but decreased in nonmoribund, recovering C3H/RV mice (*dashed line*). **B:** Cultures of C3H/He primary embryofibroblasts (*closed circles*), C3H/RV primary embryofibroblasts (*open circles*), and baby hamster kidney cells (BHK) (*closed triangles*) were infected with WNV, Eg101, at a mutiplicity of infection of 10 PFU/mL. Virus titers were measured by plaque assay in BHK cells. Data are from reference 1.

M. m. castaneus indicated that these mice also possessed the *Flv* gene.[9] Two inbred strains established from wild mice, CASA/Rk and CAST/Ei, are flavivirus resistant and appear to have the same *Flv* resistance allele found in the resistant mouse strains previously studied.[10] However, the inbred Mold/Rk strain, appears to have a different allele at the *Flv* locus that confers an intermediate level of resistance.[10] The *Flv* gene has been shown to confer resistance to the mosquito-borne flaviviruses, St. Louis, yellow fever, West Nile, Murray Valley, Banzi, Japanese encephalitis, and dengue virus as well as to the tick-borne viruses, Russian-spring-summer virus and louping ill.

Although resistant mice are resistant to flavivirus-induced disease, they are not resistant to flavivirus infection. However, resistant mice consistently produce lower virus titers after infection with flaviviruses than do susceptible mice or cell cultures[7,11,12] and the spread of a flavivirus infection in resistant mice is slower. For instance, after an intraperitoneal inoculation of WNV, strain Eg101, or an intracerebral inoculation of attenuated yellow fever virus,17D vaccine strain, 100% of adult susceptible mice develop disease and die, while none of the resistance mice show signs of disease. After an intracerebral inoculation of WNV, Eg101, virus rapidly replicates to very high titers in the brain tissues of susceptible mice, and 100% of them die by four days after infection (FIG. 1A). By contrast, this virus replicates much less efficiently in the brains of resistant mice. Although about 50% of the resistant mice died after intracerebral inoculation with a high dose ($10^{5.5}$ PFU) of WNV, Eg101, their brain titers on the day of death were still significantly lower that those observed in the susceptible mouse brains and the day of death was delayed (FIG. 1A). While virus-specific antibodies and cytotoxic T cells have been shown to be important for the clearance of flaviviruses,[13] studies with immunosupressed, resistant mice indicated that these mice also produced significantly lower titers of flaviviruses than did comparably treated susceptible mice.[14] Flavivirus resistance was also shown not to be dependent on the presence of alpha/beta interferon,[15] since treatment with anti-interferon antibody did not abrogate flavivirus resistance in animals or cell cultures.[16] These data indicate that although the host defense systems are important for clearing flavivirus infections, they do not play a specific role in reducing the yield of flaviviruses from infected resistant animals and cells. The *Flv* resistance allele functions intracellularly to reduce the amount of virus produced, and the lower production of virus results in a slower spread of the virus in the host. Both the decreased amount of virus produced and the slower spread give the host defense systems sufficient time to effectively eliminate the infection.

Lower virus yields (100- to 1000-fold) are consistently observed after infection of cell cultures prepared from various resistant mouse tissues, such as brain, kidney, embryo fibroblasts, and macrophages as compared to the yields from comparable cultures prepared from susceptible mice[11,12,15,17,18] (FIG. 1B). By contrast, these cultures produce equivalent yields of other types of viruses. After infection of cultures of resistant and susceptible embryofibroblasts at the same multiplicity of infection, comparable numbers of cells in both cultures were infected, indicating that the *Flv* resistance allele does not affect virus attachment or entry. Recent RNase protection studies indicated that the level of nascent WNV genome RNA in resistant cells at early times after infection is significantly lower than in susceptible cells, while the level of the complementary minus strand is similar in the two types of cells (Y. Li and M.A. Brinton, unpublished data). WNV defective–interfering virus particles are produced upon serial undiluted passage in both resistant and susceptible cells but interfere much more effectively in resistant cells.[15,17] These data suggest that the product of the *Flv* allele functions intracellularly at the level of viral RNA synthesis or turn over.

MAPPING AND IDENTIFICATION OF THE FLV GENE

The *Flv* gene has been mapped to a region of mouse chomosome 5 via recombination analyses in mice.[19–22] Our lab has used a positional cloning approach to identify the *Flv* gene within the region on chromosome 5 to which the *Flv* gene was mapped (Perelygin, Scherbik, and Brinton, unpublished data). The majority of genes identified from this region of chromosome 5 did not differ in their sequences between resistant and susceptible mice. However, one of the few genes that did show a sequence difference between resistant and susceptible mouse strains is a novel gene and is considered the most likely candidate. Alleles of this gene are currently being functionally tested in transgenic mice to confirm whether or not this is the *Flv* gene. Homologues of the alleles of the murine *Flv* gene may also affect susceptibility to flavivirus-induced disease in other host species.

FLAVIVIRUS INTRACELLULAR REPLICATION CYCLE

Flaviviruses bind to a specific, but as yet unknown, cell protein on the surface of target cells and then enter cells in a vesicle by a process much like endocytosis. After fusion between the viral and cell vesicle membranes, the genome RNA is released into the cytoplasm where it undergoes translation. Because the flavivirus genome functions as an mRNA, flaviviruses are designated as positive strand RNA viruses. The genome encodes a single open reading frame from which a single large polyprotein is translated. The ten mature viral proteins are produced from the polyprotein by proteolytic cleavage. The viral RNA replication complex proteins assemble and copy complementary minus strand RNAs from the genomic RNA. The complementary minus strand RNAs, in turn, function as templates for the transcription of nascent genome RNAs. The viral structural proteins that are produced assemble with the nascent genome RNAs in association with endoplasmic membranes. Progeny virions then travel to the cell surface inside vesicles and are released.

Flavivirus genomic RNA synthesis is 10 to 100 times more efficient than complementary viral RNA synthesis. The mechanisms used for the initiation and differential regulation of the two types of flavivirus RNA synthesized during infection are not well understood. The 3′ terminal regions of both the genome RNA and the complementary minus strand RNA contain structures that are conserved among divergent flaviviruses[23–26] (FIG. 2). Although the terminal RNA structures are conserved, only short sequences within these structures are conserved.[23,24] Data from studies in which the terminal regions were deleted or mutated in flavivirus infectious clones (cloned cDNA copies of the viral RNA) have indicated that the terminal regions are essential for virus replication.[27,28] Although the 3′ terminal structures are thought to contain both sequence and structural elements that function in the initiation and regulation of RNA transcription and translation, the individual elements have not yet been mapped.

There is a large, stable stem loop followed by a second short stem loop at the 3′ terminus of the genome RNA[24] (FIG. 2). The loop of the second stem loop can pair with nucleotides in the 3′ terminal stem to form a tertiary interaction (pseudoknot)[26] (FIG. 2, indicated by dashed lines). Three cell proteins (p105, p84, and p52) have been reported to interact specifically with the 3′ terminal genomic RNA structure as demonstrated by competition gel mobility shift, Northwestern, and UV-induced cross-linking assays[29] (FIG. 2). Although initial studies were done with a WNV 3′ (+) RNA probe, subsequent studies with yellow fever, dengue, or tick-borne enceph-

---

FIGURE 2. Cell proteins that bind specifically to the 3′ terminal RNAs of WNV. The 3′ terminal regions of the WNV genomic RNA (*top line*) and the complementary minus strand RNA (*bottom line*) form unique structures that are conserved between divergent flaviviruses. The cell proteins that interact with these terminal RNAs are indicated by *circles*. Competition gel mobility shift data suggest that p108 and p105 are the same protein (*astericks*).

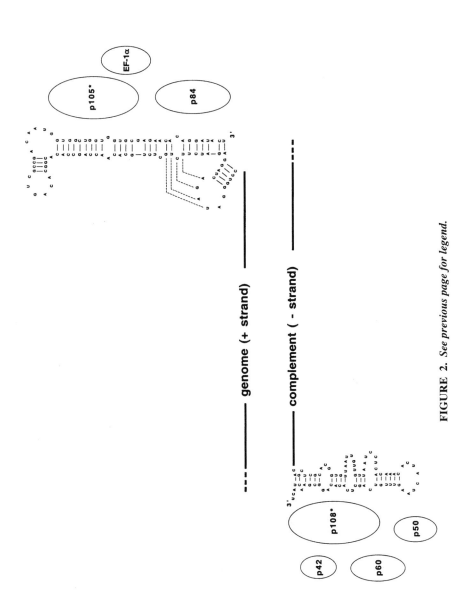

FIGURE 2. *See previous page for legend.*

alitis 3' RNA probes detected proteins of the same molecular masses (Blackwell and Brinton, unpublished data). These data suggest that all flaviviruses use the same set of cell proteins during their replication cycles.

The structure of the terminal stem loop located at the 3' end of the flavivirus complementary minus strand RNA differs both in size and shape from the one at the 3' end of the genomic RNA[24–26] (FIG. 2). Four cell proteins (p108, p60, p50, and p42) were previously shown to interact specifically with the WNV 3' (–)RNA[25] (FIG. 2). Competition studies showed that only one of these proteins, p108/p105, interacted with the 3' RNAs from both the genome and the complementary minus strand.[29]

EVIDENCE FOR THE INVOLVEMENT OF HOST PROTEINS IN FLAVIVIRUS VIRUS REPLICATION

The cell proteins that bind specifically to the flavivirus 3' (+) SL RNAs must be identified before studies can be done to determine whether they are functionally important during virus replication. Although several of the proteins that bind to the flavivirus 3' RNAs have been identified to date (Li, Emara, and Brinton, unpublished data), only the p52 protein will be discussed here. p52 was purified to near homogeneity by serial chomatography.[30] Six peptides generated from the purified protein were sequenced, and the sequences obtained identified the protein as elongation factor-1 alpha (EF-1α). The primary function of EF-1α in cells is to carry charged tRNA into ribosomes. EF-1α binds specifically to all of the charged tRNAs as well as to its docking site on the ribosomal RNA.[31] The dissociation constant (K_d) of the interaction between the WNV 3' (+) RNA and EF-1α is 10^{-9} M, which is similar to that for the interaction between EF-1α and charged tRNA.[31] The 3' (+) SL RNAs of WNV, yellow fever virus, tick-borne encephalitis virus, and dengue virus each bound to purified EF-1α with similar affinities (Blackwell and Brinton, unpublished data). The sequence of EF-1α is highly conserved between different host species, and the WNV 3' (+) RNA was shown to bind to EF-1α in mammalian, chicken, and mosquito cell extracts (Blackwell and Brinton, unpublished data). These data suggest that EF-1α is used in different host species by all flaviviruses.

The binding sites for EF-1α on the viral RNA were previously mapped.[30] An RNase footprinting assay showed that EF-1α protected a four nucleotide region on the 5' side of the 3' terminal stem loop (FIG. 3). Mutations in this site reduced the ability of the WNV 3' (+) SL RNA to bind to EF-1α in filter-binding studies by 60%, indicating that this was the major binding site for EF-1α. Two additional minor binding sites located at the top and bottom of the 3' terminal stem loop were also identified, and each accounted for about 20% of the total binding activity.[30]

The four nucleotides of the major binding site for EF-1α were mutated within a WNV infectious clone.[32] Although the sequence of the protein binding site was changed, the structure of the stem loop was preserved. The mutant progeny virus obtained grew more slowly and to significantly lower titers than the wild type virus and produced plaques that were 100 times smaller than the wild type plaques. After two passages of the mutant virus, some wild type–sized plaques appeared. Sequence analysis showed that these plaques were formed by partial reversion at the EF-1α binding site (Davis, Perelygin, and Brinton, unpublished data). These data suggest

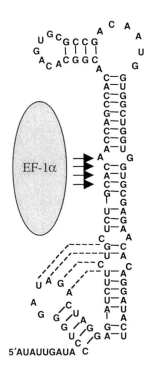

FIGURE 3. The major binding site for EF-1α on the WNV 3′ stem loop RNA. The location of the binding site was determined by footprinting and filter binding assays and is indicated by *arrows*. Data are from reference 30.

that the binding of EF-1α to the WNV 3′ SL RNA is functionally important for virus replication.

EFFECT OF THE VIRAL 3′ (+) SL RNA ON TRANSLATION

The WNV genome is an mRNA as well as a genome. Cell mRNAs form a closed loop complex via interactions between the polyA binding protein that binds to the 3′ poly A tract and proteins that interact with the 5′ cap binding complex.[33] The formation of a closed loop complex by an mRNA has been shown to significantly increase the efficiency of ribosome recruitment and the recycling of ribosomes. The WNV genomic RNA does not have a 3′ polyA tail and so cannot use polyA binding protein to facilitate the formation of a closed loop complex. Other types of viral mRNAs that do not have poly A tails use alternative proteins to bind to their 3′ sequences and facilitate interactions with proteins in the 5′ cap-binding complex. For instance, brome mosaic virus uses an alternative cell protein,[34] and rotavirus mRNA[35] uses a viral protein.

To determine whether the cell proteins that bound to the WNV 3′ (+) RNA could facilitate translation, the translation efficiencies of a number of chimeric mRNAs were analyzed.[36] These chimeric RNAs contained either the complete WNV 96 nts 5′ noncoding region or only the 5′ terminal stem loop (75 nts) at their 5′ ends. The central region contained the CAT reporter sequence with its own 3′ noncoding region but no poly A tract. At their 3′ ends, these RNAs had either the WNV 3′ terminal

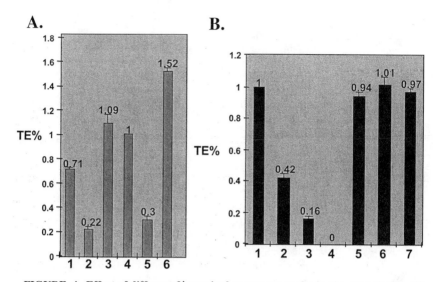

FIGURE 4. Effect of different 3′ terminal sequences on the *in vitro* **translation efficiencies of capped chimeric mRNAs. A:** Relative translation efficiency of each capped chimeric mRNA with the 3′ sequences in *cis*. All of the chimeric mRNAs used encoded the CAT reporter sequence. Lane 1, 5′ WNV 75 nt noncoding region (NCR) and CAT 3′ NCR; lane 2, 5′ WNV 75 nt NCR and WNV 3′ terminal sequence; lane 3, 5′ WNV 75 nt NCR and rubella 3′ terminal sequence; lane 4, 5′ WNV 96 nt NCR and CAT 3′ NCR; lane 5, 5′ WNV 96 nt NCR and WNV 3′ terminal sequence; lane 6, 5′ WNV 96 nt NCR and rubella 3′ terminal sequence. **B:** Effect on translation efficiency of WNV or rubella 3′ terminal sequences added in *trans*. The chimeric mRNA translated in each reaction contained a 5′ WNV 96 nt NCR and CAT 3′ NCR. Lane 1, No added 3′ RNA; lane 2, 0.5 µg of WNV 3′ RNA; lane 3, 1 µg of WNV 3′ RNA; lane 4, 5 µg of WNV 3′ RNA; lane 5, 0.5 µg of rubella 3′ RNA; lane 6, 1 µg of rubella 3′ RNA; lane 7, 5 µg of rubella 3′ RNA. TE, relative translation efficiency. Data are from reference 36.

stem loop, the 3′ region of rubella virus (a togavirus), which included an 18-mer poly A tract, or no additional 3′ sequence. The translation efficiencies of the chimeric mRNAs with the longer 5′ noncoding region were somewhat more efficient than those with the shorter 5′ noncoding region (FIG. 4A). However, the type of 3′ sequence present on a chimeric RNA had a more dramatic effect on its translation efficiency. The WNV 3′ sequence significantly decreased the translation efficiency, while the rubella 3′ sequence enhanced the translation efficiency of the chimeric mRNAs. The WNV 3′ sequence reduced the translation efficiency of chimeric mRNAs both in *cis* and in *trans* and of both capped and uncapped chimeric mRNAs.[36]

One explanation for the observed inhibitory effect of the 3′ stem loop on translation is that one or more of the cell proteins that bind to the WNV 3′ (+) RNA may normally be involved in translation and that the 3′ RNA competes with the translation machinery for these proteins. The observation that the WNV 3′ (+) RNA reduced translation efficiency rather than enhanced it suggests that the cell proteins that bind to the WNV 3′ (+) RNA do not facilitate the formation of a 3′–5′ closed loop complex. It is likely that a 3′–5′ interaction for flavivirus genomic RNA is instead facilitated via RNA–RNA interactions between short complementary sequences located near the 5' and 3' ends of the RNA.[37]

CONCLUSION

A growing body of experimental literature supports the importance of cell proteins in all phases of viral replication cycles and indicates the intimate and varied nature of the intracellular virus–host interactions. However, our current understanding of these complex host–virus interactions is still limited. The flavivirus resistance gene provides a unique system for identifying a host protein that can alter the efficiency of flavivirus replication. The existence of the *Flv* gene demonstrates that the products of different alleles of a single host gene can differentially affect the outcome of a flaviviral infection. The sizes of the proteins encoded by the candidate *Flv* genes so far identified by our positional cloning approach are different from those of the cell proteins that bind to the viral 3' RNAs, suggesting that none of the 3' RNA binding proteins are the *Flv* gene product. However, the *Flv* gene product could interact with one of these proteins via protein–protein interactions or, alternatively, with another region of the viral RNA.

The flavivirus genome RNA has multiple functions during the viral replication cycle. It functions as a template for the synthesis of minus strand RNA, an mRNA for translation of the viral polyprotein, and interacts with the structural proteins to assemble progeny virions. Both the conserved 3' terminal RNA structure of the genomic RNA and the three cell proteins (p105, p84, and EF-1α) that bind to it may play essential roles in regulating viral RNA transcription and translation. Since transcription and translation initiate from opposite ends of the genome RNA, there must be crosstalk between the 3' and 5' ends of the genomic RNA and mechanisms that block the initiation of transcription when translation begins and vice versa so that collisions between ribosomes and viral replication complexes do not occur. The mechanisms for switching a particular genome RNA between translation and transcription functions are likely to be complex.

REFERENCES

1. BRINTON, M.A. 1997. Host susceptibility to viral disease. *In* Viral Pathogenesis. N. Nathanson, Ed.: 303–328. Lippencott-Raven Publishers. Philidelphia, PA.
2. SCHERER, W.F., E.L. BUESCHER & E.H. MCCLURE. 1959. Ecological studies of Japanese encephalitis. Am. Trop. Med. Hyg. **8:** 644–722.
3. OGATA, A.K., K. NAGASHIMA, W.W. HALL, *et al.* 1991. Japanese encephalitis virus neurotropism is dependent on the degree of neuronal maturity. J. Virol. **65:** 880–886.
4. WEBSTER, L.T. 1923. Microbic virulence and host susceptibility in mouse typhoid infection. J. Exp. Med. **37:** 231–244.
5. WEBSTER, L.T. 1933. Inherited and acquired factors in resistance to infection. I. Development of resistant and susceptible lines of mice through selective breeding. J. Exp. Med. **57:** 793–817.
6. WEBSTER, L.T. 1937. Inheritance of resistance of mice to enteric bacterial and neurologic virus infections. J. Exp. Med. **65:** 261–286.
7. DARNELL, M.B., H. KOPROWSKI & K. LAGERSPETZ. 1974. Genetically determined resistance to infection with group B arboviruses. I. Distribution of the resistance gene

among various mouse populations and characteristics of gene expression in vivo. J. Infect. Dis. **129:** 240–247.

8. GROSCHEL, D. & H. KOPROWSKI. 1965. Development of a virus-resistant inbred mouse strain for the study of innate resistance to arbo B viruses. Arch. Gesamte Virusforsch. **17:** 379–391.

9. SANGSTER, M.Y. & G.R. SHELLAM. 1986. Genetically controlled resistance to flaviviruses within the house mouse complex of species. Curr. Top. Microbiol. Immunol. **127:** 313–318.

10. SANGSTER, M.Y., D.B. HELIAMS, J.S. MACKENZIE & G.R. SHELLAM. 1993. Genetic studies of flavivirus resistance in inbred strains derived from wild mice: evidence for a new resistance allele at the flavivirus resistance locus (Flv). J. Virol. **67:** 340–347.

11. VANIO, T. 1963. Virus and hereditary resistance in vitro. I. Behavior of West Nile (E-101) virus in the cultures prepared from genetically resistant and susceptible strains of mice. Ann. Med. Exp. Biol. Fenn. **41:** 1–24.

12. GOODMAN, G.T. & H. KOPROWSKI. 1962. Macrophages as a cellular expression of inherited natural resistance. Proc. Natl. Acad. Sci. USA **48:** 160–165.

13. BRINTON, M.A., I. KURANE, A. MATHEW, et al. 1998. Immune mediated and inherited defences against flaviviruses. Clin. Diagn. Virol. **15:** 129–139.

14. BHATT, P.N. & R.O. JACOBY. 1976. Genetic resistance to lethal flavivirus encephalitis. II. Effect of immunosuppression. J. Infect. Dis. **134:** 166–173.

15. DARNELL, M.B. & H. KOPROWSKI. 1974. Genetically determined resistance to infection with group B arboviruses. II. Increased production of interfering particles in cell cultures from resistant mice. J. Infect. Dis. **129:** 248–256.

16. BRINTON, M.A., H. ARNHEITER & O. HALLER. 1982. Interferon independence of genetically controlled resistance to flaviviruses. Infect. Immun. **36:** 284–288.

17. BRINTON, M.A. 1983. Analysis of extracellular West Nile virus (WNV) particles produced by cell cultures from genetically resistant and susceptible mice indicates enhanced amplification of DI particles by resistant cultures. J. Virol. **46:** 860–870.

18. WEBSTER, L.T. & M.S. JOHNSON. 1941. Comparative virulence of St. Louis encephalitis virus cultured with brain tissue from innately susceptible and innately resistant mice. J. Exp. Med. **74:** 489–494.

19. JERRELLS, T.R. & J.V. OSTERMAN. 1981. Host defenses in experimental scrub typhus: inflammatory response of congenic C3H mice differing at the Ric gene. Infect. Immun. **31:** 1014–1022.

20. SANGSTER, M.Y., N. UROSEVIC, J.P. MANSFIELD, et al. 1994. Mapping the Flv locus controlling resistance to flaviviruses on mouse chromosome 5. J. Virol. **68:** 448–452.

21. SHELLEM, G.R., N. UROSEVIC, M.Y. SANGSTER, et al. 1993. Characterization of allelic forms at the retinal degeneration (rd) and β-glucuronidase (Gus) loci for the mapping of the flavivirus resistance (Flv) gene on mouse chromosome 5. Mouse Genome **91:** 572–574.

22. UROSEVIC, N., J.P. MANSFIELD, J.S. MACKENZIE & G.R. SHELLEM. 1995. Low resolution mapping around the flavivirus locus (Flv) on mouse chromosome 5. Mamm. Genome **6:** 454–458.

23. BRINTON, M.A. & J.H. DISPOTO. 1988. Sequence and secondary structure analysis of the 5′ terminal region of flavivirus genome RNA. Virology **162:** 290–299.

24. BRINTON, M.A., A.V. FERNANDEZ & J.H. DISPOTO. 1986. The 3′-nucleotides of flavivirus genome RNA form a conserved secondary structure. Virology **153:** 113–121.

25. SHI, P.Y., W. LI & M.A. BRINTON. 1996. Cell proteins bind specifically to West Nile virus minus-strand 3′ stem-loop RNA. J. Virol. **70:** 6278–6287.

26. SHI, P.Y., M.A. BRINTON, J.M. VEAL & W.D. WILSON. 1996. Evidence for the existence of a pseudoknot structure at the 3′ terminus of the flavivirus genomic RNA. Biochemistry **35:** 4222–4230.

27. MEN, R., M. BRAY, D. CLARK, et al. 1996. Dengue type 4 virus mutants containing deletions in the 3′ noncoding region of RNA genome: analysis of growth restriction in cell culture and altered viremia pattern and immunogenicity in rhesus monkeys. J. Virol. **70:** 3930–3937.

28. ZENG, L., B. FALGOUT & L. MARKOFF. 1998. Identification of specific nucleotide sequences within the conserved 3'-SL in the dengue type 2 virus genome required for replication. J. Virol. **72:** 7510–7522.
29. BLACKWELL, J.L. & M.A. BRINTON. 1995. BHK cell proteins that bind to the 3' stem-loop structure of the West Nile virus genome RNA. J. Virol. **69:** 5650–5658.
30. BLACKWELL, J.L. & M.A. BRINTON. 1997. Translation elongation factor-1 alpha interacts with the 3' stem-loop region of West Nile virus genomic RNA. J. Virol. **74:** 6433–6444.
31. RIIS, B., S.I. RATTAN, B.F. CLARK & W.C. MERRICK. 1990. Eukaryotic protein elongation factors. Trends Biochem. Sci. **15:** 429–424.
32. YAMSHCHIKOV, V.F., G. WENGLER, A.A. PERELYGIN, *et al.* 2001. An infectious clone of the West Nile flavivirus. Virology **281:** 294–304.
33. SACHS, A.B., P. SARNOW & M.W. HENTZE. 1997. Starting at the beginning, middle, and end: translation initiation in eukaryotes. Cell **89:** 831–838.
34. DIEZ, J., M. ISHIKAWA, M. KAIDO & P. AHLQUIST. 2000. Identification and characterization of a host protein required for efficient template selection in viral RNA replication. Proc. Natl. Acad. Sci. USA **97:** 3913–3918.
35. VENDE, P., M. PIRON, N. CASTAGNE & D. PONCET. 2000. Efficient translation of rotavirus mRNA requires simultaneous interaction of NSP3 with eukaryotic translation initiation factor eIF4G and the mRNA 3' end. J. Virol. **74:** 7064–7071.
36. LI, W. & M.A. BRINTON. 2001. The 3' stem loop of the West Nile virus genomic RNA can suppress translation of chimeric mRNAs. Virology **287:** 49–61.
37. KHROMYKH, A.A., H. MEKA, K.J. GUYATT & E.G. WESTAWAY. 2001. Essential role of cyclization sequences in flavivirus RNA replication. J. Virol. **75:** 6719–6728.

Structure and Seasonality of Nearctic *Culex pipiens* Populations

ANDREW SPIELMAN

*Department of Immunology and Infectious Diseases, Harvard School of Public Health,
Boston, Massachusetts 02115, USA*

ABSTRACT: The abundance and structure of urban autogenous and anautogenous populations of *Culex pipiens* mosquitoes were documented systematically in Boston, MA, during three successive years. Autogenous larvae become abundant mainly in enclosed sites and anautogenous larvae in sites that provide free access and egress. Both populations begin to proliferate when the water temperature exceeds 15 °C during June. Larval anautogenous mosquitoes increase in abundance 10-fold in two weeks and autogenous in three weeks. Although anautogenous larvae rapidly disappear after mid-August when winter diapause commences, the abundance of autogenous larvae continues to increase until mid-October. The forms generally are reproductively isolated in nature but occasionally hybridize during August and thereafter. Anautogenous females feed mainly on birds; autogenous females generally never feed on blood; and hybrid females appear to feed indiscriminately on avian or mammalian hosts. Such northern *C. p. pipiens* mosquitoes range as far south as 33°N. Taken together, these observations suggest that *C. p. pipiens*–borne pathogens may proliferate in the northern United States until mid-August and affect human hosts thereafter. Intensity of transmission decreases toward the south.

KEYWORDS: West Nile virus; *Culex pipiens* populations; autogenous populations; larval anautogenous mosquitoes

INTRODUCTION

The recent introduction of West Nile virus into urban sites in eastern North America has directed public health attention toward the members of the *Culex p. pipiens* complex of mosquitoes,[1] the main presumed vectors of this infection. These insects appear to transmit this arboviral pathogen among birds because they are ornithophilic, competent as hosts for the pathogen,[2] frequently infected in nature, and are the main species of mosquito present where and when human infection is most frequent.[3] Efforts to protect the public health frequently involve intensive insecticidal applications directed against these mosquitoes.

The environmental factors that influence the abundance and host-seeking behavior of mosquitoes in the *C. p. pipiens* complex of populations were subjects of in-

Address for correspondence: Andrew Spielman, ScD. Department of Immunology and Infectious Diseases, Harvard School of Public Health, 665 Huntington Avenue, Boston, MA 02115. Voice: 617-432-2058; fax: 617-432-1796.
aspielma@hsph.harvard.edu

tense study during the mid-twentieth century. Mattingly assembled a series of reports on the subject in 1951 that inspired numerous additional studies,[4] including my own early contributions, and an international conference on this subject that was convened by the World Health Organization in 1964. Interest in these insects subsequently declined because their populations in the temperate zone appeared to feed on people only rarely and because their public health importance seemed minimal. Vinogradova's recent monograph on these insects, for example, cites relatively few publications dating to the 1990s.[5] This treatment focuses on the Eurasian experience, while devoting little attention to the structure and seasonal dynamics of *C. p. pipiens* populations in North America, where West Nile virus has become endemic. Although it attracted much media attention, a 1998 English study on the structure of these populations omitted discussion of the relevant North American experience.[6] A biological rationale for antivector interventions against this emergent disease in northeastern North America, therefore, is lacking.

To provide a public health rationale for anti-West Nile interventions in this newly endemic Nearctic region, I shall synthesize information that I published nearly a half century ago concerning the structure and seasonal dynamics of *C. p. pipiens* populations infesting a site in Boston, MA, located 2 km from the epicenter of the outbreak of West Nile virus infection that occurred in 2000. In particular, I shall identify conditions that appear to lead toward virus amplification and transmission to human hosts. At the time that this work was performed, these mosquitoes appeared to be harmless to the inhabitants of this urban environment. This experimental design cannot now be reapplied because these insects no longer can be considered innocuous.

GENERAL METHODS

The study site was located on the Harvard Medical School campus in an urban section of the city of Boston. Larvae were sampled systematically at least once a week throughout a three-year period from three sites, designated as the "catch basin," "air shaft" and "pit." Larval density and water temperature were recorded. A sample of the larvae were reared through to the adult stage and the resulting females individually confined over water without food. Those that failed to oviposit were dissected in order to determine the degree of ovarian development. Adults were sampled from the nearby "phone booth" and "tunnel" sites. The contents of their abdomens was judged by their external appearance and classified as "distended with blood" or "hypertrophic fat," and those that were slender were considered to be "flat." A sample of flat females was induced to gorge from capillary tubes on defibrinated chicken blood. Others were dissected to ascertain the developmental stage of their ovaries. A sample of blood-gorged females were dissected, the gut contents smeared on a microscope slide and stained with Giemsa stain.

Density of larvae was estimated by dipping a pair of 300 mL containers alternately into the water in a breeding site in a manner calculated to derive the greatest possible number of larvae. After each dip, the contents of the dipper was compared to that of the previous dip. The dipper containing fewer larvae was then discarded and the other retained. The process was repeated 10 times, and the larvae in the last remaining dipper were counted and the total recorded.

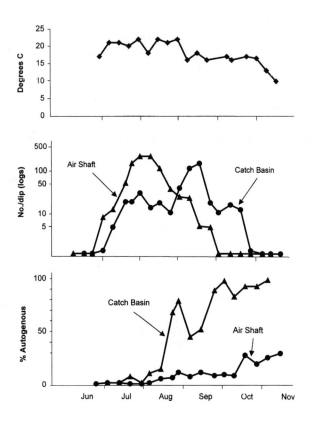

FIGURE 1. Seasonal abundance and proportion of autogenous larval *C. p. pipiens* breeding in the air shaft and catch basin sites in Boston, MA (part of a figure in Ref. 9; reproduced with permission). Larvae were reared to the adult stage and tested individually.

OBSERVATIONS

Characteristics of Autogenous Populations

Samples derived from laboratory colonies of autogenous *C. p. pipiens* differ genetically from those comprised of anautogenous mosquitoes. Genes regulating autogenous development are located on both autosomes.[7] When isolated in a container containing a little water, virtually all female pupae taken from an autogenous colony develop into adults that develop mature eggs when deprived of food. Virgin females would generally fail to oviposit. The ovaries of females derived from pupae isolated from an anautogenous colony fail to develop beyond the yolk-competent stage of development. Such an ovarian follicle contains an oocyte that is covered by a well-developed oolemma, including a mature microvillar coat.[8] F1 hybrid progenies include similar numbers of females that (1) produce mature eggs (stage V), (2) commence vitellogenesis but cease egg maturation before the eggs are mature (stage III or IV), or (3) cease ovarian development in the yolk-competent stage (stage IIb). Genetically autogenous females can thereby be distinguished from anautogenous females as well as from hybrid females by examining their offspring.

Seasonal Abundance

The density of larvae in the air shaft and catch basin sites was recorded as well as the proportion of the derived adults that commenced vitellogenesis in the absence of food.[9] Larvae first became evident in the catch basin and air shaft sites in June or July when the water temperature came to exceed 15°C and were most abundant in August. They were no longer evident in these exposed sites after the beginning of October, when the water cooled to less than 15°C (FIG. 1, illustrating the second of three similar years of observation). Larvae in the air shaft were consistently more autogenous than were those in the catch basin, and their density rose more rapidly. Larvae in the relatively autogenous catch basin became most abundant in September, more than a month after those in the air shaft began to decline. More autogenous larvae develop in the relatively open air shaft site than in the enclosed catch basin site; the density of anautogenous larvae begins to wane on 10 August at 42° latitude, when day length decreases to about 14 h 15 minutes.

The rate of increase of autogenous larvae was compared to that of anautogenous larvae by analyzing the ascending segments of the curves representing the growth of the populations infesting the catch basin and air shaft sites in each of three years of observation.[9] The anautogenous components in each of these sites during each of these years multiplied far more rapidly than did the autogenous populations (FIG. 2). Anautogenous larvae increased 10-fold in two weeks while the autogenous larvae did so in three weeks.

The density and degree of autogeny in adult mosquitoes sampled by aspirator from the phone booth site were recorded throughout the three-year period of study.[9] The first mosquitoes that appeared there were noted in June, and autogenous mosquitoes predominated among them (FIG. 3, illustrating the second of three similar years of observation). Anautogenous females and somewhat fewer males (autogenous status not determined) were most abundant at the end of July and early in August. Autogenous mosquitoes became most numerous there in September. The abundance of mosquitoes in this semisheltered resting site reflects the emergence of mosquitoes in the nearby air shaft site.

Winter Diapause

In a series of laboratory experiments, the degree of ovarian development was described in mosquitoes exposed to a short diel.[10] Specimens from autogenous as well as anautogenous laboratory colonies isolated in the catch basin and air shaft study sites were used in these experiments. Mature larvae were reared at 18°C and cohorts subjected to a graduated series of diels. The ovaries of virtually all anautogenous females that were limited to 8 h of light per day developed only to the previtellogenic stage. Primary follicles are about as long as secondary follicles. The oolemma of the oocytes in such females is devoid of microvilli.[8] Further development (to the yolk-competent stage) requires juvenile hormone stimulation.[11] By contrast, the ovaries

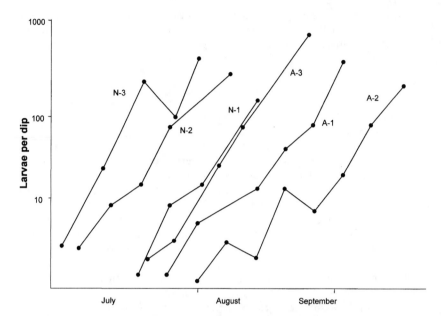

FIGURE 2. Development of larval autogenous (A) and anautogenous (N) *C. p. pipiens* breeding in the air shaft and catch basin sites in Boston, MA (part of a figure in Ref. 9; reproduced with permission). Adults were fed blood from capillary tubes and permitted to deposit eggs; their larvae were reared, and a sample of the resulting adults were tested individually.

TABLE 1. Degree of ovarian development in food-deprived adult *C. p. pipiens* mosquitoes derived from autogenous or from anautogenous larvae that were reared under short day length (8 h/day) and under long day length (16 h/day) conditions[13]

Kind	No. of hours light/day	No. females	Percent in diapause
Anautogenous	8	33	97.0
	16	36	8.3
Autogenous	8	19	0
	16	14	0

of almost all females exposed to 16 h of light per day developed to the yolk-competent stage (TABLE 1).[12] About a third of the adults that emerged from larvae held at 14 h 15 m developed into adults whose ovaries remained in the previtellogenic (FIG. 4). Ovaries of diapausing *C. pipiens* mosquitoes ceased development in response to a short diel and had yolk-incompetent ovarioles that had not been stimulated by juvenile hormone.

External evidence of hibernation was sought by examining the abdomens of adult females captured while they were resting in the phone booth site.[13] Resting adults were most abundant there late in October (FIG. 5). Freshly blood-gorged females ini-

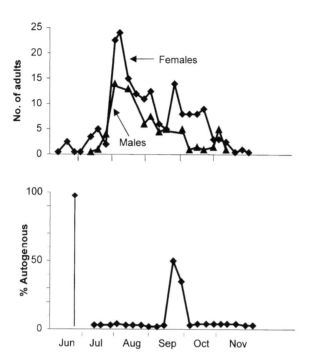

FIGURE 3. Seasonal abundance and proportion autogenous adult *C. p. pipiens* resting in the phone booth site located in Boston, MA (part of a figure in Ref. 9; reproduced with permission). Adults were fed blood from capillary tubes and permitted to deposit eggs; their larvae were reared, and a sample of the resulting adults were tested individually.

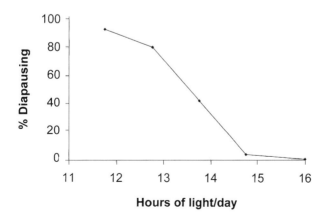

FIGURE 4. Effect of photoperiod on the development of gonoactive ovaries in larval *C. p. pipiens* derived from an anautogenous colony isolated in Boston, MA.[10]

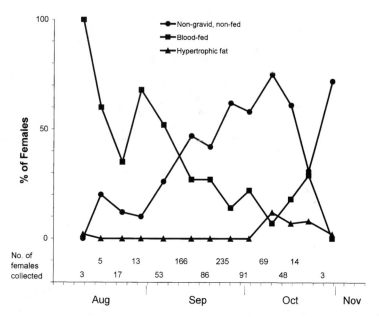

FIGURE 5. Condition of adult *C. p. pipiens* resting in the phone booth site located in Boston, MA (part of a figure in Ref. 13; reproduced with permission).

tially predominated, and some were present throughout October. A few females whose abdomens were distended with hypertrophic fat bodies became evident in October. Evidence of diapause was more evident in females taken in the underground tunnel site in October (data not shown). Half of the fat-containing females were dissected and their ovaries examined microscopically. The ovaries of these females were invariably arrested in stage 0. Blood-gorged females are most abundant early in the fall and diapausing females late in the fall.

Evidence of ovarian diapause was sought in mosquitoes captured in the tunnel site.[13] Female mosquitoes with previtellogenic ovaries first appeared in August, and the proportion of females expressing this sign of diapause increased with the onset of winter (FIG. 6). The proportion of females in this site whose abdomens were distended with fat increased rapidly during the month of September, and virtually all mosquitoes contained hypertrophic fat bodies by the end of that month. The ovaries of many of these mosquitoes contained scars that suggested previous deposition of eggs. Ovarian diapause is characterized by previtellogenic ovaries and hypertrophic fat bodies, and many females appear to enter diapause after developing and depositing their first clutch of eggs.

To determine whether autogenous *C. p. pipiens* mosquitoes would breed continuously throughout the winter, larvae were sampled systematically from the pit site.[9] Temperature of the water contained in this subterranean reservoir of stagnant water remained above 18°C between October and April. Adults reared from larvae sampled from this site generally produced eggs autogenously (FIG. 7). Anautogenous females were reared from larvae that were sampled mainly before the onset of winter.

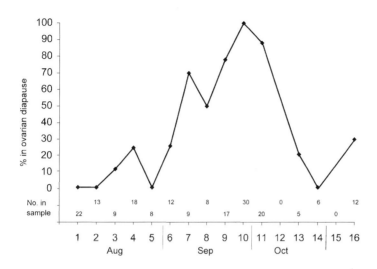

FIGURE 6. Proportion of female *C. p. pipiens* captured in the tunnel site whose ovaries were considered to be in the diapause stage (stage 0) (part of a figure from Ref. 13; reproduced with permission[13]).

Mixed progenies containing autogenous as well as anautogenous individuals were discovered mainly during midwinter. These were considered to be the progeny of heterozygous females. The ovaries of these females commenced vitellogenesis but ceased maturation before their eggs had matured (stage V). In sheltered sites, winter-breeding mosquitoes tend to be autogenous or heterozygous for this characteristic.

Blood-feeding Behavior

To determine whether these mosquitoes were parasitizing human hosts, blood-gorged females collected in the phone booth and tunnel sites were subjected to serological testing.[13] Of 184 females tested in this manner, only five contained human blood. These human-feeding mosquitoes were found during one week of observation (in September) when a guard stationed nearby complained of an episode of mosquito bites. In addition, fresh blood found in the midguts of 40 additional specimens was smeared on slides, stained with Giemsa, and examined microscopically. Each specimen contained nucleated, avian blood, and many contained red cells infected by *Plasmodium* sp. Birds provide the main source of vertebrate blood for these mosquitoes.

An additional episode of human biting occurred during the course of this study, in the pit during midwinter.[14] Females that fed on a human host were permitted to engorge and to produce progenies. Of these 13 blood-gorged mosquitoes, seven produced wholly autogenous progenies, and six produced progenies that appeared to be heterozygous. Some of the resulting first generation females matured their eggs, while others failed to undergo vitellogenesis or produced partially developed eggs. These mosquitoes appeared to be autogenous-anautogenous heterozygotes. Epi-

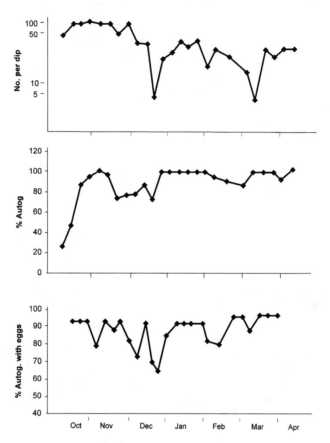

FIGURE 7. Density of larval *C. p. pipiens* and proportion autogenous throughout the winter in water contained in the pit site located in Boston, MA (part of a figure in Ref. 9; reproduced with permission).

sodes of human biting appear to be associated with episodes of interbreeding between these *C. pipiens* variants.

Population Structure

To determine whether adult mosquitoes found resting in the phone booth and tunnel sites were derived from panmictic but separate autogenous or anautogenous populations, a sample of flat adult mosquitoes found resting there during the summer and fall were fed blood from capillary tubes and their progenies reared through to the adult stage.[14] Of the 353 females that were subject to progeny tests, most were homozygous anautogenous (304) and some homozygous autogenous.[43] Only a few (6) gave rise to families that included autogenous as well as anautogenous mosqui-

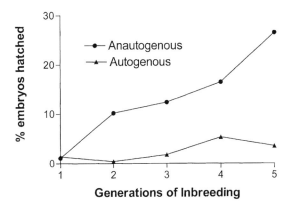

Generations of Inbreeding

FIGURE 8. Effect of successive generations of brother–sister inbreeding on the embryonic development of autogenous and of anautogenous *C. p. pipiens* captured in various sites located in Boston, MA (part of a figure in Ref 15; reproduced with permission).

toes. All of those mosquitoes that contained ingested blood when they were captured gave rise to anautogenous offspring. The autogenous mosquitoes in this site interbreed only infrequently with anautogenous mosquitoes.

To determine whether autogenous populations tend to be more clonal than are anautogenous populations, progenies were reared from females sampled in the phone booth and tunnel sites and subjected to a regimen of continuous brother–sister inbreeding.[15] Autogenous mosquitoes lines were maintained readily through the sixth filial generation, while anautogenous lines generally were lost before this level of inbreeding was complete. Embryonated eggs derived from anautogenous females, for example, failed to hatch increasingly with successive generations (FIG. 8). Anautogenous progenies are more sensitive to inbreeding than are those derived from autogenous parents, thereby indicating that autogenous populations in nature tend to be more clonal than are anautogenous populations.

DISCUSSION

In general, autogenous *C. p. pipiens* mosquitoes are associated with breeding sites that provide only limited access and egress for these insects. The catch basin and pit sites in the present study have those characteristics. The catch basin drains water from the street through a narrow slit in the curb, and that opening frequently is clogged by debris. The reservoir of water within the site is not visible from the street itself. The pit is located in the basement of an institutional building. The set of windows that provides ventilation for this space is left open, except during midwinter. The air shaft, by contrast, is located out-of-doors, and its reservoir of contained water is visible from the street. Indeed, degree of access and egress of a site correlates strongly with anautogeny, because these mosquitoes mate in association with male swarms and must leave the site in order to find vertebrate hosts.

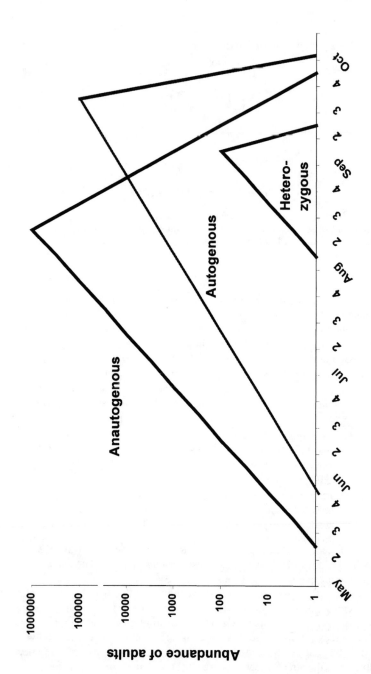

FIGURE 9. Conceptual model of the pattern of increase in the abundance of larval autogenous and of anautogenous *C. p. pipiens* in Boston, MA. The model assumes that anautogenous mosquitoes increase 10-fold in two weeks, that autogenous mosquitoes do so in three weeks, that development commences when the water temperature exceeds 15°C, and that anautogenous females fail to reproduce when day length is less than 14 h 15 m.

Although autogenous *C. p. pipiens* mosquitoes generally coexist sympatrically with anautogenous mosquitoes, and they intermate readily in the laboratory, they generally remain genetically isolated in nature. In part, this isolation is due to differences in their breeding sites. In addition, anautogenous mosquitoes are said to be "eurygamous," meaning that their mating requires a space large enough to permit unrestricted flight.[16] "Stenogamous" autogenous mosquitoes can mate in containers that are so small that opportunity for flight activity is denied. Genetic isolation between these populations is further insured by the reproductive inhibition that is evident in the progeny resulting from hybridization events. About a third are functionally autogenous and a third anautogenous. Vitellogenesis commences in the remaining third of hybrid females but without formation of mature eggs.[7] Such mosquitoes are functionally sterile.

New infestations of autogenous *C. p. pipiens* mosquitoes appear to be founded by fewer females than are anautogenous infestations. They are capable of mating and producing eggs without leaving the site and are likely to produce clonal populations. Indeed, the relative insusceptibility of autogenous mosquitoes to inbreeding depression confirms their essentially inbreeding mode of perpetuation. The effective population size of anautogenous mosquitoes, on the other hand, appears to be much larger. We have applied allozyme technology to populations of these mosquitoes and find that loci of autogenous mosquitoes are far more likely to be fixed than are those of anautogenous *C. pipiens* (unpublished). Each autogenous infestation would be unique.

A model designed to represent these autogenous-anautogenous relationships is presented in FIGURE 9. The representation is based on the observation that eggs fail to embryonate when the water temperature falls below 15°C, that anautogenous mosquitoes generally fail to produce eggs when day length falls below 14 h 15 m, that anautogenous density generally increases 10-fold in two weeks and autogenous density in three weeks, and that intermating between the populations commences mainly when anautogenous males most outnumber autogenous males. Episodes of human biting appear to accompany episodes of interbreeding, and such events might be most likely when anautogenous males most outnumber autogenous males. If these considerations are correct, a complex of *C. p. pipiens* vector populations at latitude 42° would provide a seasonal "window" for amplifying West Nile virus among birds mainly during mid-May through mid-August, assuming favorable weather conditions. The same complex of mosquitoes would provide the "bridge vector" population that would carry the agent between its avian reservoir population and human hosts. The model (FIG. 9) suggests that antimosquito interventions or flushing rains occurring during June or July would reduce the force of transmission among birds while also reducing the likelihood that intermating events might induce the resulting mosquitoes to feed on people.

These considerations also suggest that latitude may profoundly limit the force of transmission of West Nile virus in North America. When reared at a short diel,[12,10,13,17] the ovaries of anautogenous *C. p. pipiens* lack the juvenile hormone signal[11] that stimulates formation of a yolk-competent oolemma.[8] To the extent that anautogenous *C. pipiens* mosquitoes enter diapause in response to a short diel, the duration of the permissive breeding season will become progressively shorter with proximity to the equator. The length of the period that includes days that are 14 h 15 m long decreases sharply in the Middle Atlantic states and becomes nil at 32°N (FIG. 10). The duration of the permissive

Light >14.5h15m/day

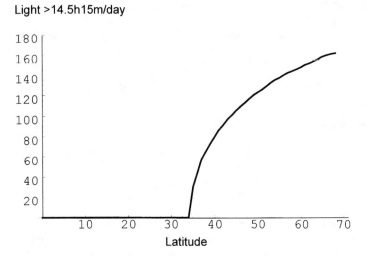

FIGURE 10. Effect of latitude on the number of days each year that include at least 14 h 15 m of daylight.

period, however, decreases as latitude increases. This consideration suggests that the force of transmission of West Nile virus may increase toward the north of the New York City epicenter of this outbreak and decrease toward the south. An extension of the range of West Nile virus into more southern parts of North America remains in doubt.

Byrne and Nichols' allozyme analysis confirms,[6] without citation, my prior finding that autogenous populations tend to perpetuate by inbreeding, anautogenous populations by outbreeding, and that interbreeding is infrequent.[15] I demonstrated that individual breeding sites frequently contain autogenous as well as anautogenous larvae and that autogeny predominates as the season progresses. In my opinion, their observations are flawed because they characterized their study subjects by mass-examining samples of larvae from various breeding sites, without regard to season. They considered an entire population to be autogenous if any mosquito reared from the site at any time of year produced even a single egg raft. If the sampled mosquitoes deposited no eggs, the site would be characterized as anautogenous. Without evidence, they assumed that any autogenous mosquito would be anthropophilic and incapable of diapause.

In the course of this work, I established the biological basis for the hormonomimetic insecticide that is now used most extensively for eliminating sources of C. pipiens breeding.[18,19] Mosquitoes, for the first time, were exposed to the preparation that later served as the model for synthesizing methoprene, then known as the Williams-Law mixture. I discovered that mosquitoes were vulnerable to this insecticide during their fourth larval instar, that nonviable juvenilized pupae would develop from treated larvae, and that adult ecdysis and terminalic rotation would be inhibited. The first semifield trials were conducted, and slow-release, plaster of paris formulations were field tested.[20,21]

Populations of *C. p. pipiens* mosquitoes are structured in a complex manner, with genetically isolated autogenous populations coexisting sympatrically with sibling anautogenous populations.[22] Anautogenous populations enter diapause in response to a photoperiodic cue and are almost exclusively ornithophilic. These vector mosquitoes and the force of transmission of West Nile virus may increase as latitude increases and may wane at lower latitudes. Transmission of West Nile virus may increase as anautogenous *C. p. pipiens* proliferate, and occasional episodes of interbreeding between these mosquitoes may provide the epidemiological bridge that results in human infection and disease.

ACKNOWLEDGMENTS

This work was supported in part by National Institutes of Health Grant #RO1 AI 44064.

REFERENCES

1. CARTTER, M. 2001. Human West Nile virus surveillance—Connecticut, New Jersey, and New York, 2000. Morb. Mortal. Wkly. Rep. **50:** 265–268.
2. TURRELL, M.J., M. O'GUINN & J.A. OLIVER. 2000. Potential for New York mosquitoes to transmit West Nile virus. Am. J. Trop. Med. Hyg. **62:** 413–414.
3. ANDERSON, J.F., T.G. ANDREADIS, C.R. VOSSBRINCK, *et al.* 2000. Isolation of West Nile virus from mosquitoes, crows, and a Cooper's hawk in Connecticut. Science **286:** 2331–2333.
4. MATTINGLY, P.F. 1951. The *Culex pipiens* complex. Trans. R. Entomol. Soc. Lond. **102:** 331–382.
5. VINOGRADOVA, E.B. 2000. *Culex pipiens pipiens* mosquitoes: taxonomy, distribution, ecology, physiology, genetics, applied importance and control. Pensoft. Sofia-Moscow. 250 pp.
6. BYRNE, K. & R.A. NICHOLS. 1998. *Culex pipiens* in London underground tunnels: differentiation between surface and subterranean populations. Heredity **82:** 7–15.
7. SPIELMAN, A. 1957. The inheritance of autogeny in the *Culex pipiens* complex of mosquitoes. Am. J. Hyg. **65:** 404–425.
8. ANDERSON, W.A. & A. SPIELMAN. 1973. Incorporation of RNA and protein precursors by ovarian follicles of *Aedes aegypti* mosquitoes. J. Submicrosc. Cytol. **5:** 181–198.
9. SPIELMAN, A. 1971. Studies on autogeny in natural populations of *Culex pipiens*. II. Seasonal abundance of autogenous and anautogenous populations. J. Med. Entomol. **8:** 555–561.
10. SPIELMAN, A. & J. WONG. 1973(a). Studies on autogeny in natural populations of *Culex pipiens*. III. Mid-summer preparation for hibernation in anautogenous populations. J Med. Entomol. **10:** 319–324.
11. SPIELMAN, A. 1974. Effect of synthetic juvenile hormone on ovarian diapause of *Culex pipiens* mosquitoes. J. Med. Entomol. **11:** 223–225.
12. ELDRIDGE, B.F. 1968. The effect of temperature and photoperiod on blood-feeding and ovarian development in mosquitoes of the *Culex pipiens* complex. Am. J. Trop. Med. Hyg. **17:** 133–140.
13. SPIELMAN, A. & J. WONG. 1973(b). Environmental control of ovarian diapause in *Culex pipiens* mosquitoes. Ann. Entomol. Soc. Am. **66:** 905–907.
14. SPIELMAN, A. 1964. Studies on autogeny in *Culex pipiens* populations in nature. I. Reproductive isolation between autogenous and anautogenous populations. Am. J. Hyg. **80:** 175–183.
15. SPIELMAN, A. 1979. Autogeny in *Culex pipiens* populations in nature: effects of inbreeding. Ann. Entomol. Soc. Am. **72:** 826–828.

16. ROUBAUD, E. 1929. Cycle autogène d'attente et generations hivernales suractives inapparentes chez le moustique commun, *Culex pipiens* L. C.R. Acad. Sci. Fr. **188:** 735–738.
17. SANBURG, L.L. & J.R. LARSON. 1973. Effect of photoperiod and temperature on ovarian development of *Culex pipiens pipiens.* J. Insect. Physiol. **19:** 1173–1190.
18. SPIELMAN, A. & C.M. WILLIAMS. 1966. Lethal effects of synthetic juvenile hormone on larvae of the yellow fever mosquito, *Aedes aegypti.* Science **154:** 1043–1044.
19. SPIELMAN, A. & V. SKAFF. 1967. Inhibition of metamorphosis and of ecdysis in mosquitoes. J. Insect. Physiol. **13:** 1087–1095.
20. SPIELMAN, A. 1970. Synthetic juvenile hormones as larvicides for mosquitoes. Industry Trop. Health **7:** 67–70.
21. SPIELMAN, A. & E. ST. ONGE. 1974. Stability of exogenous juvenile hormone: effect of larval mosquitoes. Env. Entomol. **3:** 259–261.
22. SPIELMAN, A. & J.G. KITZMILLER. 1967. The genetics of populations of medically important Arthropods. J.R. Wright & R. Pal, Eds.: 459–485. Elsevier. Amsterdam.

Interventions: Vector Control and Public Education

Panel Discussion

ROGER S. NASCI , *Moderator*
Division of Vector-Borne Infectious Diseases,
Centers for Disease Control and Prevention, Fort Collins, Colorado 80522, USA

NOLAN H. NEWTON, *Moderator*
Public Health Pest Management Section,
North Carolina Department of Environment and Natural Resources,
Raleigh, North Carolina 27699-1613, USA

GREGORY F. TERRILLION
Nassau County Mosquito Control, Roosevelt, New York 11575, USA

RAY E. PARSONS
Harris County Mosquito Control,
Public Health and Environmental Services, Houston, Texas 77021, USA

DAVID A. DAME
American Mosquito Control Association, Gainesville, Florida 32605, USA

JAMES R. MILLER
Vector-Borne Disease Surveillance and Control,
New York City Department of Health, New York, New York 10013, USA

DOMINICK V. NINIVAGGI
Vector Control, Suffolk County Department of Public Works,
Yaphank, New York 11980, USA

ROBERT KENT
Office of Mosquito Control Coordination,
New Jersey Department of Environmental Protection,
Trenton, New Jersey 08625-0402, USA

ROGER S. NASCI: We've assembled a panel of people with a wide variety of experiences and expertise. The topics that we've been asked to address in the next ninety minutes are quite broad: education and behavior modification, mosquito habitat modification, biological intervention, chemical intervention, and novel approaches. I'm an entomologist with the Centers for Disease Control. My co-moderator, at the other end of the table, is Dr. Nolan Newton. He's the chief of the Public Health Pest Management Section in the North Carolina Department of Environment and Natural

Resources, and he also brings with him a large body of experience with public health issues, including mosquitoes and other vectors. Each of our panelists will be given a few minutes to describe their experience with West Nile virus, or their experience and perspectives in general with vector control. Then we'll launch into a discussion of several of these topics and open up the floor for discussion from the attendants. Nolan Newton will now introduce the panelists.

NOLAN H. NEWTON: Thank you, Roger. Starting on my right is Mr. Gregory Terrillion with the Nassau County Mosquito Control Program in Roosevelt, New York. Next is Dr. Ray Parsons, Director of the Harris County Mosquito Control Program in Houston, Texas. Next to him is Dr. David Dame, President of the American Mosquito Control Association. Then comes Dr. Jim Miller from the Vector-Borne Disease Surveillance and Control with the New York City Department of Health. And, finally comes Mr. Dominick Ninivaggi, with Vector Control, Suffolk County Department of Public Works. Dominick will lead off.

DOMINICK V. NINIVAGGI: Suffolk County is a large suburban mosquito control district. We have a lot of different mosquito habitats, which gives us about 43 species of mosquitoes. We had the dubious distinction of having something like 25% of the 480 virus isolations of mosquitoes in 2000. We also assisted in 1999 in the New York City response. Our mosquito control program includes a lot of salt marsh and natural areas, and we have a very extensive water management program, which is going on right now. We have a great deal of larval control, visiting mosquito breeding sites due to the larviciding, and we have a small, but necessary, component for adult control.

In 2000, we were able to evaluate the bird data that were coming in and combine that with our experience with what we do about mosquitoes in Suffolk County and the surveillance that we did, and we were able to have a relatively localized response to West Nile virus. We were able to identify a part of the county that was particularly hot with the virus, and, while in most of the county, we did minimal treatments, for instance with adulticides and many areas that didn't require larviciding, in that area that we identified that did have intense virus activity, we used the full spectrum of interventions, ranging from ground larviciding, aerial larviciding, ground adult control, and aerial adult control. I think that this is the way we're going to have to respond to this virus in the future. Of course, we did conduct an extensive public education program, and we worked with the public to reduce their exposure to mosquitoes. As our understanding of this virus develops, it comes as no surprise that we're able to be a lot more focused and pointed when we need to do interventions. The key thing is the good surveillance program that we were able to put together. I will be very interested to see what happens in 2001, because I can almost guarantee that it'll be very different from the previous couple of years. That much we know about mosquito-borne virus. But as the season comes on, our main focus is to make sure we have good surveillance in place.

NEWTON: Thank you, Dom. Jim?

JAMES R. MILLER: I want to touch on five points of the issue of vector control and public education as it applies to New York City. I will quickly summarize the progression of mosquito control efforts that have taken place in New York City. As our knowledge about West Nile grows, we'll be able to better define periods of increased risk for human health effects. To summarize just briefly along the lines of what Dominick said about the whole issue of larval control, the public's participation in this process is related to another issue that is part of the environment, which is the deep mistrust of pesticide use in the United States.

The progression of mosquito control in New York City is one of having seen in 1999 an unexpected outbreak where there was emergency control of adult mosquitoes by the aerial application of adulticides over a large area. In 2000, having now anticipated the return of arboviral disease, we were able to begin with the traditional foundation type work that Dominick again described—the whole issue of larval control. We were able to begin to do that work in 2000, but it's not something that any locality is going to learn how to do effectively overnight. You can go into New York City, you can buy the American Institute of Architect's guide to buildings in New York, you can buy the Zagat's Guide to the restaurants in New York, but you can't get a guide to the mosquito breeding places in New York. We had to basically write that book ourselves last year. And then in place of aerial application, which I'm not trying to say would not work in New York City, we were able to do focal adult control of mosquitoes using trucks last year.

As we move forward into 2001, clearly we want to emphasize expanded larval control. If and when adult control is needed, it should be done in areas where there is demonstrated evidence of increased risk, which is the second point. Have we learned enough so that we can better define areas of increased risk? In 2000, adult mosquito control took place in New York City in proximity, often a two-mile radius, around a positive finding: a dead bird or an infected mosquito pool. A report would be followed 48–72 hours later by the application of adulticides in a two-mile radius. When one looks at the distribution of dead birds throughout the eastern portion of the United States, one realizes that that area was much greater than the area where human cases occurred. So the presence of a bird in an area, an infected bird, is not equivalent to extreme risk for adverse human impact. So we try to learn from our experience in 2000.

Using dead bird density, as Millie Eidson described, as well as mosquito surveillance findings in terms of anthropophilic infection, we think that mosquitoes that are infected with West Nile are at increased infection rates. We use that information to recognize what areas are at increased risk and at what time, and then conduct effective control of urban mosquitoes. I think it was very valuable to begin the discussion that started Thursday night, regarding efficacy monitoring in a systematic way, so that a number of localities can participate, because that's certainly an area about which we have questions. Again, larval control is going to be really important for us. When we started, Varuni Kulasekera, who is our entomologist, started to redescribe the spectrum of mosquitoes in New York; we didn't know when we started this time last year the species list for New York City mosquitoes, and there were certainly some surprises as the year went on in terms of what species were there, some not previously recorded.

Mapping larval habitats had to begin, and we have certainly natural areas that are easy to find, but then the enormous number of artificial containers required some effort as well. We have over 150,000 street corner storm drains. And when one looks into them, they basically all have a well that has two to three feet of water at the bottom. They're designed to hold water to keep floatables, those cans and styrofoam cups, from clogging the sewer lines. While the drains do that very well, they also provide a habitat for larval development to occur. You saw pictures in the presentation by Dennis White of swimming pools in Queens that were neglected. We estimate that about 10% of the swimming pools in New York City are not being cared for and are suitable for breeding mosquitoes. I think there was also a picture of used tires, and as Varuni and I drove up here this morning, we found yet another pile of tires in our own neighborhood.

The public's participation is really manifold. There are at least three ways in which we rely on the public to help with important issues. We talked about using dead bird density; those reports of dead birds that are used to come up with that rate of dead birds per week is largely a reflection of the public's participation. We have a data system that can collect that information, that can actually record where those dead birds are. As we go into 2001, we hope that we'll be able to use real time GIS mapping to be able to create the maps that show on a weekly basis what the density of dead birds is. We also rely on the public to report where there is standing water, which will hopefully be either eliminated or, if not, treated with larvicide. The third area is that we have asked the public to report when they suspect there have been adverse health affects due to pesticide spraying.

Again, let me close then on this final point, which is, again, this deep mistrust of pesticides. Certainly beginning in 1962 with Rachel Carson's *Silent Spring* on up through the presentation on PBS two weeks ago called *Trade Secrets: A Moyers Report*, chemicals are characterized in the United States as guilty until proven innocent. There is a great mistrust of pesticides. People feel that adverse health affects have been concealed from them and that industry has only reluctantly reported them. The New York City Department of Health is conducting an environmental impact study, and pesticide manufacturers have refused to disclose to us the inert ingredients because they are a "trade secret." In the report on the serosurveys that were done, one described by Tara McCarthy yesterday in Connecticut, there are nearly as many people afraid of pesticides as there are afraid of infection with West Nile. I think we have not yet devoted sufficient resources to gathering data to help answer the question of health effects. They may be much less than people fear, but without a dedicated effort to document what health affects there are, without the data, we're left with a lot of fearful people. I'm hopeful that we will be able to do more systematic surveillance for health effects monitoring at times when pesticides are used.

NEWTON: Thank you, Jim. David?

DAVID A. DAME: I'd like to address two subjects. One follows on what Jim had to say: the public anxiety over the use of public health pesticides, and the other topic is risk reduction by modification of human behavior, by community restriction on activities during epidemic times. The public animosity towards what I consider now to be the safest and most effective mosquito adulticides that we have is depressing in many ways. These pesticides have been selected over the last forty years out of perhaps two or three hundred different pesticides. The bad ones have been legislated out by state and federal legislatures. They've been taken off the market because of market strategy and because of bad results, and we're now down to just six adulticides that are available for public health use against mosquitoes. These six pesticides have been assessed by the EPA, which is our national agency for documenting the safety of these products for health and environmental purposes. These six products have been assessed as being at the level of no concern to the public and the environment. This level of no concern includes a minimum of a one hundred–fold safety factor between laboratory results and field exposure. These six compounds range between a one hundred–fold and a ten thousand–fold safety factor against the laboratory results.

The dichotomy in public response is interesting. In those areas in the United States that have experienced two or three decades of mosquito control, there is very little anxiety over the use of pesticides. In the areas where we are now introducing for the first time, in large scale, the use of these techniques, there is public anxiety. Much of the anxiety as I see it—and I've been exposed quite a bit during the last two years in my association with the American Mosquito Control Association—is coming from misinformation that is put out and orchestrated, I believe, by people who have a definite agenda. Press releases come out as a result of misinformation, which is being dispersed. I'm very fearful that the end result of the misinformation and the public perception of pesticide risk will eventually lead to the loss in use of these very safe compounds. And I can assure you, the industry will not replace them. They do not make a lot of money for industry; they're a side product; they exist because they do serve a public health purpose. Industry can make a small profit from them, but if we put too much pressure on industry, legally or otherwise, they won't produce these products, and we will not have them. There are no safe, inexpensive, probable molecules coming down the line for public health use. If we lose what we've got, we'll have to fall back on something else. I know that most mosquito control agencies want to use mosquito adulticides as their last resort. The best resort for mosquito control is starting at the beginning with source reduction, with larval control, and when that does not work either ground or aerial ULV [ultralow volume] applications are used. In many cases, the ground and aerial ULV application is necessary and is used.

I would like to make another point. The definition of a vector includes both an insect that annoys people and animals, and an insect that transmits disease. A vector by federal law is not just a transmitting insect. It's an annoying insect, and this is why these different procedures for controlling public health pests are used throughout the country. The definition fits this use. It's legal and appropriate. I think that we have to become very proactive in getting into the news and into the media the safety of the pesticides we're using, the rationale behind the safety, and the fact that probably none of us has the capacity to decide and determine, with available data, which pesticides are safe and which are not. This has been done by the process of selection over the years and done federally by the Environmental Protection Agency. There is documentation, and if the subject comes up, we can deal with that.

A second subject I'd like to deal with is the reduction of risk to individuals through personal protection and through community action. Yesterday Tara McCarthy showed results of a survey done in Connecticut indicating the public response to public service announcements. At the Charlotte West Nile virus meeting held by the CDC in February, the Florida group led by Lisa Conti gave a presentation on the impact of public service announcements in Florida. It's obvious that public service announcements can provide a great deal of help in reducing the risk during epidemic seasons. In Florida, on a regular basis, they use many different methods to control nuisance insects. When epidemic periods come along, public service announcements are put into effect, and they are very effective. They come through TV regularly; they come through the media and the newspapers, and they are continually in that area.

Additionally, Florida asks communities to be responsible regarding activities during epidemic seasons. Public service announcements, of course, ask people to use repellents, stay indoors during the active mosquito period, and wear clothes that protect them—a variety of different things to reduce their exposure to mosquitoes. In addition to that, the communities restrict outdoor activities. They call off baseball games; they stop outdoor exhibits. Disney World, you remember, shut down after 6:30 PM during the last SLE outbreak. When Disney World shuts down in the evening for an epidemic, they potentially lose a lot of money. They feel that this particular approach is very good, and the Florida and state and community public health departments are very supportive of this. They are the ones who initiate this activity. I would like to finish by saying that communities should organize community events so that the risk does not increase.

NEWTON: Thank you, Dave. Ray?

RAY E. PARSONS: I'd like to briefly tell you a little bit about Harris County Mosquito Control, which is in Houston, Texas. The program was started in 1965 in response to a St. Louis encephalitis outbreak that occurred in 1964. It was one of the few programs in the country up until West Nile virus hit up here where the mission was primarily vector control rather than nuisance mosquito control, and this is still the case. Most of our time, effort, and money is spent on the prevention and control of St. Louis encephalitis. When you send us West Nile virus down there, we'll be involved with that also. Probably we'll need a little more funding at that time. Our program is based primarily on surveillance; we have 248 locations in the county that we sample for mosquitoes. We have our own virology labs, and we can do the work in-house and get the information back to our control operation regarding active mosquito control. What I would like to do is throw out some questions or ideas that people can be thinking about regarding types of programs.

Before it slips my mind, something that Dave said during his presentation about misinformation reminded me of a situation that I just found out about. I got a call from a woman in Ohio, and she was wondering how we control mosquitoes in Harris County without using any insecticides, because the national coalition against some issues of pesticides apparently has on their web page that we did mosquito control without insecticides and that we'd saved a million dollars by doing this. I have no idea how they got that information, except that when people call or ask, what we tell them is that we do not do any adulticiding until we find positive mosquitoes. And at that time, we go in with a very intensive adulticide program. In 1998 when we had St. Louis encephalitis pop out in the Harris County area, in about 20% of the county, we treated over a million acres. There was a lot of repeating of applications in that area. I think it goes around up here sometimes that we're doing mosquito control in Texas without using insecticides, and I just want to make it clear that this is definitely not the case. We'd like to. I think everybody in mosquito control would like to be able to control mosquitoes without using adulticides or even larvicides, but at the present time, that's just not possible. When you have a disease situation and you've got infected mosquitoes flying around, the only recourse we have at the present time is using adulticides, because that's the only way that we're able to kill them. In the future there might be some options that we can look at, but at the present time we don't have them. And, as Dave said, we may not have our adulticides too much longer either.

What I'd like to do is go through some of the basic mosquito control programs that just about everybody uses—something on adulticides because that seems to be the thing that everybody thinks about and it's the most critical. I understand that Paul Reiter is going to be doing some work up in the Boston area on evaluation of methods that are used for adult mosquito control. I think this is going to be real essential for everybody in the country. We don't really know how to effectively measure the effect of adulticiding or larviciding on mosquito populations. You might be surprised when I say larviciding because if you go out and treat an area with just about anything and go back and sample it, you'll find that you can control those mosquito larvae, but that doesn't mean that you've reduced the overall adult population in your area. That's what I think we need to start looking at too.

A challenge to those of you in mosquito control is to develop a way to evaluate the effect of the adult population when you larvicide, because if you can't get enough larvicide done to reduce that adult population, then you're not controlling mosquitoes, especially the *Culex* that actually emerge as adults. Ninety-five percent die before they actually start flying. So you can tell everybody in your area that you get 95% control without insecticides. One of the things that I'd like to see them look in Boston—that we're going to be looking at a little bit in Harris County—is dosage rate associated with adulticiding. Everybody has a little different way of doing it in mosquito control. County to county, it's done differently, and that'll probably never change because of political boundaries. Anticipating West Nile virus getting into Harris County, we just did a little study to see what it might cost us, assuming that we would have to spray seven nights a week with twenty trucks, and probably even more. The dosage rate that we're using now, 0.003 pounds per acre of Scourge, would cost us about $300,000 per month just for insecticide to treat like that. If we upped the rate to 0.006, which I think Paul is going to be doing in Boston, the cost would jump up to about $500,000. That's about a $200,000 difference. But if that 0.006 rate increases your kill, your mortality, it's probably worth it. But we don't know. You don't have to use any particular rate according to the EPA label, except you can't go over the max rate. You can cut it in half or by three-fourths, but if you lower that rate you really lower the potential for controlling mosquitoes.

We need to look at treatment methodology, something that people usually don't think about, the training associated with the actual spraying, whether it be larviciding or adulticiding. I've told some people around here that what we do in our programs, for the most part—and we do it in Harris County also—is take all this really scientific information from surveillance collections, laboratory work. We take all this information and we find a positive in the area, positive mosquitoes, and go out and treat with an adulticide; we take the least trained, the least motivated person in the whole system and send them out to kill the mosquitoes. This needs to be worked on also. I think there are better ways to do it, and we need to start looking at that— a little bit on public education and source reduction.

We have three full-time people in our public education program. We have, I think, an outstanding school program. We have media contacts all the time, but how effective is public education in reducing the potential for transmission. I'm not sure it's very effective at the present time. We all do it, and I think we have to do it, but we're looking at going into an area and developing what we call a community-based program. These programs are usually used in other health programs right now, and I think if you're going to do public education and *really* get people to change their behavior, you have to do it on a community-by-community basis. First you've got to be able to find what that community is. We have found in the Houston area, especially, that the people on one side of the street consider themselves in one community; on the other side it's a different community. So if you're going to do public education at what you're considering a community level, you really have to know what that community is. We're getting some of the other people in the health department in public education involved with us on this.

I want to talk briefly about novel approaches to mosquito control, and I think that this is something that we're going to need to look at in the future. There are some trap systems that are coming out now that—I won't say that they'll really reduce mosquitoes in an overall area—do collect a lot of mosquitoes and kill them. I think we're going to have to look at some of these novel approaches in the future, even to supplement maybe our adulticiding program, because as we start doing some tests with adulticides, we'll find—and I'm sure this is true in New York City and in the larger urban areas like Houston and Boston—that there may be areas within the city where mosquitoes do not respond to adulticides. It's not because the insecticides are not killing the mosquitoes, but the insecticides just don't get to them. And how we're going to get around this I think is one of the research projects that we need to look at. Right now, I think there's a lot of research that's being started and that will continue, but what we're really lacking in the mosquito control community is the research information. Unfortunately, the academic community's job ends when this information is published, but it doesn't get the information to us in the mosquito control agency. One of the things I think we're lacking in this country, and even in the world, is a translation agency to take the material from the academic stage into the real world.

NEWTON: Thank you, Ray. Gregory?

GREGORY F. TERRILLION: I work in Nassau County, which is nestled between New York City and Suffolk County. Nassau County has had a program since 1916 that was in response to a malaria outbreak at the time. The Nassau County Health Department has become a partner with us in our mosquito control program, and their help has enhanced the well-run program that we have today. We have extensive salt marsh and approximately one thousand miles of salt marsh beaches that need to be maintained and monitored on a weekly basis. We have 650 recharge basins that at any time can hold water. We have 200 miles of upland streams that need to be monitored, and with that we have 70,000 street basins that can transmit rainwater into any one of these retention areas that need to be treated and monitored also. We have approximately 50 ponds in Nassau County and 12 preserves that need to be monitored. Over the years of experience, we have made predictive models with rain incidents. We know some areas will retain water at different levels of rain, whether it's a quarter inch, half inch, or one inch. We know which sumps our recharge basins hold water year-round. We know which ones retain fish that we can restock into other areas—our Gambusia.

Our county is broken into sectors, and our sanitary inspectors are responsible for their own area. They get to know the area. I've had this position for thirty years. What's very important is the need to know the topography of your county and interpret that with the environmental conditions that may occur any time during the season.

What we did in 2000, knowing that we had a good program—a lot of this information is already on our GIS—was ask ourselves what we could do to enhance our program. We concentrated on earlier larviciding in these areas, to knock the *Cx. pipiens* population down. That was very successful. With our light traps, we had to double and triple up just to get enough mosquitoes for pools. The feedback from the communities was that mosquito biting was down from past years.

The other issue that we concentrate on is public education. In Nassau County, we have 19 legislative districts for the county, and we probably did somewhere between three and four town meetings for each district. During the meetings, the legislators would introduce us and then they'd go out into the audience. As the public started to come on board with our message about removing stagnant water around their properties, the legislators would come right up there with us and stand side-by-side with us when we discussed educational issues and sanitary issues around the home. The legislators and public came on board; it was a very good program on education. I also provided educational programs to our golf course superintendents throughout Long Island, statewide, and for personnel of the Nassau County Parks Department. We went into the sewer plants and discussed issues related to stagnant water.

We kept the public informed with taped messages. We informed them when we had dead crows, when we had positive dead crows, when we had positive mosquito pools, and we told them what was going to be happening. When we had mosquitoes breeding on our salt marshes, we used a helicopter to larvicide. A lot of people misunderstood and thought that we were adulticiding. We tried to correct that notion on our taped message. We would indicate, for example, that on August 16th between the hours of 7 AM and 12 noon Nassau County would be larviciding along the Jones Beach salt marsh. Then I would call the health department and they would change that message to announce that the larviciding that was scheduled had been completed. We also have a website to keep people informed.

Something new that we're going to do this year is a public service announcement. We run a 15-second radio blurb after a rain incident in Nassau County. I announce on a taped message that it's just recently rained: "Please go into your backyard, check your property, look for standing water, and eliminate the problem." We had eighty-eight positive crows last year as well as seven positive mosquito pools and four positive horses. We only did one evening treatment and that was for two positive mosquito pools. The reason why we only treated two areas was because of the risk to human health. It was in a highly populated area, and we used natural boundaries. We used railroad tracks, a parkway, and a preserve, which was roughly just under three-quarters of a mile radius for each treatment area.

NEWTON: Thank you, Gregory. I'd like to take a few minutes and talk about North Carolina's mosquito and vector control program. In North Carolina, we have about ninety local mosquito control programs. About a quarter of those are run by county health departments, a quarter of them are run by county public works departments, and the other half are run by cities and towns. We have approximately fifty-three species of mosquitoes in North Carolina. Our local programs run from about $900,000 per year to $300 per year. We figured about $5.5 million are spent annually on mosquito control in North Carolina by organized programs. All of the mosquito control in North Carolina is local. The state doesn't do any mosquito control except during emergency situations. The two major examples of that were Hurricane Fran in 1996 and Hurricane Floyd in 1999. We sprayed about 4.3 million acres with adulticide after Hurricane Fran. After Hurricane Floyd in 1999, we sprayed something like five million acres with adulticide, with 90% FEMA reimbursement for this work. Our major diseases in eastern North Carolina are eastern equine encephalitis—we had three cases and one death from that last year; LaCrosse encephalitis in western North Carolina—in the mountainous areas, we had one death from that last year; and several years ago we had, to my knowledge, the only new death from Cache Valley encephalitis in the United States. Our programs are integrated. They use a number of methodologies: ground ULV is used extensively, larviciding, and a lot of educational work from the state program and from local programs. Generally, we get very good press coverage, very positive press coverage on mosquito control activities. Our media are very interested in mosquito control and are very supportive of it in North Carolina.

By the way, our main pests are albopictus in the urban areas and, of course, in the salt marshes, salt marsh mosquito species. Container cleanup is something we push a lot because of the albopictus problem in North Carolina; the worst we're expecting is *Oc. japonicus* to get there if it's not already there. So we'll be pushing that even more as well as the tie in with West Nile. We do put out some information on the use of repellents and avoidance of mosquito areas, or personal protection. There's quite a bit of water management, mostly the maintenance of existing drainage in North Carolina. There's very little new drainage being done. And our grid spoil islands in the intercoastal waterway in eastern North Carolina when mud's pumped out of the intercoastal waterway to deepen it, it's put on spoil islands. That mud can crack and produce enormous numbers of *Oc. sollicitans* and *Oc. taeniorhynchus*. The state does provide some financial aid to local programs. About 10% of the local spending, on average, comes from state financial aid. We also provide technical assistance to our local programs through eight medical entomologists. For some twenty years, we've been running sentinel flocks for EEE detection and to advise local programs when they need to take some action on EEE. Last year, we had about sixty sentinel flocks, mostly in eastern North Carolina. We do educational work. We distribute press releases; we publish quite a number of pamphlets that we provide without charge to county health departments and others who want them; we have web pages with our pamphlets on them and a lot of other information on mosquito control in North Carolina.

In terms of efficacy, we've been doing landing rates before and after spraying for about twenty years or so. If you average all these things out, you see about an 80% control from a ground view of the application. We do quite a bit of light trapping for arbovirus surveillance and isolation. Of course, our contained animal facilities are a concern. Much of the manure that comes out of these facilities goes into lagoons. Those lagoons, of course, are highly organic, and the following year we have *Culex pipiens* and *quinquefasciatus*, and all sorts of hybrids between the two. The following year, those lagoons produce tremendous numbers of *Culex* mosquitoes. We're working with an extension service in North Carolina. According to our legal folks, that means anything, under the law, from a hundred thousand acre lake down to a retention/detention pond or anything else. So we can make rules regarding impounded water mosquito control. Mistrust of pesticides is not the major problem in North Carolina. It's of course an agricultural economy to a large extent; pesticides are used extensively over many areas of the state, except in the urban areas. Of course our experience with West Nile virus so far has been one dead crow we found in the fall of 2000. Roger?

NASCI: Thank you. I want to say a couple of things before we open up the panel for discussion. It's become apparent from this series of short presentations that mosquito abatement programs are much more than what the usual resident sees, which is the guy driving down the street with the yellow light going and the plume of aerosol spewing from the back of his truck. These programs are truly integrated pest management programs in the complete sense of that philosophy: the understanding of the ecology of the pests, the establishment of action thresholds, and the use of a variety of intervention mechanisms when and where they're necessary. So, in many ways, the concept of integrated pest management has been simplified to the point where people think it's just using larvicides and adulticides or a couple of different larvicides. Someone on the first day of the conference said, "Make it simple but not too simple." Integrated pest management is not simple. It's a very complicated process, and mosquito abatement programs—all the modern mosquito abatement programs that are in place—fully adopt this philosophy. We need to keep this philosophy in mind as public health educators. Education of the residents in our areas is a major function of public health that helps them understand what the risks are and what the appropriate interventions are. We need to make this piece of information available to them as well.

At this time, I'd like to open the floor for discussion and comments from the audience.

MARC PALADINI (*Bergen County Department of Health Services, Paramus, NJ*): This is a question for any of the panelists who have had counties or communities with a history of vector-borne disease outbreaks. What change have you noticed in the public and media response over time as subsequent outbreaks have been identified, and what do you think the reaction will be if and when West Nile virus is introduced into those communities? Will you see a similar response as we have here from the public and the media?

NINIVAGGI: We have the dubious distinction in Suffolk County of not only dealing with West Nile virus, but we've had a couple of years when we've also had to deal with eastern equine encephalitis, particularly in 1994 and also in 1996. I found that very interesting because the media coverage for the eastern virus made us into heroes. Basically, the message that was coming out was that there was a deadly virus on the loose but that the Suffolk County Vector Control was on the case. I hope that that was true; I'd like to think it was! I think that one of the things that we've seen here with West Nile virus is that we have the misfortune of having the virus show up in an area that was not used to seeing mosquito control, was not mosquito aware. And there are a lot of people who are philosophically opposed to the use of pesticides. One organization has as its goal to eliminate the use of pesticides as a tool for control of West Nile virus. I think a lot of misinformation was presented, and some of it was very close to the point of disinformation. We need to do a better job of explaining ourselves and what we do, because often what goes out to the general public, as Dr. Nasci was saying, is a caricature of what we actually do as mosquito control agencies. There has been a change in perception in some ways, but on the other hand, what I find in my own county is a microcosm of that. We have some communities where mosquitoes, on a year-to-year basis, are a serious problem for the people living in those communities. When the mosquitoes get out of hand, they literally can't go out of their houses without having twenty or thirty salt marsh mosquitoes start to bite them. Needless to say, those folks tend to be a lot more supportive of all the things we do to control mosquitoes. Areas that traditionally haven't had high mosquito populations were extremely concerned when we started to use pesticides in those areas. The only answer we have is to try and get the best information out to the public and, again, try to get the idea out that we are trying to be as judicious as we can be in all our control measures. A lot of the things that we've been asked to do—like using biologicals and source reduction—we already do. As everybody gets smarter, this will help the situation.

NASCI: Ray, could you say a few words about how you think the response to West Nile virus will be received in Harris County?

PARSONS: I don't think it'll be quite as dramatic as it was up in this area, but the media will pick it up, and for a while they'll really play it up. Now, what we're going to try to do is start this year. I don't anticipate that West Nile is going to be in Texas this year. Roger has predicted that it will take two years.

NASCI: I never said that (laughter).

PARSONS: This was in a Louisiana meeting and I've got a recording (laughter)! I've been telling everybody in Texas that Roger Nasci said this too! We'd like to get a proactive program going with the media; they can really help you, especially TV stations. And we've got—I don't know how many—probably six to ten programs in Houston. When we started having a problem, such as St. Louis encephalitis, or even severe pest mosquito problems that we really didn't address ourselves, we had them lining up in our office to wait their turn to get an interview. We're going to try to gradually work them into being able to help us, because as I said before, I'm not sure how effective public education is, that is, in actually reducing mosquito populations. To inform the public about what your programs are doing is something that public education does quite well in mosquito control. As far as getting a community to clean up and reduce the overall mosquito population, I'm not sure we're there yet. But we're expecting the media is not going to leave us alone in Harris County, either, when West Nile gets there.

NASCI: Tom?

THOMAS MONATH (Acambis Inc., Cambridge, MA): I'd value some discussion from the group about an idea that we discussed many years ago at the CDC, and that is the focus on one of the weakest links in mosquito biology, which is a hibernating mosquito as the focus for control efforts. Obviously, Culex overwinters in the adult stage, and it should be feasible, at least in part, to map out the hibernacula, just as you pay attention to the larval breeding site. It's obvious that the population that overwinters is small compared to the population in the summer—also the container, overwintering, infected mosquitoes. So, I wonder whether treatment of large hibernacula and promotion of public health education to treat basements and so on during the winter wouldn't have a dramatic impact, at least on delaying the emergence of Culex. Spraying pushes it from May to June—that might have a dramatic effect on virus transmission. I wonder whether this is feasible or whether it's ever been a thought that perhaps we've overlooked.

NASCI: That's exactly a point that was discussed last year at some hearings after the first season of West Nile virus and actually preceding our investigations to find if the virus was in the hibernating mosquitoes. I think it's hypothetically possible, but applying it would be extremely difficult. In our searches through the city, for example, to find hibernating mosquitoes, we found a few large hibernacula, but in general, we found a mosquito here, a mosquito there, widely distributed through a number of habitats. I think the logistics of finding all those sites to begin with, or a representative sample that would make a biological difference—and then actually finding some mechanism of control that would work in conditions where the temperature is low, air movement is very minimal—would be difficult. I don't think it's something that we should dismiss out of hand. It needs some investigation and some development work, but it poses problems that are not addressed by current mosquito control technology.

NEWTON: I was noting some of the information that Dr. Spielman gave yesterday. It seems that the *Culex* populations that he studied were building up much faster than we see *Culex* mosquito populations building up. I wonder in the urban areas whether there aren't more, say, hibernacula than we have in many of our rural areas.

DEBORAH ASNIS (*Flushing Hospital Medical Center, Flushing, NY*): You mentioned that there were six adulticides. Part of the concern is that one county might be using, for instance, a safer adulticide than another. The other comment I had is a practical one. We all are homeowners; do you have advice on how we should conduct ourselves during this summer when barbecuing? Are there commercial products that we can purchase that would minimize exposure to mosquitoes during our summer events?

DAME: The six insecticides that are used for controlling adult mosquitoes fall into two insecticide classes: the organophosphates and the pyrethroids, or the natural pyrethrins. Communities have the task of deciding which pesticide works best in its circumstance for the species that they have a problem with. These pesticides are not equally effective against all species. In the United States, we have over 150 mosquito species, probably about 25 or 30 that are pest species around the country, and some are pest species everywhere, like *Culex*. The cost is different with the pesticides; the type of application will make a difference in the cost as well. So there are many judgment calls that are involved in a selection of pesticide, and some mosquito populations have developed a resistance to those pesticides. That factors into this particular decision making too. I only mentioned the adulticides, but there are several larvicides that are available, and communities have an opportunity to select those too. They are selected based on their efficacy against the target species, and that efficacy varies with the target species. The EPA sets up a level of maximum application rate, and then as Ray Parsons said a few minutes ago, many of the mosquito control agencies elect to use less than the maximum and still get control. One of the problems in using less than the maximum to achieve mosquito control is that you're likely to give sublethal doses to some parts of the mosquito population, and, therefore after two, three, or four replications of exposure, start to create resistant populations. So for the most part, it's advantageous to use the higher amounts, and if you use the higher amounts, it's more costly. This factors into the decision by the community. What was the second part of your question?

ASNIS: Residential protection.

DAME: Residential protection. First of all, for all of these adulticides that are being used, the EPA has decreed that human exposure to these adulticides is not deleterious. However, they do realize that there are people who are chemically sensitive to pesticides and to other types of organic materials. In most organized mosquito control operations, these chemically sensitive people have been identified. They are notified ahead of time when spraying is going to occur through a telephone answering machine connection. The spray is different than agricultural spray. When we use a ULV, we use a spray with a small droplet running from ten to twenty-five microns. It tends to stay airborne, does not deposit, and that's why we get good mosquito control because it stays airborne to get the flying insects. Agricultural sprays use droplet sizes of one hundred microns to five hundred microns, or larger, and they're meant to deposit; they're meant to go to the ground and to stay on the ground and the insect comes in and meets the deposit. With ULV sprays, these deposits don't occur. So after the spray, there's no real hazard for people going out into the yard and being exposed to anything that's left behind because there's not enough left behind to do any damage. There are products on the market that you can buy at any of the stores that you can apply in your backyards with a handheld machine to reduce the mosquito population for two to three hours. They're available for homeowner use, and they are effective.

NINIVAGGI: One thing that I would like to mention is that protecting an individual backyard from mosquitoes is a very difficult thing, because mosquitoes fly from a lot of different sources. Some of the measures that Dr. Dame was talking about, such as even residual sprays on vegetation, can't help, but the fact that an individual homeowner can't really do much, particularly if there are large sources of mosquitoes, is ultimately why control organizations like mine exist. It's the realization that mosquito control needs to take place on a area-wide, community-wide basis to be truly effective. There's a good, sound biological reason why this needs to be attacked on a broad scale.

NASCI: Even though there are limitations to what you can do to protect your backyard, we do know that DEET-based repellents, the personal repellent products, are quite effective, and quite safe, and have been proposed and promoted quite widely for nuisance protection as well as for prevention of bites during the outbreaks. Keeping your window screens in good repair and using personal repellents is also effective.

PAUL REITER (*CDC Dengue Branch, San Juan, Puerto Rico*): What we're anticipating, what we're hoping for, is to try some collaborative efforts to look at the efficacy of these particular space spraying efforts against West Nile vectors. We're still open to suggestions. We have a draft program called "Anyone who's interested, please come to me and we'll discuss that later." Let me start with the premise that *we're* starting from, that is, that we know very little about the real efficacy of aerosols, of ULV—ground-based ULV—against these species. Yes, we know its susceptibility and we've done a lot of trials, particularly using bioassay cages, but the real impact of the sprays on the mosquito in the environment is something that we feel has been very rarely monitored, or very little evaluated. Ray Parsons is always complimenting me that we did good work in Memphis, Tennessee. A group of us with the Memphis and Shelby County Health Departments first of all developed two very simple methods for monitoring the *Culex* species. We've decided simply for reasons of triage to concentrate this season on the *Culex* species that are considered to be the epizootic vectors. We use egg raft collections, and also we use the gravid trap. I haven't got time to go into all of this, but I want to expand the concept of these trials, to ask really what the questions are that we really need to ask. Obviously, we want to know what the impact is, what the reduction of the female mosquito population is. What is the percent reduction? And I've heard numbers bandied around that are supposed to be objective—30%, some people say, or 60%, 90%. How much is that reduction and of what population is that reduction? If a bird is being bitten by ten mosquitoes per night, and we reduce that to three mosquitoes per night, is that epidemiologically significant over the long term? How long does that impact last? How quickly is the population being regenerated? In other words, our trials will be designed to look before and after at the population.

What we basically envisage is looking at paired areas—one area will be treated, and the untreated group will be monitored. We'll start at least four or five days before treatments and will continue for at least as long as we see that there appears to be a decrease in the population. In other words, in which population and of how long does it take? How much did we reduce it by? How long is that impact going to last? The fundamental question is, What is the epidemiologic impact of what we're doing? In Puerto Rico, we've been doing similar studies with *Aedes aegypti*. We then started a trial of dengue transmission. We did actually find, very disappointingly, that the impact of even a 90% reduction from a single ULV treatment was relatively limited—less than 5% in our modeled population in the overall reduction of dengue cases. I don't want to go any further into that except to say that some of the basic parameters that go into the dynamics of transmission are really unknown to us. What do we know about the longevity of a vector in the field? What do we know about other aspects—even, for example, Tom Monath brought up hibernacula? What do we know about the true resting sites, the true places where the mosquitoes are secluded? There are an awful lot of questions that we want to answer, but the basic thing that we're going to look at is, By how much do we reduce the *Culex* population and for how long? And how is this likely to influence other transmissions?

NASCI: Paul will be developing this program over the next few weeks, and we urge anyone who has an interest or comments or some input to contact him about the possibility of interacting with this study.

NINIVAGGI: I've talked to Dr. Reiter about his coming to Suffolk County to look at some of our work, and I approach that with some trepidation, because we'll finally have the CDC looking over our shoulders and seeing how good a job we actually do. I think a lot of his remarks are also addressed particularly to control of *Culex* mosquitoes. I wouldn't want anybody to leave with the idea that we have no idea whether the things we do to control mosquitoes really work. That's far from the case. For instance, when we introduced methoprene to our larvicide program, our salt marsh numbers and our light traps went down 70 to 90%. That's a good indication of efficacy. Particularly with the human biting species, as a control program, you can be sitting in your office answering a couple of hundred phone calls a day—"The mosquitoes are eating us alive!" You send out the trucks or the helicopter; you do the ULV application, and the next day the phones are quiet except for a couple of people calling to thank you. So I don't think that we should paint too dim a picture of the efficacy of these things. But I do agree that very often the *Culex* species are particularly difficult to control with ULV, so I'll be very eager to see how this program works out, and we hope to improve our methods.

REITER: Can I please say to Dominick and to anyone else in this room that I approach this with much more trepidation than you do? I'm entering into your territory. This is a collaborative effort. I really want to stress that. I've done some work with

Culex in Memphis, Tennessee. I think you'll agree that if we're simply focusing on the final solution, which we all go to when we do have evidence of transmission—the aerosols, the ULVs—there is relatively little information on the *Culex* species, but it's a combined effort.

NINIVAGGI: Yeah, I think there's also a bit of irony here in that our program traditionally hasn't paid a tremendous amount of attention to *Culex pipiens* and *restuans* and species that seem to be important for West Nile virus for the main reasons that they're not aggressive biting species, so they generally don't create a large nuisance problem. Up until West Nile virus, they weren't really important from the disease control point of view. So, in general, we really haven't paid that much attention to those particular species. And I think that as we direct new attention, from a science and control point of view, to these species, we're certainly going to learn a lot. I think it's going to be very exciting.

NASCI: Duane?

DUANE GUBLER (*Centers for Disease Control and Prevention, Fort Collins, CO*): I think this discussion underscores a major problem that we have. No matter how much we discuss mosquito control, the discussion always comes back to emergency adulticiding. I can tell you up front—I think most people will agree with this—that if you wait for an epidemic to occur or a transmission to occur, and then try to respond in an emergency fashion, you end up losing the battle. You'll never be able to effectively prevent vector-borne diseases that way. The key is sitting at the table. We just have heard from several of the best mosquito control programs in the country. There are others, but these people make a tremendous effort. The thing they have in common is that they're locally funded and they're locally controlled. They place the emphasis on larval mapping and larval control. They have good community relations. They have support from their local politicians, and they use the adulticiding only as a last resort, when they really, really need to.

I think we need to somehow bring the discussion back to how you effectively control mosquitoes to prevent disease. The way to do it is to follow the lead of the local mosquito control programs that are so effective in doing this. In our West Nile guidelines for the last two years—last year and now, again, in the revision this year—we have made a strong recommendation that we focus on local mosquito control, local mosquito abatement districts. The question I have for Ray or one of the others is how your program is funded. How do you maintain that funding year after year after year so that you have the professionals out there that know where the mosquitoes are breeding, when they're breeding, and how to control them. How do you prevent getting your budget pulled and moved to other competing priorities? I think it's very important for those areas that are trying to address this question, and how do you set up a program like this?

TERRILLION: Well, I describe the Nassau County perspective. We have significant salt marsh in Nassau County. I explained we have one thousand miles of salt marsh ditches that need to be maintained and monitored, and generally, at different times during the season, batches will get off. We are very highly urbanized on the south shore where these salt marshes are, so we're influencing a good portion of our population—ten to fifteen percent of our county population at any given time during the summer. To give you an example of the dynamics of mosquito control, last year was the first year we never adulticided for salt marsh mosquitoes. It's the first time I can remember that ever happening. We have nineteen legislative districts; six of them are on the south shore, so these legislators are going to make sure we're properly funded.

To give you an example, back in 1991 we had some budgetary constraints. The program was scaled back a little bit. We stopped salt marsh maintenance, and we had salt marsh mosquitoes picked up in our Jersey traps. I don't know how familiar you are with Long Island—as far north as the Southern State Parkway, we're talking a mile or two miles off the salt marsh. When people cannot enjoy their backyard barbecue, when people cannot have their children wait at the bus stop, when the kids can't go out for daytime recreation during lunch in June, it's a big problem. These people remember that. We got funded quite quickly the following season with more money than we needed. It works when we have these types of problems. We're very fortunate that our mosquito habitats are right up against people's backyards, and they're aware of it year after year.

GUBLER: What if you don't have that kind of a pest mosquito? What if you have a program that runs routinely? How does the Harris County program work?

PARSONS: We're talking about two different things here. We're talking about nuisance mosquito control and vector control. As I said before, our program is primarily set up for vector control. Over the years, the program has been in and out of nuisance mosquito control, and we don't have a real good system in Harris County for nuisance mosquito control. It's fragmented. Most of it is actually done by pest control companies on a neighborhood-by-neighborhood basis. We don't have any control; the only input we have is through public education. Homeowners' associations will ask us to come out and make a presentation, and I have some information I give them, and if they're going to contract work what they should ask their contractor to do. We don't have nuisance mosquitoes most of the year because of the dry weather down there, but we've been able to maintain the disease vector part, mainly through educating the politicians on the importance of keeping a strong surveillance program.

Harris County, I think, is the third most populous county in the country, and we only have about two million dollars a year, and most of that is taken up with personnel costs. If we get into a St. Louis encephalitis outbreak or West Nile, we don't budget yearly very much for insecticide, because there's no need for storing thousands of gallons of it when you're not going to use it that year. But I have no doubt that if West Nile comes to the area that if we go to our local politicians, and say we need a million dollars or two million dollars, that they will provide it as we need it. So we've got a pretty constant budget on a year-to-year basis.

We do have a new program that strictly addresses nuisance mosquitoes and salt marsh mosquitoes in the channel area created partially by the corps of engineer's pumping into spoils. We were able, through one of the politicians from that area, to get about another $300,000 just to work on that. But it's very important to work with the political groups in an area, to let them understand what you're doing. I think all the larger programs in the country probably are able to do that pretty well. What happens on a nuisance basis if you have one or two years where your nuisance population goes down for some environmental reason, then you might have a little trouble. But with nuisance mosquitoes, every year they're always out there biting people, and they remember it so they say don't cut that budget. With vectors it's a little different.

DAME: In many communities that have mosquito control, the mosquito control has been requested by the citizens. It has been set up by public referendum. Independent taxing districts are set up, and people are assessed. Once this has been approved by the public, then they are taxed each year a certain amount of money. This is very popular throughout the country. It's an indication that the people want and need this service, that they're willing to pay for it, and then they do pay for it. They hire professionals to run the operation. This works extremely well. You brought up a question of what kind of approaches we use for mosquito control. We discussed many, but I would like to direct you all to the American Mosquito Control Association's website, which is www.mosquito.org. At that website we discuss all the types of activities that are used for mosquito control, and there's a great deal of information there that may be helpful to you.

NASCI: I'll take one more comment from the panel and then we'll take some other questions.

MILLER: In New York State, although one cannot get state aid for nuisance control, one can get it for disease surveillance. We've got different jurisdictions; we've got to gather funds from different ways, but in New York State, at least, we have vector surveillance funding.

DURLAND FISH (*Yale University School of Medicine, New Haven, CT*): In a former life, I used to set up, develop, and operate mosquito control programs, concentrating on public health, and I can remember the typical procedures that were involved in taking a municipality with virtually no experience with mosquito biology or mosquito problems and trying to implement a mosquito surveillance control program based on larval control. It took a good four or five years to go around and map all these larval breeding sites, visit them monthly, inventory mosquitoes that were coming out, and apply larvicides to try to reduce the numbers of adults. So when I hear or read about how the municipalities are going to reduce the risk of West Nile virus or reduce the need for using adulticides based on larval control, I'm a little skeptical of this, knowing the difficulties that are involved, especially for municipalities that haven't had any previous experience. It's a challenge enough for experienced mosquito control programs to do an effective job of eliminating larval breeding sites. I also have to disagree with my former mentor, Dave Dame, on the role of the public in reducing West Nile virus risk and personal protection. I think with Lyme disease, we've learned that personel protection has not been particularly effective in reducing cases of Lyme disease for various sociological reasons. I don't think it's going to have much of an impact on West Nile either. Furthermore, I think it's kind of a cop-out for government agencies to push the responsibility on to the public to protect themselves from being bitten by an infected mosquito. To me, that's a government responsibility—to keep infected mosquitoes out of the environment. And then the last option we have is adulticiding, and we hear the problems with the likelihood that adulticiding is not going to be very effective in reducing West Nile virus risk, either. So, my question to the panel is, What impact do you think—even with the fifty or one hundred million dollars that's going to be spent this summer—we are going to have on reducing the risk of West Nile virus? Would it be any different from the impact, say, the weather might have?

DAME: I'd like to respond, since I've taken a few hits. What we're advocating is that the public be aware of the risk and that they help themselves by doing protective things to reduce that risk. We're aware that there shouldn't be mosquitoes out there biting them, but there are and therefore they need that advice. I think that there's a reason why there are mosquitoes out there when you think they should not be. Several species lend themselves to excellent control with larval approaches, and the *Ochlerotatus sollicitans* and *Ochlerotatus taeniorhynchus* are species that can be addressed by mosquito control agencies. Some of the *Culex*, like *Culex nigripalpus* that breeds in fresh water ponds, temporary ones, they can be addressed quite directly. Those species that are difficult to address with larviciding are the peridomestic types that breed in containers, which are found by the thousands in neighborhoods—those are very difficult to control by larviciding. Those are the ones that we're dealing with in West Nile, in many respects. *Culex quinquefasciatus* breeds both in open water, if it's suitable for them, and in small containers. And it's much more difficult for mosquito control agencies to get to the breeding sites for those particular targets.

NASCI: I'd also like to disagree very strongly on your perception of government role. Public health is a shared responsibility, and if you look at all the other public health programs, there is a role for government. There is a role for the public health institutions, for example, in the development and proofing of vaccines. But the decision to use that vaccine comes from the public. With regard to the dissemination of HIV and the message to use a condom, no one's proposing that the government has the responsibility to install those devices (*laughter*). So I also disagree that personal protection measures or the involvement of the public has no role. I believe this is a significant role that should be promoted very strongly. We know that we can reduce the biting of mosquitoes by use of personal repellents. We know that window screens keep mosquitoes out of people's houses. Our job is to determine what the risk factors are and determine what the best mechanisms are. Then if they involve public investment or public buy in, we have to do the best education job we can to make that happen.

NEWTON: I have a question for the audience. How many of your jurisdictions have laws requiring that all openable windows be screened? There's a simple, legal way for the government to take responsibility.

DALE MORSE (*New York State Department of Health, Albany, NY*): Can the panel elaborate on larviciding agents and timing or monitoring after heavy rains?

NINIVAGGI: It's more labor intense; it's a more difficult proposition than just identifying that you've got flying mosquitoes and then treating a broad area for adult mosquitoes. You have to literally get down in the mud and see where the mosquitoes are breeding, and, of course, with West Nile we have a particular problem with the peridomestic mosquitoes. Suffolk County Vector Control is never going to be able to go into everybody's backyard and pump off pool covers and have them empty all their flowerpots. That's something that we need the public's help on. As far as the mosquitoes that breed in the general community, in the drainage areas and in the wetlands, *that* we recognize is our responsibility as a government agency. But, it's more labor intensive; it costs more. Also, there are additional restrictions and considerations that go into that.

Mosquitoes have a habit of liking to breed in environmentally sensitive habitats and legally protected habitats. There are a whole series of additional measures that you have to consider when you're dealing with those sorts of habitats. In New York State, fresh water and tidal wetlands are highly regulated. Any pesticide that you put in water is highly regulated—even the bacterials. This is necessary and worthwhile but it does make the job of mosquito control a bit more complicated, and that's one reason why we realize that it's better to get the mosquitoes in the larval stages. What we have to recognize is that that's not always going to be possible. No matter what we do, some of them are going to get away from us. In some cases, habitats are out right protected where absolutely no larval control is allowed. I have hundreds of acres of salt marsh in Suffolk County where we're not allowed to do any mosquito prevention. Needless to say, those mosquitoes don't stay home all the time, and when they come out into the residential areas, we don't have a lot of choices. But with adult control, we're telling people to stay in their houses. Again, this is why the integrated approach is important.

Use of Live and Inactivated Vaccines in the Control of West Nile Fever in Domestic Geese

M. MALKINSON,[a] C. BANET,[a] Y. KHINICH,[a] I. SAMINA,[a]
S. POKAMUNSKI,[b] AND Y. WEISMAN[a]

[a]Kimron Veterinary Institute, Beit Dagan, Israel 50250

[b]Israel Veterinary Services and Animal Health, Beit Dagan, Israel 50250

ABSTRACT: The recent epizootic of West Nile fever in Israel affected predominantly young domestic geese between three and eight weeks old. Clinically, the birds presented paralytic signs while morbidity and mortality were severe in affected flocks. The condition was encountered from early September through late November on goose farms located throughout the country. Losses incurred by goose flocks were sufficiently great as to warrant investigation of ways to protect young geese against the neurological form of the disease. We have conducted a series of vaccination trials in which three-week old geese were immunized with an attenuated, commercial flavivirus vaccine derived from Israel turkey meningoencephalitis virus (TME). Birds were challenged two weeks later with a low Vero cell passage of West Nile virus by the intracerebral route. In a second group of experiments, inactivated and live TME vaccines were given in tandem at an interval of two weeks and challenged two weeks later. The third vaccination trial was based on West Nile virus (WNV) harvested from infant mouse brain, inactivated with formalin and oil adjuvanted. A single injection given either subcutaneously or intramuscularly resulted in 75% protection of the vaccinated groups, while two injections spaced two weeks apart resulted in 94% protection. Groups of geese, vaccinated at the farms and challenged under controlled conditions in the laboratory, showed levels of protection ranging from 39% to 72% for TME vaccine and 52% and 80% for WNV vaccine. The lower levels of protection are attributable to flocks being affected with intercurrent infections at the time of vaccination.

KEYWORDS: West Nile virus; turkey meningoencephalitis virus; domestic geese

INTRODUCTION

We have briefly reported isolating West Nile viruses in November 1997 from the brains of young domestic geese aged between 5 and 9 weeks presenting a neuroparalytic disease.[1] This was the first West Nile virus (WNV) isolate from a series of outbreaks that were to appear in the late summer and fall months on Israeli goose farms in 1997 through 2000.

In November 1997, four commercial flocks of 2000–2500 birds each, located in one village, were affected. High morbidity and mortality in these flocks were record-

Address for correspondence: Mertyn Malkinson, Ph.D., Kimron Veterinary Institute, Beit Dagan, Israel 50250. Voice: +972.3.968.1691; fax: +972.3.968.1739.

martinm@moag.gov.il

ed and reached 40% on one farm. On another farm, 400 geese died between 5 and 14 weeks of age from a flock of 2200 birds. Histopathological findings of perivascular cuffing typical of a viral encephalitis were seen. In the following year, the disease was diagnosed in 17 goose flocks distributed among 9 villages, while in 1999, 12 flocks raised in 8 villages were affected. In 2000, however, the disease was diagnosed in 7 flocks in 4 villages. This lower incidence is a possible reflection on the introduction of vaccination in young goose flocks in 2000. Most of the flocks were 5 to 8 weeks old, but flocks as young as 3 weeks and as old as 12 weeks were also affected. In contrast to 1997, the outbreaks in 1998 and 1999 followed a similar seasonal pattern; the first cases were in mid-August or September, and the last ones occurred in mid- to late November. The 2000 season was remarkably shorter: the first case was reported on August 15 and the last on September 21.

The financial damage to the flocks themselves and the annual appearance of the disease over four successive years (1997–2000) prompted an investigation of the efficacy of vaccinating young goose flocks as they become exposed to infected mosquitoes in July and August. Based on epidemiological considerations, flocks should be actively immunized before exposure to seasonal biting-insect activity and before one month of age. Vaccination should be continued through November when cold nights gradually reduce mosquito activity. In Israel, a flaviviral disease of domestic turkeys known as Israeli turkey meningoencephalitis (TME) has been recognized for many years. It was first described in 1960, with most of the outbreaks occurring seasonally between August and December.[2] Both viruses are arthropod borne; WNV belongs to the Japanese encephalitis group, while TME virus is classified serologically within the Ntaya group.[3] In contrast to West Nile fever of geese, turkeys younger than 10 weeks are seldom affected, and rarely have outbreaks occurred in successive years. There is no evidence that TME is in any way infectious for humans. A live attenuated vaccine in its present formulation has been available commercially since 1975.[4]

In addition to laboratory and field studies with TME vaccine in goose flocks, we have investigated the efficacy of an inactivated WNV vaccine prepared from suckling mouse brains. This type of vaccine resembles most closely one used in protecting humans against Japanese encephalitis.[5]

MATERIAL AND METHODS

Geese

Commercial out-bred geese between three to four weeks old were used in most laboratory experiments. In some field trials, day old goslings and seven-day-old birds were vaccinated.

West Nile Virus

The 1998 isolate was passaged three times in Vero cells, and a stock of virus was aliquoted and stored at $-70°C$. Its titre was $10^{6.3}$ $tcid_{50}/mL$. For challenge, the virus was inoculated intracranially into geese at a dose of $10^{2.7}$ $tcid_{50}/0.1$ mL. This was shown by titration to be equivalent to $10^{2.7}$ goose lethal $dose_{50}$.

A batch of suckling mouse brain virus was prepared by inoculating litters of two-day old mice and harvesting their brains four to five days later when they showed neurological signs.[6] The titer of the batch was $10^{9.8}$ mouse LD_{50}/mL. To inactivate the virus, 0.01% (v/v) formalin was added to the brain extract in 2% fetal bovine serum and the mixture stirred constantly at $4°$ C for four days. Thereafter the mixture was blended with mineral oil to form a stable adjuvant mixture, which was stored at $4°$ C.

Turkey Meningoencephalitis (TME) Vaccine

A commercial live vaccine manufactured in specific pathogen-free eggs was used in these studies. The vaccine dose was $10^{3.0}$ EID_{50}/goose, injected intramuscularly. In some experiments, a formalin-inactivated, oil-adjuvanted product was used. In this case, the concentration of the virus was $10^{5.8}$ EID_{50}/mL before inactivation.

Protection Experiments

In most experiments, the geese were vaccinated at 19–21 days old with either live TME vaccine or killed WNV. In some experiments, the geese were boosted with a second dose of killed WNV three weeks later. Intracranial challenge was performed two to three weeks after injecting either the live vaccine or the second injection of inactivated WNV. In some field trials, killed TME vaccine was injected at one day old and revaccination with live TME at three weeks of age. After challenge the geese were inspected daily for clinical signs and mortality for 14 days. On a number of occasions goose flocks were vaccinated on the farm, and then groups of 20–25 geese were transported to the laboratory for intracranial challenge under controlled conditions.

Serology

Geese were bled on the day of vaccination and at weekly intervals thereafter, including the day of challenge. Sera were separated and stored at $-20°$ C. To determine virus-neutralizing (VN) antibody titers, the sera were diluted two-fold, commencing at 1:10 in 96-well microtiter plates. An equal volume of $10^{2.7}$ $tcid_{50}$ of WNV/0.1 mL was added to each well and the virus-antibody mixture held at room temperature for one hour. Thereafter, 10^4 Vero cells/0.1 mL were added to each well and the plates placed at $37°$ C in an atmosphere of 5% CO_2 for 72 hours. The VN titer of the serum is the highest dilution that neutralized 50%–100% of the cytopathogenic effect of the virus.

RESULTS

Vaccination of Geese with Killed WNV Titration of Mouse Brain Extract

In this experiment groups of seven-day-old geese were inoculated intramuscularly with either undiluted, ten-fold, or hundred-fold dilution of inactivated brain extract. A second injection was given two weeks later. All the groups were challenged intracranially three weeks later.

TABLE 1. Vaccination of 7- and 21-day-old geese with serial dilutions of a single batch of inactivated West Nile virus vaccine. The groups were challenged at 6 weeks of age

Dilution	Number challenged	Number survived	Percent protection
undiluted	27	24	89
1:10	30	22	73
1:100	29	13	45
1:1000	20	7	24
Control	20	0	0

TABLE 2. Protection against intracranial challenge of 18-day-old geese vaccinated with inactivated WNV vaccine of mouse brain origin

Vaccine dose	Number of injections	Number challenged	Number survived	Percent protection
Single	One	12	5	42
Double	One	8	5	63
Single	Two	16	15	94
None	None	14	0	0

TABLE 3. Effect of the route of immunization on the duration of immunity

Route	21-day challenge	Percent protection	42-day challenge	Percent protection
Subcutaneous	7/22[a]	58	12/13	92
Intramuscular	9/12	75	8/10	80

[a]Number surviving/number challenged.

TABLE 1 summarizes the levels of protection produced by each dilution. The protective dose (PD_{50}) of this batch was estimated to be 1:50. This estimate is of considerable interest in determining the potency of a batch before embarking on a field trial.

In the second experiment, groups of 18-day-old geese were immunized once or twice (21 days later) with a single or a double dose of inactivated vaccine. All the groups were challenged intracranially three weeks postvaccination.

TABLE 2 shows that even one immunization with a vaccine dose of 0.5 mL resulted in 42% protection. When the volume of inoculum was increased to 1.0 mL, 63% protection was achieved. As seen in TABLE 2, two injections of vaccine spaced three weeks apart resulted in 94% protection in this trial.

In an attempt to determine the duration of immunity following immunization with two doses of inactivated vaccine three weeks apart, groups of birds were challenged three and six weeks postvaccination. TABLE 3 shows that the route of immunization (subcutaneous or intramuscular) had a minor effect on the level or duration of protection.

TABLE 4. TME vaccine: Effect of route of inoculation, age of bird, and vaccine dose on level of protection

Age (days)	Dose	Route	No. survivors/ no. challenged	Percent protection
7	0.5	im	10/12	84
7	0.5	sc	13/14	93
7	1	im	14/17	82
7	1	sc	12/17	71
18	1	im	14/15	93
18	1	sc	10/13	77

TABLE 5. Protection in commercial flocks challenged intracranially under controlled conditions

Flock	Vaccine	No. Survivors/No. challenged	Percent Protection
A	WNV (1x)	13/25	52
	WNV (2x)	16/20	80
B	TME	11/18	61
C	TME	14/25	56
D	TME	14/25	56
E	TME	11/25	44
F	TME	16/24	67
G	TME	17/24	71
H	TME	14/25	56
I	TME	18/25	72
J	TME	9/23	39
K	TME	17/25	68

Efficacy Studies with TME Vaccine

Several parameters, including the immunizing dose, age at vaccination, route of administration, and duration of immunity were investigated. TABLE 4 shows that the level of protection established by TME vaccine was between 71% and 92%. In addition, it was possible to achieve good protection in birds as young as seven days of age.

In a further experiment when groups of birds were challenged 3 and 6 weeks after intramuscular vaccination at 18 days of age, levels of protection were 92% and 95%, respectively. Injection of inactivated TME vaccine at one day of age followed by live vaccine administered either intramuscularly or subcutaneously at 21 days and challenged at 42 days old resulted in 100% protection.

Levels of Immunity Attained in Commercial Flocks following Immunization of WNV and TME Vaccines under Field Conditions

Groups of 18 to 25 geese were brought to the laboratory from designated farms where they had been inoculated with either TME or WNV vaccine. In this trial the

TABLE 6. Level of protection and serological response of geese vaccinated at seven days of age with TME or WNV vaccine

Vaccine	No. surviving/ no. challenged	Virus neutralizing antibody (No. positive/No. tested)			
		Day 0	+21 d	+42 d[a]	Chall +14 d
TME	13/17	4/9	9/17	1/17	9/9
WNV	17/19	4/6	9/19	16/19	17/17

[a] Day of challenge.

geese were six to seven weeks old when challenged. Groups of unvaccinated geese of the same age were challenged together with the farm-derived birds. TABLE 5 shows that under farm conditions of vaccination there was a wide variation in the level of protection among the birds vaccinated with TME. Nevertheless with the exception of farms E and J, over 50% of the birds survived intracranial challenge. In all these protection studies, all the nonvaccinated birds died following challenge.

Investigation of Virus-neutralizing Antibody Levels in Vaccinated and Challenged Geese

In this study groups of geese were immunized at seven days old with either live TME or inactivated WNV vaccine. They were bled on the day of vaccination, at 21 and 42 days old when they were challenged, and two weeks later at the termination of the experiment.

TABLE 6 shows the results of intracerebral challenge. Of the 17 birds receiving TME vaccine, 4 died after challenge. Only one bird in this group had virus-neutralizing (VN) antibodies on the day of challenge. By contrast, 2 of the 19 geese vaccinated with WNV succumbed to challenge, while all but 3 had VN antibodies on the day of challenge.

DISCUSSION

In this study, we have described the incidence of West Nile fever among young goose flocks on Israeli farms from 1997 to 2000. This is the first report of the marked susceptibility of the domestic goose to WNV and parallels that observed among crows in New York in 1999 and 2000. Goose mortality is also remarkable, because human outbreaks of WNV have been reported on several occasions in Israel. In the past, there were no observations involving geese or other domestic fowl. This is in contrast with the report of four WNV isolates from turtle doves (*Streptopelia turtur*) in 1964.[7] The only other domestic animal known to be clinically affected by WNV is the horse, and in 2000 isolates were made from four horses in Israel.[8]

Because of the high fatality rate among goose flocks, we have conducted laboratory and field trials with the heterologous TME vaccine and found that in the laboratory it effectively protected geese against intracerebral challenge with a virulent field isolate of WNV. In this respect, this cross-protection is another example of that demonstrated previously in hamsters immunized with dengue virus and challenged with West Nile virus.[9] In their report, Price and Thind showed that an anamnestic neutralizing antibody response to WNV was detected following challenge of hamsters immunized with dengue 2 virus. In our experiments, the level and duration of protection in the geese was high and long enough to extend through the period of maximal susceptibility of the birds as observed in the field outbreaks. Nevertheless, it was found that production of WNV neutralizing antibodies was not correlated with TME vaccination. The reasons for this enigmatic finding are possibly related to the antigenicity of nonstructural viral proteins, notably NS1, that are also involved in stimulating immunity or in the possible generation of a cell-mediated response that is cross-reactive.[10] By contrast, the antigenicity of the inactivated mouse brain extract was demonstrated both serologically and by protection studies. Because of difficulties involved in its preparation and its cost, the inactivated vaccine would require careful evaluation before mass production is initiated. However, a possible advantage of an inactivated WNV vaccine is that it is less likely to induce postvaccinal reactions in the young geese. Follow-up studies on TME vaccine in the field showed that some flocks reacted unfavorably following vaccination and showed neurological signs and appreciable mortality. In most of these cases, the flocks were affected with intercurrent bacterial infections and may have been aggravated by needle transmission, and other flocks were incubating West Nile fever.

In conclusion, the use of WNV vaccine seems to be the best alternative against West Nile Fever in young geese. In the coming season, precautions will be taken to avoid immunizing flocks experiencing nonspecific mortality.

REFERENCES

1. MALKINSON, M., C. BANET, S. MAHANY, et al. 1998. Virus encephalomyelitis of geese: some properties of the viral isolate [Abstract]. Isr. J. Vet. Med. **53:** 44.
2. KOMAROV, A. & E. KALMAR. 1960. A hitherto undescribed disease—turkey meningoencephalitis. Vet. Rec. **72:** 257–261.
3. CALISHER, C.H., N. KARABATSOS, et al. 1989. Antigenic relationships between flaviviruses as determined by cross-neutralization tests with polyclonal antisera. J. Gen. Virol. **70:** 37–43.
4. IANCONESCU, M., K. HORNSTEIN, et al. 1975. Development of a new vaccine against turkey meningo-encephalitis using a vaccine passaged through the Japanese quail. Avian Pathol. **4:** 119–131.
5. AIZAWA, C., S. HASEGAWA, et al. 1980. Large-scale purification of Japanese encephalitis virus from infected mouse brain for preparation of vaccine. Appl. Environ. Microbil. **39:** 54–57.
6. GOULD, E.A. & J.C.S. CLEGG. 1985. Growth, titration and purification of togaviruses. In Virology: A practical approach. B.W.J. Mahy, Ed.: 43–79. IRL Press. Oxford, UK.
7. NIR, Y., R. GOLDWASSER, et al. 1967. Isolation of arboviruses from wild birds in Israel. Am. J. Epidemiol. **86:** 372–378.
8. BANET, C., A. BRILL, et al. 2001. Phylogenetic relationships of West Nile viruses isolated in Israel from 1997 to 2000. J. Gen. Virol. Submitted.
9. PRICE, W.H. & I.S. THIND. 1972. The mechanism of cross-protection afforded by dengue virus against West Nile virus in hamsters. J. Hyg. (Lond.) **70:** 611–617.
10. CHAMBERS, T.J., T.F. TSAI, et al. 1997. Vaccine development against dengue and Japanese encephalitis: report of a World Health Organization meeting. Vaccine **15:** 1494–1502.

Current Status of Flavivirus Vaccines

ALAN D. T. BARRETT

*Department of Pathology and Center for Tropical Diseases,
University of Texas Medical Branch, Galveston, Texas 77555-0609, USA*

ABSTRACT: Although there are approximately 68 flaviviruses recognized, vaccines have been developed to control very few human flavivirus diseases. Licensed live attenuated vaccines have been developed for yellow fever (strain 17D) and Japanese encephalitis (strain SA14-14-2) viruses, and inactivated vaccines have been developed for Japanese encephalitis and tick-borne encephalitis viruses. The yellow fever live attenuated 17D vaccine is one of the most efficacious and safe vaccines developed to date and has been used to immunize more than 300 million people. A number of experimental vaccines are being developed, most notably for dengue. Candidate tetravalent live attenuated dengue vaccines are undergoing clinical trials. Other vaccines are being developed using reverse genetics, DNA vaccines, and recombinant immunogens. In addition, the yellow fever 17D vaccine has been used as a backbone to generate chimeric viruses containing the premembrane and envelope protein genes from other flaviviruses. The "Chimerivax" platform has been used to construct chimeric Japanese encephalitis and dengue viruses that are in different phases of development. Similar strategies are being used by other laboratories.

KEYWORDS: West Nile virus; flavivirus vaccines; DNA vaccines; yellow fever

INTRODUCTION

The *Flavivirus* genus of the family Flaviviridae consists of approximately 68 viruses. The majority of the viruses in the genus have been associated with either diseases in humans and/or animals or been responsible for one or more laboratory infections. However, a few flavivirus diseases are of major public health importance, including dengue, Japanese encephalitis, tick-borne encephalitis, West Nile, and yellow fever. Commercial vaccines are used to control Japanese encephalitis, tick-borne encephalitis, and yellow fever and have been reported in recent reviews.[1–5] There are no human vaccines currently available to control dengue or West Nile (see TABLE 1).

Address for correspondence: Alan D.T. Barrett, Department of Pathology and Center for Tropical Diseases, University of Texas Medical Branch, Room 4.128A Keiller Building, 301 University Blvd., Galveston, TX 77555-0609. Voice: 409-772-6662; fax: 409-747-2417.
abarrett@utmb.edu

TABLE 1. Current and Experimental live attenuated and inactivated flavivirus vaccines

	Vaccine			
	Current		Experimental	
Virus	Live	Inactivated	Live	Inactivated
Dengue 1	No	No	Yes[a]	No
Dengue 2	No	No	Yes[a]	Yes
Dengue 3	No	No	Yes[a]	No
Dengue 4	No	No	Yes[a]	No
Japanese encephalitis	Yes (China only)	Yes	Yes	No
Tick-borne encephalitis	No	Yes	No	Yes
Yellow fever	Yes	No	Yes	No

[a]Experinental tetravalent dengue vaccine being tested in clinical trials

LIVE ATTENUATED VACCINES

Yellow Fever

Historically the development of live attenuated vaccines has been empirical. The yellow fever (YF) 17D vaccine is one of the finest vaccines ever developed. Wild-type YF virus was first isolated in 1927: strain Asibi was isolated in Ghana, while the French viscerotropic virus (FVV) was isolated in Senegal. Great efforts were made to develop a vaccine, and two approaches were successful. Wild-type FVV was given 128 passages in mouse brain to develop an attenuated variant termed French neurotropic vaccine (FNV). This virus was given additional passages in mouse brain, such that passage 238 was used to vaccinate humans. The vaccine was used in Franco-Africa and proved to be highly immunogenic. Unfortunately, FNV had enhanced neurotropic potential that made it unsuitable for use in children. It was found that 3 in every 1000 children had postvaccinal complications with a case fatality rate of 40%, such that the World Health Organization decided that the vaccine could not be used in children under 14 years of age. This resulted in FNV losing popularity, with the last doses of vaccine used in 1981.

Wild-type Asibi virus was given 176 passages in chicken tissue by Max Theiler and coworkers, and the attenuated variant 17D was isolated. It is interesting to note that other variants were generated at passage 176 and were named 17A, 17B, etc. Only 17D had the phenotypic properties of attenuation and immunogenicity, and Theiler and coworkers were never able to repeat the generation of 17D. Subsequently, strain 17D was given additional passages in chicken tissue, and two substrains were derived. 17D-204 is a substrain derived from passage 204, while 17DD was derived from passage 195. Substrain 17D-204 is used as a vaccine at passages 235-241, while 17DD was given extensive passaging in Brazil, such that the vaccine is used at passages 286-288. Both vaccine substrains are used as vaccines and are manufactured in embryonated chicken eggs. The 17D vaccine has proved to be very safe and highly efficacious. Over 300 million doses of vaccine have been administered, with only 21 cases of reversion reported and only one death (a three-year-old girl in 1965). Reversion to virulence involves vaccine viruses acquiring a neurovirulent phenotype in contrast to the viscerotropic phenotype of wild-type YF virus. One dose of vaccine, that is given by subcutaneous inoculation to those over nine months of age, contains 5000 to 50,000 plaque-forming units of virus. An IgM response is seen within 5–7 days postvaccination, and IgG is present by day 10 postvaccination. Vaccine-induced immunity lasts for at least 10 years and may be 45 years, as demonstrated by studies with U.S. Army volunteers. The World Health Organization certifies vaccination at 10 days postvaccination for a period of 10 years and publishes criteria for the manufacturing of 17D vaccine.

The molecular basis of attenuation of YF virus has been investigated. Comparison of the wild-type Asibi and attenuated 17D-204 virus genomes revealed 61 nucleotide differences that encoded 31 amino acid substitutions. Following the nucleotide sequencing of the genome of the 17DD substrain virus, it was found that the two 17D vaccine substrains shared 19 amino acid substitutions. Over 40% (i.e., 8 of 19) of the amino acid substitutions were in the envelope protein, suggesting that the envelope protein may make an important contribution to the attenuated phenotype. Wild-type FVV differed from the attenuated FNV by 77 nucleotides that encoded 35 amino acid substitutions. The attenuation of Asibi and FVV share a number of common phenotypic features: both viruses have lost their viscerotropic phenotype and are not vector competent (i.e., cannot be transmitted by mosquitoes). Comparison of the mutations in the two attenuation processes reveals two common amino acid substitutions: one at residue 36 of the membrane protein and the other at residue 95 of the nonstructural protein NS4B. The membrane protein is found on the surface of virions closely associated with the envelope protein, while the function of NS4B is unknown other than it is part of the replication complex in virus-infected cells. The significance of the two common amino acid substitutions is unclear, except that it is surprising that two very different attenuation processes, Asibi through chicken tissue and FVV in mouse brain, both result in identical amino acid substitutions. Additional studies have shown that six passages of wild-type strain Asibi in human HeLa cells results in an attenuated variant that has the phenotype of 17D and FNV vaccine viruses, namely loss of viscerotropism and no vector competence. Interestingly, comparison of the genomes of Asibi virus with Asibi HeLa passage six virus reveals only 10 amino acid substitutions, including a substitution at residue 95 of NS4B.[6] Thus, there is indirect evidence that NS4B is involved in attenuation of virulence, but this remains to be confirmed using reverse genetics.

Japanese Encephalitis

The only other live attenuated flavivirus vaccine is Japanese encephalitis (JE) vaccine, strain SA14-14-2, that was developed in the People's Republic of China. This vaccine strain was developed by passage of wild-type strain SA14 in primary hamster kidney cell culture. Following 114 passages of SA14 in primary hamster kidney cell culture, an attenuated derivative, 12-1-8, was isolated. This virus was given additional passages in primary hamster kidney cell culture in different laboratories to generate two substrains, SA14-2-8 and SA14-5-3. The former was used as a veterinary vaccine in horses (see below), whereas the latter was evaluated in humans. Although both viruses were attenuated, neither was sufficiently immunogenic with seroconversion rates below 50% following one dose of vaccine. Subsequently, SA14-5-3 was given additional passages in primary hamster kidney cell culture to derive strain SA14-14-2. This virus has proved to be highly attenuated yet immunogenic. It has been successfully used as a vaccine in the People's Republic of China with over 100 million children vaccinated. Currently, the vaccine is administered as a two-dose regimen, one year apart, with the first dose given at one year of age. The World Health Organization is currently developing criteria for the manufacturing of live attenuated JE vaccines that will, we hope, result in the vaccine's use outside the People's Republic of China. This virus is very attenuated; there is no clinical disease, there are no lesions following direct inoculation into the brains of monkeys or mice, and the virus is nonvector competent. There are no reported cases of reversion to virulence. The molecular basis of attenuation of SA14-14-2 has been investigated by comparing the nucleotide sequence of the genomes of wild-type SA14 and SA14-14-2. The two viruses differ by 57 nucleotides encoding 24 amino acid substitutions. Reverse genetics studies indicate that the envelope protein is a major determinant of the attenuation, in particular, amino acid 138.[7,8]

Tick-borne Encephalitis

Attempts to generate a live attenuated tick-borne encephalitis (TBE) vaccine have investigated the use of the Langat virus, a member of the TBE serogroup of the *Flavivirus* genus that was isolated from a rat in Malaysia. Although the virus is serologically related to Russian spring summer encephalitis and is attenuated in rodents and monkeys, compared to TBE viruses (Russian spring summer encephalitis and central European encephalitis), it did not perform well in human trials involving over 600,000 persons and caused clinical disease in 1 in 18,570 volunteers.[9]

INACTIVATED VACCINES

Owing to problems in generating attenuated yet immunogenic viruses, inactivated vaccines have been developed to control JE and TBE.

Japanese Encephalitis

For Japanese encephalitis, the aim of vaccination is the induction of circulating neutralizing antibodies that prevent invasion of the central nervous system during the viremic phase of JE virus infection. Knowledge of the role of cell-mediated immunity in protective immunity induced by JE vaccines is very limited. The first inactivated vaccines were prepared in 1954 and based on formalin-inactivated strain Nakayama, grown in adult mouse brain. Three- to five-week-old mice were chosen as the system to grow the virus, as virus yields were very high and cell culture systems were very limited at that time. Each mouse brain produced the equivalent of 4–10 doses of vaccine. Current vaccines are still produced in mouse brain, but the technology involved in manufacturing has continually improved. Protamine sulfate precipitation was introduced in 1958 to remove lipids, and sucrose density gradient centrifugation was introduced in 1968 to concentrate and purify the virus to decrease the quantity of mouse brain–derived material administered, especially myelin basic protein. The vaccine is used both as a liquid or lyophilized product and has been available in Japan since 1973.

JE virus antigenic variation has been considered to be an important issue, as the ability of neutralizing antibodies to be effective against all virus strains has given variable results. Some studies have identified differences in the ability of antibodies to neutralize wild-type strains from different geographic locations in Asia, while other studies have failed to show any differences. Accordingly, inactivated vaccines have been produced incorporating different wild-type strains of JE virus. As stated above, the first vaccines were based on strain Nakayama, while more recent vaccines in Asia have used strain Beijing-1 (Nakayama and Beijing-1 strains are considered to be prototypes of the two major immunotypes of JE virus). Interestingly, the Nakayama-based vaccine is still used in the United States. In the People's Republic of China, inactivated vaccine is based on strain P3 that is grown in primary hamster kidney cell culture. Manufacturing of inactivated vaccine is required to meet minimum standards published by the World Health Organization in 1988.

All JE vaccines are given as multiple doses to generate protective immunity. Travelers are given two doses of vaccine by the subcutaneous route 1–3 weeks apart, whereas residents of endemic countries are given a booster dose at one year after the second dose and subsequent boosters every 3–4 years. The seroconversion rate is 90–100% after two doses of vaccine with a protective efficacy of 80%.

The acceptability of the inactivated Japanese encephalitis mouse brain-derived vaccine in the twenty-first century has resulted in vaccine manufacturers developing cell culture–derived vaccines. The acceptability of monkey kidney Vero cells as a substrate to produce vaccine has resulted in candidate inactivated Vero cell-derived vaccines undergoing clinical trials.

Tick-borne Encephalitis

A formalin-inactivated TBE vaccine is based on a central European TBE virus, strain Neudorfl, to control central European TBE (also known as western subtype TBE). Initially, in the 1970s, virus was grown in embryonated chicken eggs; however, transferring manufacture to primary chick embryo fibroblast cell culture and using continuous-flow zonal centrifugation to purify the virus subsequently improved the vaccine. A second vaccine has been developed based on strain K23 (another central European subtype strain) that is also grown in primary chick embryo cell culture. Two doses are given two weeks to three months apart followed by a booster given nine months to one year after the second dose. Boosters are recommended every three years. The seroconversion rate is >95% after two doses of vaccine. The vaccine has proved to be very efficacious with few adverse reactions and has resulted in the near elimination of TBE in Austria. It is unclear if the vaccine is efficacious against the related Russian spring summer encephalitis (also known as the Far Eastern subtype of TBE). A formalin-inactivated vaccine is produced in Russia against Russian spring summer encephalitis. This involves growth of strain Sofjin in chick embryo cell culture.

VETERINARY VACCINES

Live attenuated vaccines have been used to immunize pigs against JE in Japan and the People's Republic of China, as the pig is an amplifying host and causes still-births. In Japan, the ML-17 strain, derived from wild-type strain JaOH066 by passage in monkey kidney cell culture, has been used, while vaccine strains SA14-2-8 and SA14-14-2, derived from wild-type strain SA14, have been used in the People's Republic of China. Neither vaccine virus is able to replicate or be transmitted by mosquitoes.

In the 1960s an inactivated vaccine was developed to control louping ill, a member of the TBE serogroup, in Great Britain. This vaccine was subsequently discontinued in the 1970s.

Wesselsbron is a mosquito-borne flavivirus that was originally isolated in South Africa in 1955 and infects sheep, goats, and cattle in Africa. A live attenuated vaccine was developed to control Wesselsbron by 145 intracerebral passages of a wild-type strain in newborn mice. The vaccine is manufactured in BHK-21 cells, and one dose of vaccine appears to give life-long immunity. There is little published information about this vaccine. Similarly, Israel turkey meningoencephalitis was first reported in turkeys in Israel in 1958 and subsequently in South Africa. Again a live attenuated vaccine was developed to control the disease, but there is little information available on the vaccine.

CANDIDATE VACCINES

There are a number of experimental and/or candidate flavivirus vaccines undergoing development. These are summarized in TABLE 2 and described below.

Poxvirus-vectored Vaccines

Recombinant poxviruses have been studied as potential JE vaccines. The pre-membrane, envelope, NS1, and NS2A protein genes have been expressed using recombinant poxviruses. Initial studies used vaccinia virus, whereas subsequent studies have used the highly attenuated host range defective derivative of the Copenhagen strain of vaccinia virus (known as NYVAC). Recombinant NYVAC expressing JE antigens were shown to protect pigs from JE virus viremia, and the viremia was too low to allow transmission to feeding mosquitoes. More recent studies have used recombinant ALVAC (a plaque-purified isolate of an attenuated vaccine strain of canarypox virus). The advantage of ALVAC is its limited host range that potentially overcomes safety concerns of recombinant vaccinia viruses. These recombinants have been successfully used to protect mice and nonhuman primates. However, in human trials only 1 of 10 vaccinees receiving recombinant ALVAC induced JE neutralizing antibodies, and none of the vaccinia-immune individuals seroconverted.[10] Thus, these results have tempered additional studies using the poxvirus approach to vaccine development. Recently, the attenuated, replication-deficient modified vaccinia Ankara (MVA) strain has been used to immunize nonhuman primates against dengue-2 and dengue-4 viruses. Although there was moderate protec-

TABLE 2. Candidate vaccines

Inactivated virus
Recombinant poxviruses
Infectious clone-derived Live attenuated
Chimeric viruses
Subunit
Yeast
E. coli
Baculovirus
subviral particles
DNA/RNA

tion with one dose of vaccine, booster doses resulted in a protective immune response.[11]

Live Attenuated Dengue Vaccines

Dengue (DEN) is a disease caused by four serologically related viruses known as DEN-1, DEN-2, DEN-3, and DEN-4. Accordingly, a DEN vaccine will need to be tetravalent and include components that induce protective immunity simultaneously against all four DEN viruses. This has proved to be a major stumbling block in the development of a dengue vaccine. Characteristics of a live vaccine are attenuated for neurotropism in the mouse model, and attenuated for dengue disease in nonhuman primates and humans, plus nonvector competence. Two groups have developed candidate live attenuated vaccines. A Thai group in collaboration with Aventis-Pasteur have taken DEN-1 (strain 16007, PDK13), DEN-2 (strain 16681, PDK53), DEN-3 (strain 16562, PGMK 30, FrhL 3), and DEN-4 (strain 1036, PDK 48) and passaged each virus in primary dog kidney (PDK) cell culture to attenuate the viruses. Passage of DEN-3 virus in PDK cells did not attenuate the virus, and so the virus was attenuated by passage in primary green monkey kidney (PGMK) cells and fetal rhesus lung (FrhL) cells. A tetravalent vaccine is undergoing clinical trials.[12] The genomic sequences of wild-type dengue-2 strain 16681 and its attenuated derivative, PDK 53, have been compared, and, interestingly, there are no amino acid differences in the envelope protein, suggesting that this protein is not involved in the attenuated phenotype.[13]

The U.S. military have also developed a candidate tetravalent live attenuated vaccine incorporating DEN-1 (strain 45AZ5, PDK20), DEN-2 (strain S16803, PDK50), DEN-3 (strain CH53489, PDK20), and DEN-4 (strain 341750, PDK20). As with the Thai vaccine, this vaccine is also undergoing clinical trials.[14]

Reverse Genetics/Infectious Clone Technology

Flavivirus molecular biology was revolutionized in 1989 when Rice and coworkers developed technology to rescue YF 17D vaccine virus from complementary DNA.[15] Since flaviviruses have a positive-sense RNA genome, transcription of a cDNA copy of the virus genome will result in an mRNA that is equivalent to the virus genome. Thus, transfection of cells with the mRNA will result in the recovery of infectious virus. Currently, there is no technology to genetically manipulate RNA while genetic manipulation of DNA is straightforward. Therefore, genetic manipulation of a flavivirus cDNA enables mutations to be subsequently recovered in virus. These procedures are known as reverse genetics or infectious clone technology.

Early studies by Lai and coworkers demonstrated that it was possible to construct chimeric flaviviruses (i.e., a "backbone" of one flavivirus with replacement of one or more genes from a different flavivirus). This group used DEN-4 virus as a backbone and showed that the structural protein genes of DEN-4 virus could be replaced with the equivalent genes of other DEN or TBE viruses.[16] Reverse genetics has also been used by a number of laboratories to investigate the molecular basis of attenuation of flaviviruses by introducing specific mutations into a genome and investigating the effects of the mutation(s) of the phenotype of the recovered virus.

Clearly, reverse genetics has great applications to the development of live attenuated flavivirus vaccines. The major issue is the availability of an attenuated virus backbone. One obvious candidate is the YF 17D vaccine virus. Chambers, Monath, and coworkers have used the 17D-204 vaccine virus backbone, exchanging the premembrane and envelope protein genes of YF virus with other flaviviruses to generate chimeric flaviviruses that induce neutralizing antibodies to the heterologous flavivirus.[17] This has been termed the ChimeriVax™ platform. The initial studies involved incorporation of the premembrane and envelope protein genes of the live attenuated JE vaccine virus SA14-14-2. The chimeric YF-JE virus was shown to be highly attenuated and very immunogenic in mice and nonhuman primates. This was not surprising, inasmuch as the chimera included the attenuated backbone of YF 17D and the envelope protein of the live attenuated JE vaccine virus SA14-14-2. The same group and another group have also generated chimeras incorporating the premembrane and envelope protein genes of DEN-2 virus,[18,19] demonstrating that the technology has applicability for a number of flaviviruses, including, potentially, West Nile virus.

The reverse genetics approach, using an attenuated backbone, has also been developed for two other flaviviruses. Lai and coworkers have developed an attenuated backbone for DEN-4 virus,[16] while Huang and coworkers have taken the DEN-2 16681 PDK53 candidate vaccine virus and used this as their attenuated backbone to generate chimeric dengue viruses.[20] The live attenuated JE vaccine virus SA14-14-2 is an attractive candidate as an attenuated backbone to generate chimeric vaccine viruses, but this has not been reported in the literature.

DNA/RNA Vaccines

In recent years "DNA vaccines" have attracted much attention. This involves immunization with a plasmid containing the gene of an immunogen plus a promotor, such that the immunogen is expressed in cells of the host. DNA vaccines have been developed for a number of flaviviruses, including dengue and JE.[21,22] In the case of both viruses, this approach has generated protective immunity in mice and nonhuman primates. A novel variation of this approach was demonstrated for tick-borne encephalitis virus, where immunization with viral RNA also induced a protective immune response.[23] The DNA vaccine approach will not be considered further in this chapter, as it is the subject of the chapter by Chang *et al.* (this volume).

Recombinant Immunogens

Recombinant antigens, in particular those based on the envelope protein being the major target of neutralizing antibodies, have been examined as potential vaccine candidates for JE and DEN. Baculovirus and *E. coli*–expressed envelope protein have given variable results in mice and nonhuman primate models; researchers have lost interest in this technique in recent years. However, the advent of DNA vaccines may see a resurrection in recombinant immunogens, as a number of DNA vaccines have had improved efficaciousness following booster immunizations with protein.

CONCLUSIONS

Vaccines against YF, JE, and TBE have proved to be very effective. Although live attenuated vaccines give superior immunity due to replication of virus in the vaccinee, inactivated vaccines against JE and TBE have been successful but require booster immunizations to maintain immunity. In comparison, development of dengue vaccines has proven to be very difficult due to the requirement to induce protective immunity simultaneously against the four dengue viruses. Development of recombinant vaccines using reverse genetics has great potential. The recent outbreak of West Nile virus in the northeast United States has instigated a push for the development of a vaccine against West Nile virus. Development of a live attenuated West Nile vaccine will be very difficult, as the only successful attenuated flavivirus vaccines were derived empirically following many years of research. A live vaccine will need to be attenuated in humans and be nonvector competent. In the twenty-first century, regulatory authorities require detailed information on the genotype and phenotype of candidate live vaccines, and, to date, there is very limited knowledge of molecular determinants of virulence, attenuation, and vector competence of West Nile virus. This is an area that needs research support. Furthermore, development of a West Nile infectious clone is an important step in the progress of West Nile vaccine research. An inactivated vaccine is the most straightforward route to a vaccine and can follow the process used for JE and TBE viruses. However, our knowledge of West Nile virus–induced immunity is poor, and a vaccine would require multiple doses (at least two doses to get immunity, plus subsequent boosters to maintain immunity) and detailed studies to measure various parameters of the immune response to West Nile virus. At the present time, the most likely candidate vaccines will come from applications of recombinant DNA technology. DNA vaccines and chimeric flaviviruses offer attractive routes to the development of a West Nile vaccine.

REFERENCES

1. BARRETT, A.D.T. 1997. Yellow fever vaccines. Biologicals **25:** 17–25.
2. BARRETT, A.D.T. 1997. Japanese encephalitis and dengue vaccines. Biologicals **25:** 27–34.
3. BARRETT, P.N., F. DORNER & S.A. PLOTKIN. 1999. *In* Vaccines, 3rd edit. S.A. Plotkin & W.A. Orenstein, Eds.: 767–780. W. B. Saunders. Philadelphia, PA.

4. TSAI, T.F., G.-J.J. CHANG & Y.X. YU. 1999. In Vaccines, 3rd edit. S.A. Plotkin & W.A. Orenstein, Eds.: 672–710. W. B. Saunders. Philadelphia, PA.
5. MONATH, T.P. 1999. In Vaccines, 3rd edit. S.A. Plotkin & W.A. Orenstein, Eds.: 815–879. W. B. Saunders. Philadelphia, PA.
6. DUNSTER, L.M. et al. 1999. Molecular and biological changes associated with HeLa cell attenuation of wild-type yellow fever virus. Virology 261: 309–318.
7. SUMIYOSHI,. H., G.H. TIGNOR & R.E. SHOPE. 1995. Characterization of a highly attenuated Japanese encephalitis virus generated from molecularly cloned cDNA. J. Infect. Dis. 171: 1144–1151.
8. ARROYO, J. et al. 2001. Molecular basis for attenuation of neurovirulence of a yellow fever virus/Japanese encephalitis chimera vaccine. J. Virol. 75: 934–942.
9. SMORODINCEV, A.A. & A.V. DUBOV. 1986. Live vaccines against tick-borne encephalitis. In Tick-borne Encephalitis and Its Vaccine Prophylaxis. A.A. Smorodincev, Ed.: 190–211. Meditsina, Leningrad.
10. KONISHI, E. et al. 1998. Induction of Japanese encephalitis virus-specific cytotoxic T lymphocytes in humans by poxvirus-based JE vaccine candidates. Vaccine 16: 842–849.
11. MEN, R. et al. 2000. Immunization of rhesus monkeys with a recombinant of modified vaccinia virus Ankara expressing a truncated envelope glycoprotein of dengue type 2 virus induced resistance to dengue type 2 virus challenge. Vaccine 18: 3113–3122.
12. BHAMARAPRAVATI, N. & Y. SUTEE. 2000. Live attenuated tetravalent dengue vaccines. Vaccine 18 (Suppl. 2): 44–47.
13. KINNEY, R.M. et al. 1997. Construction of infectious cDNA clones for dengue-2 virus: strain 16681 and its attenuated vaccine derivative, strain PDK-53. Virology 230: 300–308.
14. EDELMAN, R. et al. 1994. A live attenuated dengue-1 vaccine candidate (45AZ5) passaged in primary dog kidney cell culture is attenuated and immunogenic for humans. J. Infect. Dis. 170: 1448–1455.
15. RICE, C.M. et al. 1989. Transcription of infectious yellow fever RNA from full-length templates produced by in vitro ligation. New Biol. 1: 285–296.
16. LAI, C.J. et al. 1998. Evaluation of molecular strategies to develop a live dengue vaccine. Clin. Diag. Virol. 10: 173–179.
17. CHAMBERS, T.J. et al. 1999. Yellow fever: Japanese encephalitis chimeric viruses: construction and biological properties. J. Virol. 73: 3095–3101.
18. GUIRAKHOO, F. et al. 2000. Recombinant chimeric yellow fever-dengue type 2 virus is immunogenic and protective in nonhuman primates. J. Virol. 74: 5477–5485.
19. VAN DER MOST, R.G. et al. 2000. Chimeric yellow fever/dengue virus as a candidate dengue vaccine: quantitation of the dengue virus-specific CD8 T-cell response. J. Virol. 74: 8094–8101.
20. HUANG, C.Y. et al. 2000. Chimeric dengue type 2 (vaccine strain PDK-53)/dengue type 1 virus as a potential candidate type 1 virus vaccine. J. Virol. 74: 3020–3028.
21. KOCHEL, T.J. et al. 2000. A dengue virus serotype-1 DNA vaccine induces virus neutralizing antibodies and provides protection from viral challenge in Aotus monkeys. Vaccine 18: 3166–3173.
22. KONISHI, E. et al. 1998. Induction of protective immunity against Japanese encephalitis in mice by immunization with a plasmid encoding JE virus premembrane and envelope genes. J. Virol. 72: 4925–4930.
23. MANDL, C.W. et al. 1998. In vitro–synthesized infectious RNA as an attenuated live vaccine in a flavivirus model. Nature Med. 4: 1438–1440.

Flavivirus DNA Vaccines

Current Status and Potential

GWONG-JEN J. CHANG, BRENT S. DAVIS, ANN R. HUNT, DEREK A. HOLMES, AND GORO KUNO

Division of Vector-Borne Infectious Diseases,
Centers for Disease Control and Prevention, Public Health Service,
United States Department of Health and Human Services,
Fort Collins, Colorado 80522, USA

ABSTRACT: The use of DNA-based vaccines is a novel and promising immunization approach for the development of flavivirus vaccines. This approach has been attempted in vaccine development for various virus species, including St. Louis encephalitis, Russian spring-summer encephalitis, Central European encephalitis, dengue serotypes 1 and 2, Murray Valley encephalitis, Japanese encephalitis, and West Nile viruses. However, very little is known about the factors affecting its efficacy. Recently, we demonstrated that a single intramuscular immunization of DNA vaccine of Japanese encephalitis and West Nile viruses protected mice and horses from virus challenge. Administration of these recombinant plasmid vectors resulted in endogenous expression and secretion of extracellular virus-like particles that correlated well with the induction of protective immunity. These results provided evidence that the virus-like particles composed of premembrane/membrane and envelope proteins are essential for eliciting immune responses similar to those induced by live, attenuated virus vaccines. The biosynthesis and protein processing of premembrane/membrane and envelope proteins that preserve the native conformation and glycosylation profiles identical to virion proteins could be determined by the effectiveness of the transmembrane signal sequence located at the amino-terminus of premembrane protein. The use of DNA vaccines in multivalent and/or combination vaccines designed to immunize against multiple flaviviruses is also a promising area of development.

KEYWORDS: Flavivirus; vaccine; infection; protein

INTRODUCTION

Epidemics of flavivirus infections continue to be a major public health concern worldwide. The yellow fever (YF) virus is the prototype member of the genus *Flavivirus* that includes 70 distinct virus species.[1] More than two billion people are at risk of being infected with members of this group of viruses, including Japanese encephalitis (JE) virus in Asia and Australia; YF virus in Africa and Latin America; West

Address for correspondence: G-J. J. Chang, Division of Vector-Borne Infectious Diseases, Centers for Disease Control and Prevention, Public Health Service, U.S. Department of Health and Human Services, P.O. Box 2087, Fort Collins, CO 80522-2087. Voice: 970-221-6497; fax: 970-221-6476.

gxc7@cdc.gov

Nile (WN) virus in Africa, Central Europe, and America; tick-borne encephalitis (TBE) complex viruses, including Russian spring-summer encephalitis (RSSE) and Central European encephalitis (CEE) viruses in the temporal regions of Europe and Asia; and four serotypes of dengue (DEN-1, -2, -3, and -4) viruses in the tropical and subtropical regions of the world. Conventional vaccines have contributed enormously to the improvement of human health, yet infectious diseases remain the leading cause of mortality worldwide. With the exceptions of YF, JE, and TBE, there is no vaccine available to prevent other flavivirus infection in humans or animals.

The YF 17D vaccine, available since 1936, has been widely regarded as one of the safest and most effective arboviral vaccine ever developed. However, even such a vaccine has not succeeded in controlling the outbreak of the disease. Some of the problems were the failure to implement a routine vaccination program for financial and other reasons, and inadequate public infrastructure to support the deployment of vaccine in developing countries. Significant efforts have been made to develop new and effective vaccine strategies to combat flavivirus infection in humans as well as in domestic animals.[2,3] The reverse genetic technique using infectious cDNA clones derived from 17D, PDK-53 (an attenuated DEN-2 vaccine virus) and genetic engineered, attenuated DEN-4 814669 strain, has greatly increased the potential of creating the genetic-engineered, live-attenuated chimeric flavivirus vaccine.[4–10] However, there is a potential risk of serious infection by virulent viruses that may arise by gene reversion or recombination derived from attenuated vaccine viruses, as demonstrated by the problem encountered in the polio virus eradication campaign and in vaccine development for HIV vaccine.[11–13] With infectious clone technology, it is still difficult to formulate a multivalent live-attenuated vaccine regimen due to potential homologous or heterologous interference during virus replication.

Inoculation of animals with purified plasmid vectors (DNA) represents a novel means of expressing antigens *in vivo* for the generation of both humoral and cellular responses that protect against infectious disease agents and prevent illness due to cancer and autoimmune diseases.[14,15] Plasmid DNA is stable at ambient temperature and amenable to developing a standardized generic manufacturing process. It allows a rapid screening and manipulation of gene sequence to identify and enhance vaccine potential. Plasmid DNA vaccines thus provide an invaluable alternative to attenuated, inactivated, or viral-vectored subunit vaccines.

Members of the genus *Flavivirus* have a positive-sense single-strand RNA genome approximately 11 kb in size, which encodes for a single polyprotein precursor arranged in the order of capsid (C), premembrane (prM), envelope (E), and seven nonstructural (NS) proteins (NS1, NS2A, NS2B, NS3, NS4A, NS4B, and NS5).[16,17] Processing of the N-terminal polyprotein by the host signalase and virus serine protease complex, NS2B/NS3, yields three structural proteins (C, prM, and E) that are assembled into the virion. Virus assembly occurs at the membrane of the endoplasmic reticulum (ER) and leads to formation of immature virions containing prM. The immature virions are then transported from the ER to the Golgi apparatus where the majority of prM is cleaved to M by the furin-like host protease during exocytosis.[18] The immature virions do not exhibit low-pH-induced conformational changes or fusion activity in the low-pH exocytic vesicles. Thus, the significant function of prM is to prevent irreversible conformational changes in the E protein that leads to inactivation of the virus. Some DEN virus prM-specific monoclonal antibodies have a detectable virus-neutralizing activity and are protective in mice.[19] However, E protein is believed to mediate receptor binding and membrane fusion; further, it induces a protective immunity. The importance of antibodies to E protein in antiviral protection has been demonstrated in passive transfer experiments.[20–23] In addition to infectious virions, noninfectious virus-like particles (VLPs) that contain the prM/M and E proteins, but lack the nucleocapsid, are released during virus infection. Mason and coworkers have demonstrated that similar particles can be obtained in secreted form when prM and E proteins of JE virus are coexpressed properly in the absence of the C protein and suggested that the VLPs represent capsidless empty viral envelopes.[24,25] Thus, the attention has been focused on the construction of flavivirus DNA vaccine that has a potential of expressing VLPs composed of prM and E proteins.

Flavivirus DNA vaccines for SLE,[26] RSSE and CEE,[27,28] DEN-1,[29] DEN-2,[30] JE,[31–33] MVE,[34] WN,[35] and louping ill (LI)[36] viruses have been developed. All these plasmid DNA constructs contained similar transcriptional regulators and flavivirus gene cassette, induced antibody responses, and provided full or partial protection from virus challenge in mice. In this report, we summarize the current status of flavivirus DNA vaccines and then attempt to correlate the immunogenicity and protective efficacy of various DNA vaccines with genetic constituents of the transcriptional unit. Finally, we discuss the future direction for flavivirus DNA vaccine development.

CURRENT STATUS OF FLAVIVIRUS DNA VACCINES

Expression of the gene cassette in the recombinant DNA vaccine is regulated by transcriptional and translational regulators that include the following basic components: promoter/enhancer, translation initiation sequence, translation terminator, and transcription terminator/polyadenylation signal. The characteristics of the transcriptional and translational control elements in the plasmids expressing flavivirus prM and E proteins are summarized in TABLE 1. The most commonly used transcriptional regulator is human cytomegalovirus immediate-early gene promoter (CMV IE) used in conjunction with bovine growth hormone transcription terminator/polyadenylation sequence [BGH/poly (A)]. The SV40 early promoter used in conjunction with SA40 poly (A) in the SV-PE plasmid has been used to express TBE prM and E proteins with great efficiency.[37] Expression of many genes may depend on or increase by the inclusion of an intron sequence, located at the 5′-nontranslational region of transcribed mRNA. Some of the vaccine plasmids also contain an intron sequence (TABLE 1). Experiments conducted in our lab indicated that the optimal plasmid for *in vitro* JE virus prM-E expression utilizes the CMV IE and the BGH/poly (A).[33] In addition, we demonstrated that inclusion of an intron sequence or a eukaryotic replication origin, $SV40_{ori}$, in the plasmid with CMV IE and BGH/poly (A) neither increases *in vitro* antigen expression nor enhances protective immune response.

In general, vaccine potential, measured by induction of neutralizing (Nt) antibody and protective efficacy after virus challenge, can be improved by multiple intramuscular (i.m.), intradermal (i.d.), or "gene gun" (g.g.) deliveries of DNA vaccine. The most common method is i.m. injection by which plasmid DNA, formulated in

TABLE 1. Characteristics of transcriptional and translational control elements in various eukaryotic plasmids expressing flavivirus prM and E protein

Plasmid	Virus	Promoter	Intron	Kozak sequence surrounding translation initiation site	Poly (A)	Eukaryotic origin of replication	Reference
pSLE1	SLE	CMV IE	No	?	CMV IE	No	26
pJME	JE	CMV IE	No	–9•CGGCTCAATCATCATGGC•+4	BGH	SV40$_{ori}$	31
pCJEME	JE	CMV IE	No	–9•CGAATTCACCATGGC•+4	BGH	SV40$_{ori}$	32
pNJEME	JE	CMV IE	Yes	–9•CGAATTCACCATGGC•+4	BGH	No	43
pCDJE2-7	JE	CMV IE	No	–9•CGCCGCCGCCATGGC•+4	BGH	SV40$_{ori}$	33
pCBJE1-14	JE	CMV IE	No	–9•CGCCGCCGCCATGGC•+4	BGH	No	33
pCIBJES14	JE	CMV IE	Yes	–9•CGCCGCCGCCATGGC•+4	BGH	No	33
pCEJE	JE	CMV IE	No	–9•CGCCGCCGCCATGGC•+4	SV40	OriP	33
pREJE	JE	RSV	No	–9•CGCCGCCGCCATGGC•+4	SV40	OriP	33
pRCJE	JE	RSV	No	–9•CGCCGCCGCCATGGC•+4	BGH	SV40$_{ori}$	33
pcDNA3 prM-E	MVE	CMV IE	No	–9•CTGATTTCAAATGTC•+4	BGH	SV40$_{ori}$	34
pCBWN	WN	CMV IE	No	–9•CGCCGCCGCCATGGC•+4	BGH	No	35
p1012D2ME	DEN-2	CMV IE	Yes	?	BGH	No	30
SV-PE	TBE	SV40	No	–9•CGCGGCCGCCATGGC•+4	SV40	SV40$_{ori}$	37
		CMV	No	–9•CGCGGCCGCCATGGC•+4	BGH	No	28
pWRG7077-RSSE	RSSE	CMV IE	Yes	–9•CGTAGACAGGATGGC•+4	BGH	No	27
pWRG7077-CEE	CEE	CMV IE	Yes	–9•CACGGACAGGATGGC•+4	BGH	No	27
pBK-prME	LI	CMV IE	No	–9•CATCCGCACCATGAC•+4	BGH	No	36

NOTE: SLE, St. Louis encephalitis virus; JE, Japanese encephalitis virus; MVE, Murray Valley encephalitis virus; WN, West Nile virus; DEN-2, dengue serotype 2 virus; TBE, tick-borne encephalitis complex viruses, including Russian spring-summer encephalitis virus (RSSE) and Central European encephalitis virus (CEE); Li, louping ill virus; CMV, cytomegalovirus; RSV, respiratory syncytial virus; BGH, bovine growth hormone; SV40$_{ori}$, replication origin of SV40 virus; OriP, replication origin of human papillomavirus.

phosphate-buffered saline, is taken up by muscle cells in which the genes are expressed. Subsequent transfer of expressed gene product(s) to the antigen-presenting cells stimulates proper immune responses. In the administration by g.g., DNA-coated gold particles are propelled into skin by a high-pressure device to deliver DNA to the epidermis.[38] The injected gene is expressed by the specialized antigen-presenting cells, Langerhans' cells, capable of presenting transfected antigens to the T-helper component of the immune system. The amount of DNA-coated gold particles that can be administered in a single application is limited to 2.5 µg per 1 mg of gold beads. TBE DNA vaccine trials in monkeys indicated that between 3 and 12 applications per monkey may be required to achieve an effective vaccination.[39] One study using a WN virus DNA construct demonstrated that the i.m. electrotransfer method greatly increased the vaccine efficacy in mice.[35,40]

The first flavivirus DNA vaccine demonstrating partial protection against challenge virus in mice was the plasmid DNA encoding the prM and E genes of SLE virus.[26] In the study, control mice exhibited about 25% survival, but no Nt antibody was detected in the mice immunized with double doses of the vaccine. In the mice that received three i.d. injections of a recombinant DEN-2 plasmid DNA containing prM and 92% of the E gene, all mice developed anti-DEN-2 Nt antibody.[30] However, experiments using a two-dose schedule failed to protect mice against a lethal DEN-2 virus challenge. Incorporation of the immunostimulatory CpG motif containing pUC19 plasmid in the vaccine regimen improved antibody response to the DEN-2 vaccine.[41] Sixty percent of the mice immunized with DEN-2 DNA vaccine plus pUC19 survived the challenge compared with only 10% in the control group. In other experiments, BALB/C mice inoculated i.m. with 100 µg of pcD2ME two or three times at intervals of two weeks developed a low level of Nt antibody; however, strong anamnestic responses were observed on days 4 and 8 after challenge.[42]

The three DNA vaccines each designed on a different strain of JE virus showed different characteristics of stimulating Nt antibody and of protective efficacy after virus challenge.[31–33] The most promising result among three JE studies demonstrated that a single i.m. injection of a recombinant JE virus DNA induces a long-lasting protective immunity and that the recombinant DNA vaccine is as effective as the inactivated JE vaccine currently used for humans (JE-VAX) in preventing JE in mice.[33] Another study extended the observation that JE virus DNA vaccine is more effective in inducing long-lasting Nt antibody than the licensed vaccine in swine.[43] Similarly, a single i.m. injection of a WN virus DNA construct also induced Nt antibody and provided protection in mice and horses.[35]

The quality of immune responses obtained with DNA vaccination is determined by the molecular configuration and properties of the expressed antigen that govern whether the antigen is secreted by the cell, remains bound in the cell membrane, or remains sequestered within the cell.[44] The DNA construct that expressed a secreted particular form of the prM-E antigen of TBE is far superior to the constructs that synthesize intracellular or soluble secreted forms of the same antigen in terms of the extent and functionality of antibody responses and protection against virus challenge.[28] Furthermore, this study revealed that induction of a Th1 and/or Th2 response is dependent on the route of immunization (i.m. vs. g.g.) and that it is strongly influenced by the physical properties of the antigen. The plasmid expressing the VLP is partially able to overcome the imbalance in favor of Th2 immune response that is inherent in g.g. immunization by stimulating both Th1 and Th2 immunity. LI virus DNA vaccine is not as effective as the recombinant Semliki Forest virus construct in inducing protective response in mice.[36] However, other investigators demonstrated that the g.g. route of DNA vaccination for tick-borne viruses (RSSE and CEE) not only induced protective Nt antibody, but also provided a sterile immunity in mice and monkeys.[27,39]

PARAMETERS AFFECTING GENE EXPRESSION AND VACCINE POTENTIAL OF FLAVIVIRUS DNA VACCINE

Vaccine potential and characteristics of various eukaryotic plasmids that express flavivirus prM and E proteins are summarized in TABLES 1 and 2. Nearly all constructs listed have the same transcriptional control elements and a similar viral gene cassette, with the exception of the DEN-2 plasmid, p1012D2ME, which contains prM gene and 91% of the E gene (TABLE 1). Sequences surrounding the translation initiation site and the composition of the signal peptide preceding the prM protein are the two major differences among the constructs. These differences may contribute to the differences in quantity and quality of the protein synthesized and hence vaccine efficacy. Conserved features of the Kozak sequence flanking vertebrate translation initiation sites include a strong preference for purine at the −3 position; a higher frequency of G at positions −9, −6, −3, and +4; and a preference for A or C at positions −5, −4, −2, and −1.[45] The sequence used in our JE and WN virus constructs was −9•GCCGCCGCCATGG•+4, which fits the general criteria listed above.[33,35] Although less than 1% of eukaryotic mRNA sequences exhibit this sequence, the experimental data have suggested that this sequence provides exceptionally high levels of translation potential.[45,46] In the cell lines (COS-1) transformed by pCBJE1-14 or pCBWN plasmid, secretion of prM/M and E proteins to the culture media was as efficient as in virus infection (G-J. Chang, unpublished observation). Another DNA construct fitting Kozak's general consensus sequence is TBE virus for which the NotI restriction endonuclease with recognition sequence GCGGCCGC was used to construct SV-PE plasmid.[28,47] The cell line (COS-7) transformed with SV-PE plasmid also secreted the prM and E proteins in the form of VLP to the culture medium. One other observation further supported that a single base difference in the −3 position (G to C change) abrogated the target cell recognition because of reduced surface expression of a minigene-encoded lymphocytic choriomeningitis virus T cell epitope.[48] Thus, a proper Kozak sequence is crucial for efficient recombinant protein synthesis.

Signal peptides determine translocation and orientation of inserted protein—hence, the topology of prM and E proteins. The most common feature of signal peptides of eukaryotes consists of an 8–12 stretch of hydrophobic amino acids called the h-region.[49] The region between the initiator Met and the h-region, the n-region, usually has 1–5 amino acids and normally carries positively charged amino acids. Between the h-region and the cleavage site is the c-region, which consists of 3–7 polar, but mostly uncharged, amino acid residues. During viral polyprotein synthesis, modulation of the signalase cleavage site from a cryptic to cleavable conformation at the junction of C and prM proteins depends on prior removal of the C protein by

TABLE 2. Characteristics of the signal peptides and their vaccine of potentials among flavivirus DNA vaccine constructs

Plasmid	Signal peptide sequence preceding prM protein	Signal peptide probability[a]			Immunization protocol/protection
		SP	AP	C site	
pSLE1	?LDTINRRPSKKKRGGTRSLLGLAALIGLASS/LQLLSTYQG	0.702	0.292	0.352	i.m. × 2/partial
pJME	MWLASLAVVIACAGA/MKLSNFQGK	0.998	0.000	0.778	i.m. × 2/partial
pCJEME	MNEGSIMWLASLAVVIACAGA/MKLSNFQGK	0.985	0.012	0.785	i.m. × 2/100%
pCBJE1-14	MGRKQNKRGGNEGSIMWLASLAVVIACAGA/MKLSNFQGK	0.791	0.199	0.623	i.m. × 1/100%
pcDNA3 prM-E	MSKKKRGGSETSVLMVIFMLIGFAAA/KLSNFQGK	0.721	0.277	0.622	i.m. × 4/partial g.g. × 2–4/100%
pCBWN	MGKRSAGSIMWLASLAVVIACAGA/VTLSNFQGK	0.976	0.024	0.526	i.m. × 1/100%
p1012D2ME	MNVLRGFRKEJGRMLNILNRRRRTAGMIIMLIPTVMA/FHLTTRNGE	0.165	0.778	0.164	i.d. × 2/none
SV-PE	MVGLQKRGKRRSATDWMSWLLVITLLGMTLA/ATVRKERGD	0.943	0.056	0.899	i.m. or g.g. × 2/100%
pWRG7077-RSSE	MGWLLVVVLLGVTLA/ATVRKERGD	1.000	0.000	0.912	g.g. × 2/100%
pWRG7077-CEE	MSWLLVITLLGMTIA/ATVRKERGD	0.999	0.000	0.821	g.g. × 2/100%

NOTE: Single amino acid codes are used, and charged amino acids are highlighted by underlined bold letters. The signalase cleavage site separating SP and prM is indicated by a slash. DNA vaccines were inoculated by the intramuscular (i.m.), intradermal (i.d.), or gene gun (g.g.) method.

[a]The SignalP-HMM program (http://www.cbs.dtu.dk/services/SignalP-2.0/)[51] was applied to calculate the signal peptide (SP), anchor peptide (AP), and signalase cleavage site (C site) probabilities.

the viral protease complex, NS2B/NS3.[50] Therefore, it is critical to consider the effectiveness of the viral signal sequence when prM and E proteins are to be expressed alone by an expression plasmid.

Signal peptide differences in various plasmid constructs may account for the difference in protein translocation, cleavage site presentation, and correct topology—thus, prM and E secretion and VLP formation. A machine-learning computer program using a hidden Markov model (HMM) trained on eukaryotes (http://www.cbs.dtu.dk/services/SignalP-2.0/)[51] was applied to calculate the signal peptide probability of the prM signal peptide sequences in different plasmid constructs (TABLE 2). SignalP-HMM searches correctly predicted the signal peptidase cleavage sites in all constructs. However, considerable differences in cleavage probability (ranging between 0.164 and 1.000) and in signal peptide probability (ranging between 0.165 and 1.00) were observed (TABLE 2). The cleavage site and signal peptide probabilities are influenced by the positively charged amino acids in the n-region, the length of the hydrophobic amino acids in the h-region, and amino acid composition in the c-region in the constructs (FIG. 1).[52] Three JE virus plasmid constructs each derived from a different strain of JE virus showed different vaccine potentials.[31–33] The signal peptide sequences in these constructs are different in the length of n-region that may or may not contain charged amino acids (TABLE 2). The n-region containing positively charged amino acids forms a short loop in the cytoplasmic side that causes the h-region (transmembrane helix) to be inserted in a tail orientation, exposing the signalase cleavage site. In our study, secreted VLPs containing prM/M and E proteins could be purified from culture medium of the pCDJE2-7 transformed cell line, JE4B, or the pCBJE1-14 transiently transformed COS-1 cells. The gradient-purified VLPs and virions have identical immunological and biochemical properties. Processing efficiency from prM to mature M protein, the hallmark of flavivirus morphogenesis, is also similar between VLPs and virion particles.[53] Thus, there exists a high probability that prM and E proteins expressed by pCDJE2-7 and pCBJE1-14 would be expressed as type I transmembrane proteins in the orientation similar to that of virion prM and E.[33] On the other hand, the prM protein of pcDNA3JEME could be expressed as a type II membrane protein with its transmembrane h-region inserted in a head orientation because of the absence of positively charged amino acids in its n-region.[32] Efficient protein synthesis in conjunction with correct topology of expressed prM and E would most likely enhance VLP formation and secretion, thus promoting the immunogenicity of the DNA vaccine.[33]

We have taken advantage of the predictive power of the SignalP-HMM program and applied it to design the WN virus expression plasmid (TABLE 2).[35] The pCBWN plasmid consists of a short version of JE virus signal peptide followed by WN virus prM-E gene sequence. Vaccine potential of this construct was amply demonstrated

---

FIGURE 1. Graphic presentation of the signal peptide probabilities located at the N-terminus of the prM gene of the flavivirus DNA vaccine constructs. Each *panel* represents the graph generated by the SignalP-HMM program (http://www.cbs.dtu.dk/services/SignalP-2.0/)[51] using the signal peptide sequence encoded in each DNA construct as indicated in TABLE 2. The n-, h-, and c-region of a signal peptide are represented in *panel* A by *n*, *h*, and *c*, respectively. *Panels* F and G, representing pSLE1 and p1012D2ME constructs, respectively, predict that the signal peptides in these two plasmids may contain a cryptic cleavage.

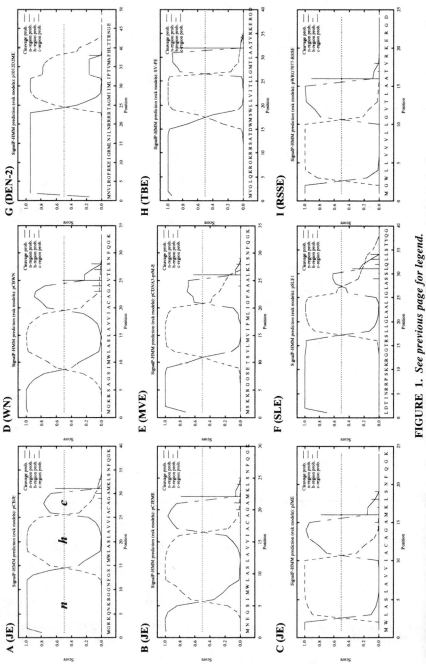

FIGURE 1. *See previous page for legend.*

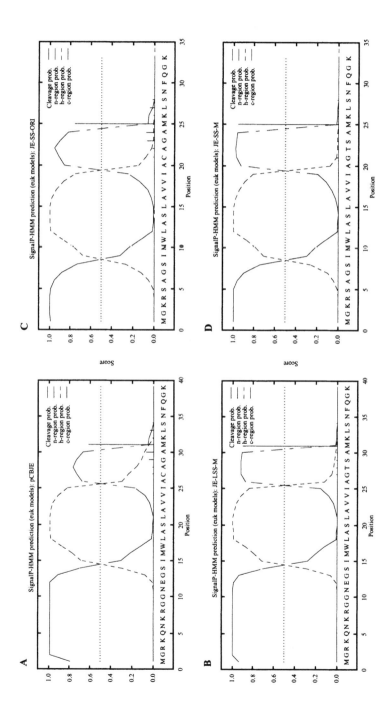

FIGURE 2. Signal peptide probability of the pCBJE1-14 (pCBJE) predicted by the SignalP-HMM program (*panel A*). The signal peptide probability can be improved by altering the c-region sequence at −4 and −2 positions (C-4G and G-2S) (*panel B*, JE-LSS-M), by shortening the n-region (*panel C*, JE-SS-ORI), or by a combination of both modifications (*panel D*, JE-SS-M).

TABLE 3. Neutralizing antibody (Nt) responses in mice immunized with different doses of the combined WN and JE virus DNA vaccines

| | pCBWN + pCBJE1-14 [dose per plasmid (µg)] | | | | pCB control |
	100 + 100	40 + 40	20 + 20	10 + 10	(100 µg/ plasmid)
Percentage of mice with Nt:					
WN virus/JE virus	100/100	100/70	70/0	60/0	0/0
Range of PRNT$_{90}$ titer:					
WN virus	1:320–1:80	1:80–1:20	1:80–<1:10	1:20–<1:10	<1:10
JE virus	1:40–1:10	1:10–<1:10	<1:10	<1:10	<1:10

NOTE: Groups of 10, 3-week-old, female ICR outbred mice were i.m. injected with a single dose of combined plasmid DNAs as indicated. The serum specimens collected 12 weeks after immunization were assayed by the plaque-reduction neutralization test (PRNT). The end-point titers against JE and WN virus were calculated based on the 90% plaque reduction using JE virus (strain SA-14) and WN virus (strain NY-6480), respectively.

because a single i.m. injection of pCBWN DNA not only induced a protective immunity, but also prevented WN virus infection in mice and horses.

FUTURE DIRECTIONS

Efficient synthesis of the immune-dominated protective antigen(s) in its native conformation is indispensable for the development of an effective DNA vaccine. Thus, designing an optimal signal sequence at the N-terminus of the prM gene is the key element and deserves more attention to achieve this objective. Virus-encoded signal sequence is, by no means, the only optimal signal peptide available. Using the signal peptide encoded in the pCBJE1-14 plasmid as an example, the signal sequence probability can be improved by shortening the n-region, altering the c-region sequence, or a combination of both modifications (FIG. 2). We have used the shortened version of JE virus signal peptide for the expression of WN virus prM and E genes.[35] Dose titration studies by single i.m. inoculation indicated that the pCBWN was at least 2- to 4-fold more immunogenic than pCBJE1-14 in mice (G-J. Chang, unpublished observation). Increased immunogenicity of the pCBWN vaccine may correlate with the observation that secretion of WN virus proteins by pCBWN plasmid was more efficient than its JE virus counterpart.

Use of multivalent and/or combination vaccines designed to immunize against multiple flaviviruses is also a promising area of development. The first step to achieve this goal is the construction of monovalent vaccine components that include all important human pathogens, such as YF, four serotypes of DEN, JE, WN, SLE, and TBE (RSSE and CEE) viruses. Use of the combination vaccine to protect immunized animals from RSSE and CEE virus infections was first demonstrated by Schmaljohn and coworkers.[27,54] Preliminary data from our group also demonstrated that i.m. injection of the combined pCBJE1-14 and pCBWN DNA vaccines induced

JE virus– and WN virus–specific Nt antibodies in mice (TABLE 3; G-J. Chang, unpublished results). Each monovalent component, constructed using an expression vector that has identical transcriptional and translational regulators, needs to be tested in the same model system to ensure its vaccine potential. A combination vaccine cocktail can then be formulated specifically for a particular geographic region. The vaccine cocktail for tropical and subtropical Asia should include four serotypes of DEN, WN, and JE virus vaccines. Likewise, four serotypes of DEN, WN, and YF virus vaccines and four serotypes of DEN, Rocio, and YF virus vaccines are included in the cocktail for Africa and Latin America, respectively.

REFERENCES

1. KUNO, G., G.J. CHANG, K.R. TSUCHIYA, *et al.* 1998. Phylogeny of the genus *Flavivirus*. J. Virol. **72:** 73–83.
2. BRANDT, W.E. 1990. From the World Health Organization: development of dengue and Japanese encephalitis vaccines. J. Infect. Dis. **162:** 577–583.
3. CHAMBERS, T.J., T.F. TSAI, Y. PERVIKOV & T.P. MONATH. 1997. Vaccine development against dengue and Japanese encephalitis: report of a World Health Organization meeting. Vaccine **15:** 1494–1502.
4. GUIRAKHOO, F., R. WELTZIN, T.J. CHAMBERS, *et al.* 2000. Recombinant chimeric yellow fever–dengue type 2 virus is immunogenic and protective in nonhuman primates. J. Virol. **74:** 5477–5485.
5. MONATH, T.P., I. LEVENBOOK, K. SOIKE, *et al.* 2000. Chimeric yellow fever virus 17D–Japanese encephalitis virus vaccine: dose-response effectiveness and extended safety testing in rhesus monkeys. J. Virol. **74:** 1742–1751.
6. GUIRAKHOO, F., Z.X. ZHANG, T.J. CHAMBERS, *et al.* 1999. Immunogenicity, genetic stability, and protective efficacy of a recombinant, chimeric yellow fever–Japanese encephalitis virus (ChimeriVax-JE) as a live, attenuated vaccine candidate against Japanese encephalitis. Virology **257:** 363–372.
7. MONATH, T.P., K. SOIKE, I. LEVENBOOK, *et al.* 1999. Recombinant, chimaeric live, attenuated vaccine (ChimeriVax) incorporating the envelope genes of Japanese encephalitis (SA14-14-2) virus and the capsid and nonstructural genes of yellow fever (17D) virus is safe, immunogenic, and protective in non-human primates. Vaccine **17:** 1869–1882.
8. BUTRAPET, S., C.Y. HUANG, D.J. PIERRO, *et al.* 2000. Attenuation markers of a candidate dengue type 2 vaccine virus, strain 16681 (PDK-53), are defined by mutations in the 5′-noncoding region and nonstructural proteins 1 and 3. J. Virol. **74:** 3011–3019.
9. HUANG, C.Y., S. BUTRAPET, D.J. PIERRO, *et al.* 2000. Chimeric dengue type 2 (vaccine strain PDK-53)/dengue type 1 virus as a potential candidate dengue type 1 virus vaccine. J. Virol. **74:** 3020–3028.
10. BRAY, M. & C.J. LAI. 1991. Construction of intertypic chimeric dengue viruses by substitution of structural protein genes. Proc. Natl. Acad. Sci. USA **88:** 10342–10346.
11. LIU, H-M., D-P. ZHENG, L-B. ZHANG, *et al.* 2000. Molecular evolution of a type 1 wild-vaccine poliovirus recombinant during widespread circulation in China. J. Virol. **74:** 11153–11161.
12. GUILLOT, S., V. CARO, N. CUERVO, *et al.* 2000. Natural genetic exchanges between vaccine and wild poliovirus strains in humans. J. Virol. **74:** 8434–8443.
13. BERKHOUT, B., K. VERHOEF, J.L.B. VAN WAMEL, *et al.* 1999. Genetic instability of live, attenuated human immunodeficiency virus type 1a vaccine strains. J. Virol. **73:** 1138–1145.
14. WANG, S., X. LIU, K. FISHER, *et al.* 2000. Enhanced type I immune response to a hepatitis B DNA vaccine by formulation with calcium- or aluminum phosphate. Vaccine **18:** 1227–1235.
15. DONNELLY, J.J., J.B. ULMER, J.W. SHIVER, *et al.* 1997. DNA vaccines. Annu. Rev. Immunol. **15:** 617–648.

16. RICE, C.M., E.M. LENCHES, S.R. EDDY, *et al.* 1985. Nucleotide sequence of yellow fever virus: implications for flavivirus gene expression and evolution. Science **229:** 726–733.
17. CHAMBERS, T.J., C.S. HAHN, R. GALLER, *et al.* 1990. Flavivirus genome organization, expression, and replication. Annu. Rev. Microbiol. **44:** 649–688.
18. STADLER, K., S.L. ALLISON, J. SCHALICH, *et al.* 1997. Proteolytic activation of tick-borne encephalitis virus by furin. J. Virol. **71:** 8475–8481.
19. KAUFMAN, B.M., P.L. SUMMERS, D.R. DUBOIS, *et al.* 1989. Monoclonal antibodies for dengue virus prM glycoprotein protect mice against lethal dengue infection. Am. J. Trop. Med. Hyg. **41:** 576–580.
20. BRANDRISS, M.W., J.J. SCHLESINGER, E.E. WALSH, *et al.* 1986. Lethal 17D yellow fever encephalitis in mice: I. Passive protection by monoclonal antibodies to the envelope proteins of 17D yellow fever and dengue 2 viruses. J. Gen. Virol. **67:** 229–234.
21. CECILIA, D., D.A. GADKARI, N. KEDARNATH, *et al.* 1988. Epitope mapping of Japanese encephalitis virus envelope protein using monoclonal antibodies against an Indian strain. J. Gen. Virol. **69:** 2741–2747.
22. ZHANG, M.J., M.J. WANG, S.Z. JIANG, *et al.* 1989. Passive protection of mice, goats, and monkeys against Japanese encephalitis with monoclonal antibodies. J. Med. Virol. **29:** 133–138.
23. KREIL, T.R., E. MAIER, S. FRAISS, *et al.* 1998. Neutralizing antibodies protect against lethal flavivirus challenge, but allow for the development of active humoral immunity to a nonstructural virus protein. J. Virol. **72:** 3076–3081.
24. MASON, P.W., S. PINCUS, M. FOURNIER, *et al.* 1991. Japanese encephalitis virus-vaccinia recombinants produce particulate forms of the structural membrane proteins and induce high levels of protection against lethal JEV infection. Virology **180:** 294–305.
25. KONISHI, E. & P.W. MASON. 1993. Proper maturation of the Japanese encephalitis virus envelope glycoprotein requires cosynthesis with the premembrane protein. J. Virol. **67:** 1672–1675.
26. PHILLPOTTS, R.J., K. VENUGOPAL & T. BROOKS. 1996. Immunisation with DNA poly-nucleotides protects mice against lethal challenge with St. Louis encephalitis virus. Arch. Virol. **141:** 743–749.
27. SCHMALJOHN, C., L. VANDERZANDEN, M. BRAY, *et al.* 1997. Naked DNA vaccines expressing the prM and E genes of Russian spring-summer encephalitis virus and Central European encephalitis virus protect mice from homologous and heterologous challenge. J. Virol. **71:** 9563–9569.
28. ABERLE, J.H., S.W. ABERLE, S.L. ALLISON, *et al.* 1999. A DNA immunization model study with constructs expressing the tick-borne encephalitis virus envelope protein E in different physical forms. J. Immunol. **163:** 6756–6761.
29. RAVIPRAKASH, K., T.J. KOCHEL, D. EWING, *et al.* 2000. Immunogenicity of dengue virus type 1 DNA vaccines expressing truncated and full length envelope protein. Vaccine **18:** 2426–2434.
30. KOCHEL, T., S.J. WU, K. RAVIPRAKASH, *et al.* 1997. Inoculation of plasmids expressing the dengue-2 envelope gene elicits neutralizing antibodies in mice. Vaccine **15:** 547–552.
31. LIN, Y.L., L.K. CHEN, C.L. LIAO, *et al.* 1998. DNA immunization with Japanese encephalitis virus nonstructural protein NS1 elicits protective immunity in mice. J. Virol. **72:** 191–200.
32. KONISHI, E., M. YAMAOKA, *et al.* 1998. Induction of protective immunity against Japanese encephalitis in mice by immunization with a plasmid encoding Japanese encephalitis virus premembrane and envelope genes. J. Virol. **72:** 4925–4930.
33. CHANG, G.J., A.R. HUNT & B. DAVIS. 2000. A single intramuscular injection of recom-binant plasmid DNA induces protective immunity and prevents Japanese encephalitis in mice. J. Virol. **74:** 4244–4252.
34. COLOMBAGE, G., R. HALL, M. PAVY, *et al.* 1998. DNA-based and alphavirus-vectored immunisation with prM and E proteins elicits long-lived and protective immunity against the flavivirus, Murray Valley encephalitis virus. Virology **250:** 151–163.
35. DAVIS, B.S., G-J.J. CHANG, B. CROPP, *et al.* 2001. West Nile virus recombinant DNA vaccine protects mouse and horse from virus challenge and expresses *in vitro* a non-

infectious recombinant antigen that can be used in enzyme-linked immunosorbent assays. J. Virol. **75:** 4040–4047.

36. FLEETON, M.N., P. LILJESTROM, B.J. SHEAHAN, *et al.* 2000. Recombinant Semliki Forest virus particles expressing louping ill virus antigens induce a better protective response than plasmid-based DNA vaccines or an inactivated whole particle vaccine. J. Gen. Virol. **81:** 749–758.

37. SCHALICH, J., S.L. ALLISON, K. STIASNY, *et al.* 1996. Recombinant subviral particles from tick-borne encephalitis virus are fusogenic and provide a model system for studying flavivirus envelope glycoprotein functions. J. Virol. **70:** 4549–4557.

38. FYNAN, E.F., R.G. WEBSTER, D.H. FULLER, *et al.* 1993. DNA vaccines: protective immunizations by parenteral, mucosal, and gene-gun inoculations. Proc. Natl. Acad. Sci. U.S.A. **90:** 11478–11482.

39. SCHMALJOHN, C., D. CUSTER, L. VANDERZANDEN, *et al.* 1999. Evaluation of tick-borne encephalitis DNA vaccines in monkeys. Virology **263:** 166–174.

40. MIR, L.M., M.F. BUREAU, J. GEHL, *et al.* 1999. High-efficiency gene transfer into skeletal muscle mediated by electric pulses. Proc. Natl. Acad. Sci. USA **96:** 4262–4267.

41. PORTER, K.R., T.J. KOCHEL, S.J. WU, *et al.* 1998. Protective efficacy of a dengue 2 DNA vaccine in mice and the effect of CpG immuno-stimulatory motifs on antibody responses. Arch. Virol. **143:** 997–1003.

42. KONISHI, E., M. YAMAOKA, I. KURANE, *et al.* 2000. A DNA vaccine expressing dengue type 2 virus premembrane and envelope genes induces neutralizing antibody and memory B cells in mice. Vaccine **18:** 1133–1139.

43. KONISHI, E., M. YAMAOKA, I. KURANE, *et al.* 2000. Japanese encephalitis DNA vaccine candidates expressing premembrane and envelope genes induce virus-specific memory B cells and long-lasting antibodies in swine. Virology **268:** 49–55.

44. VOGEL, F. & N. SARVER. 1995. Nucleic acid vaccines. Clin. Microbiol. Rev. **8:** 406–410.

45. CAVENER, D.R. & S.C. RAY. 1991. Eukaryotic start and stop translation sites. Nucleic Acids Res. **19:** 3185–3192.

46. KOZAK, M. 1997. Recognition of AUG and alternative initiator codons is augmented by G in position +4, but is not generally affected by the nucleotides in positions +5 and +6. EMBO J. **16:** 2482–2492.

47. ALLISON, S.L., C.W. MANDL, C. KUNZ, *et al.* 1994. Expression of cloned envelope protein genes from the flavivirus tick-borne encephalitis virus in mammalian cells and random mutagenesis by PCR. Virus Genes **8:** 187–198.

48. AN, L.L., F. RODRIGUEZ, S. HARKINS, *et al.* 2000. Quantitative and qualitative analyses of the immune responses induced by a multivalent minigene DNA vaccine. Vaccine **18:** 2132–2141.

49. VON HEIJNE, G. 1985. Signal sequences: the limits of variation. J. Mol. Biol. **184:** 99–105.

50. LOBIGS, M. 1993. Flavivirus premembrane protein cleavage and spike heterodimer secretion require the function of the viral proteinase NS3. Proc. Natl. Acad. Sci. USA **90:** 6218–6222.

51. NIELSEN, H. & A. KROGH. 1998. Prediction of signal peptides and signal anchors by a hidden Markov model. Proc. Int. Conf. Intell. Syst. Mol. Biol. **6:** 122–130.

52. SAKAGUCHI, M., R. TOMIYOSHI, T. KUROIWA, *et al.* 1992. Functions of signal and signal-anchor sequences are determined by the balance between the hydrophobic segment and the N-terminal charge. Proc. Natl. Acad. Sci. USA **89:** 16–19.

53. HUNT, A.R., B.C. CROPP & G.-J.J. CHANG. 2001. A recombinant particulate antigen of Japanese encephalitis virus produced in stably-transformed cells is an effective non-infectious antigen and subunit immunogen. J. Virol. Methods **97:** 133–149.

54. SCHMALJOHN, C., D. CUSTER, L. VANDERZANDEN, *et al.* 1999. Evaluation of tick-borne encephalitis DNA vaccines in monkeys. Virology **263:** 166–174.

Antibody Prophylaxis and Therapy for Flavivirus Encephalitis Infections

JOHN T. ROEHRIG,[a] LISA A. STAUDINGER,[a,b] ANN R. HUNT,[a]
JAMES H. MATHEWS,[a] AND CAROL D. BLAIR[b]

[a]*Arbovirus Diseases Branch, Division of Vector-Borne Infectious Diseases,
National Center for Infectious Diseases, Centers for Disease Control and Prevention,
United States Public Health Service, Department of Health and Human Services,
Fort Collins, Colorado 80522, USA*

[b]*Department of Microbiology, Colorado State University,
Fort Collins, Colorado 80523, USA*

ABSTRACT: The outbreak of West Nile (WN) encephalitis in the United States
has rekindled interest in developing direct methods for prevention and control
of human flaviviral infections. Although equine WN vaccines are currently
being developed, a WN vaccine for humans is years away. There is also no
specific therapeutic agent for flaviviral infections. The incidence of human WN
virus infection is very low, which makes it difficult to target the human populations in need of vaccination and to assess the vaccine's economic feasibility.
It has been shown, however, that prophylactic application of antiflaviviral antibody can protect mice from subsequent virus challenge. This model of antibody
prophylaxis using murine monoclonal antibodies (MAbs) has been used to
determine the timing of antibody application and specificity of applied antibody necessary for successful prophylaxis. The major flaviviral antigen is the
envelope (E) glycoprotein that binds cellular receptors, mediates cell membrane fusion, and contains an array of epitopes that elicit virus-neutralizing
and nonneutralizing antibodies. The protective efficacy of an E-glycoprotein-
specific MAb is directly related to its ability to neutralize virus infectivity. The
window for successful application of prophylactic antibody to prevent flaviviral
encephalitis closes at about 4 to 6 days postinfection concomitant with viral
invasion of the brain. Using murine MAbs to modify human disease results in
a human antimouse antibody (HAMA) response that eventually limits the
effectiveness of subsequent murine antibody applications. To reduce the HAMA
response and make these MAbs more generally useful for humans, murine
MAbs can be "humanized" or human MAbs with analogous reactivities can be
developed. Antiflaviviral human or humanized MAbs might be practical and
cost-effective reagents for preventing or modifying flaviviral diseases.

KEYWORDS: Passive protection; monoclonal antibodies (MAbs); flaviviruses;
cross-protection

Address for correspondence: John T. Roehrig, Arbovirus Diseases Branch, Division of Vector-
Borne Infectious Diseases, National Center for Infectious Diseases, Centers for Disease Control
and Prevention, U.S. Public Health Service, Department of Health and Human Services, P.O.
Box 2087, Fort Collins, CO 80522.Voice: 970-221-6442; fax: 970-221-6476.
jtr1@cdc.gov

INTRODUCTION

The recognition of a human outbreak of West Nile (WN) encephalitis in the late summer of 1999 has rekindled interest in developing methods to prevent and cure arboviral disease. Currently, there are commercially approved vaccines only for central European tick-borne encephalitis (TBE) and Japanese encephalitis (JE).[1-7] Both of these inactivated vaccines have a long history of efficacy and the JE vaccine has recently become available to American travelers. For the North American flaviviral encephalitides, St. Louis, Powassan, and now WN encephalitis, no human or veterinary vaccines exist. Although equine WN virus vaccines of various formulations are being developed, a human WN virus vaccine is years away. The sporadic nature of flaviviral outbreaks makes it difficult to assess the risk to humans of acquiring these infections. Additionally, flaviviral encephalitis is usually severe only in the elderly, making the potential recipient base for such vaccines small. These factors mitigate against the initiation of costly research, development, and approval processes associated with vaccine implementation in the United States and Europe.

HUMAN ANTIBODY PROPHYLAXIS FOR FLAVIVIRUSES

Applications of antibody, either prophylactically or therapeutically, continue to be evaluated and used as interventional approaches for a number of viral infections.[8-10] There are, however, no approved therapeutic agents specific for flaviviral encephalitis. Commercial anti-TBE virus immune sera have been used in nonimmunized humans following a possible tick-bite exposure to TBE virus in endemic areas of Austria. In an attempt to determine the efficacy of this practice, a telephone survey was conducted in Vienna.[11] The results from this survey revealed that the incidence of clinical TBE for unvaccinated persons in TBE virus endemic areas was reduced from approximately 1:1000 to 1:2500 by administration of TBE immunoglobulin after a tick bite. Although this analytical approach was not scientifically rigorous, the low incidence of human TBE virus infection made it difficult to use more standard epidemiological tools to answer this question. Adverse effects and failure of passive immunization of children with TBE virus immunoglobulin have been reported, but these events appear to be rare.[12-14]

MURINE MODELS OF FLAVIVIRAL ENCEPHALITIS AND THEIR USE IN EVALUATING THE EFFICACY OF ANTIBODY PROPHYLAXIS AND THERAPY

The laboratory mouse is a good animal model for flaviviral encephalitis.[15] Following peripheral inoculation of a virulent strain of St. Louis encephalitis (SLE) virus, there is a transient viremia that lasts from 4 to 5 days postinfection (FIG. 1). One to 2 days postinfection, viral replication in the spleen can be detected, with the peak splenic viral titer occurring at 4 to 5 days postinfection. Virus is first detected in the brain at 3 days postinfection, and virus titer rises dramatically, reaching a peak at 2 to 3 days later. Two days after virus entry into the brain, virus-specific morbidity and mortality can be observed, starting with ruffled fur and progressing to hind-limb

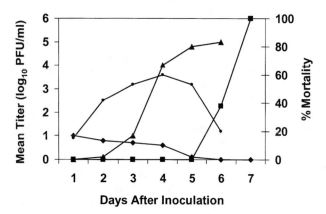

FIGURE 1. SLE virus replication in mice following i.p. inoculation. Mice were inoculated i.p. with 100 i.p. LD$_{50}$ SLE virus strain MSI-7. Tissues were harvested, homogenized in PBS, and titrated by plaque assay in PS cells. Symbols: serum (♦), spleen (●), brain (▲), and mortality (■).

paralysis and death. For a virulent flavivirus, the median survival time (MST) can be as short as 5 days.[16–20] Less virulent viruses have a more prolonged disease process. In general, mice become more resistant to flaviviral infection as they age.[16] This resistance is thought to be associated with maturation of the immune response and, therefore, many immunization-challenge studies are performed in mice younger than 21 days old. Certain strains of mice have also been shown to be genetically resistant to flaviviruses.[21,22]

Studies to define the ability of polyclonal or monoclonal antibodies (MAbs) to protect mice from virus challenge have been performed with JE,[23,24] Murray Valley encephalitis (MVE),[25,26] SLE,[27] and TBE[28–36] viruses. All of these studies have used MAbs specific for the envelope (E) glycoprotein, which is the major flaviviral antigen.

THE E-GLYCOPROTEIN: ITS ANTIGENIC STRUCTURE AND ROLE IN PROTECTION FROM ENCEPHALITIS

The 56-kDa flavivirus E-glycoprotein binds cellular receptors, mediates membrane fusion, and elicits virus-neutralizing antibodies.[25,28,37–44] Using MAb mapping, the fine antigenic structure of this protein has been shown to contain multiple epitopes of varying serologic and biologic activity. For illustration, the antigenic map of SLE virus E-glycoprotein is shown in TABLE 1.[38] Epitope specificity ranges from SLE virus–specific (E-1a to E-1d) to flavivirus group–reactive (E-4a and E-4b), as well as many other combinations in between. For all flaviviruses, including SLE virus, virus-specific epitopes (e.g., E-1c) elicit the most potent virus-neutralizing antibody. It has been shown with other flaviviruses that epitopes capable of eliciting virus-specific, neutralizing antibody can be located in either domain II or domain III of the E-glycoprotein.[41,42,44–53]

TABLE 1. Epitope mapping of the SLE (MSI-7) virus E-glycoprotein

Epitope	MAb	Specificity	PRNT[a]	% protection[b] 5–40 µg	50–200 µg
E-1a	3B4C-4	SLE	<1.7	20	40
E-1b	1B2C-5	SLE	<1.7	17	40
E-1c	6B5A-2	SLE	4.8	100	100
E-1d	4A4C-4	SLE	2.9	13	20
E-2	1B5D-1	SLE/JE	<1.7	20	47
E-3	2B5B-3	SLE/JE/MVE/WN/YF	2.3	4	38
E-4a	2B6B-2	All flaviviruses	<1.7	8	40
E-4b	6B6C-1	All flaviviruses	2.3	12	36

NOTE: Adapted from reference 38. MAbs were purified from murine ascitic fluids by ammonium sulfate precipitation and column chromatography on Sepharose 4B–protein A. Antibody concentrations were determined by BioRad protein assay and antibodies were standardized to 1 mg/mL.
[a]PRNT = plaque-reduction neutralization test.
[b]Two or more observations of 21-day-old mice (n = 10–35). Antibodies were administered intravenously 24 h prior to i.p. virus challenge with 100 i.p. LD_{50} of SLE virus strain MSI-7. Mice were observed daily for clinical signs of viral encephalitis for 15 days. Percent protection was calculated as the number of mice without symptoms/number of total mice challenged.

The ability of MAb to efficiently protect animals from virus challenge correlates directly with its ability to neutralize virus. However, some MAbs that have little or no neutralizing capacity can protect mice from virus challenge, albeit to a much reduced level (e.g., E-1a, E-1b, E-2, and E-4a for SLE virus). The ability of a protective MAb to function passively is directly related to the dose of the challenge virus and the amount of antibody administered (FIG. 2): the larger the virus challenge dose, the more antibody needed for protection. For SLE virus, mixing of MAbs does not result in a level of passive protection greater than that seen with the individual anti–E-1c MAb alone.[38]

The ability of a potent virus-neutralizing MAb to cure mice from virus infection depends on antibody dosage and the timing of antibody administration (FIG. 3). Higher levels of transferred antibody are capable of curing mice of a virulent SLE virus infection if administered no later than 3 to 4 days postinfection. If MAb is administered to the animals after this time, it cannot cure infection, regardless of the amount of MAb transferred. Not surprisingly, the protective window closes when virus is first detected in the brain (FIG. 1).

PASSIVE CROSS-PROTECTION BETWEEN FLAVIVIRUSES ANALYZED WITH MONOCLONAL ANTIBODIES

To date, most laboratory evaluations of MAb passive protection from flavivirus encephalitis have used challenge viruses homologous to the specificity of the MAbs being investigated. In reality, many of these flaviviruses cocirculate in nature. In

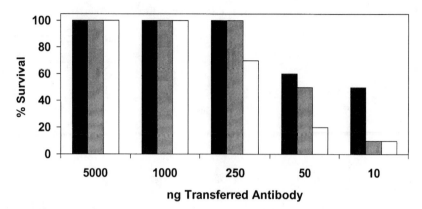

FIGURE 2. Ability of anti–E-1c MAb to protect mice from varying SLE virus challenge doses. Mice (21 days old, $n = 10$) were intravenously administered purified anti–E-1c
MAb 24 h prior to i.p. challenge with 100 i.p. LD_{50} (■), 1000 i.p. LD_{50} (☐), or 10,000
i.p. LD_{50} (☐) of SLE virus strain MSI-7. Mice were observed daily for 15 days for clinical
signs of viral encephalitis. Percent protection was calculated as the number of mice without
symptoms/number of total mice challenged. (Adapted from reference 27.)

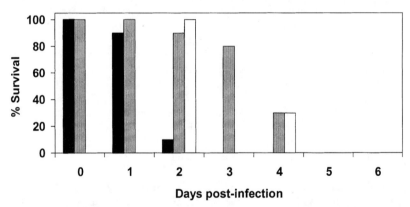

FIGURE 3. Ability of anti–E-1c MAb to cure SLE virus–infected mice. Mice (21 days
old, $n = 10$) were intravenously administered purified anti–E-1c MAb at the time of challenge or at 1, 2, 3, 4, 5, or 6 days after i.p. challenge with 100 i.p. LD_{50} of SLE virus strain
MSI-7. Amounts of transferred antibody were 1 μg (■), 20 μg (☐), and 100 μg (☐). Mice
were observed daily for 15 days for clinical signs of viral encephalitis. Percent protection
was calculated as the number of mice without symptoms/number of total mice challenged.
(Adapted from reference 27.)

North America, the geographic range of SLE and WN viruses now overlap. Because
of this, it is of interest to understand the amount of protection afforded by passive
transfer of cross-reactive antibody. Using a panel of cross-reactive MAbs elicited by
JE, SLE, or MVE viruses, we investigated cross-protection in mice between these
closely related flaviviruses. The binding and virus-neutralizing characteristics of

TABLE 2. Virus binding and neutralization characteristics of E-glycoprotein epitopes on JE, SLE, and MVE viruses

		Virus							
		JE		SLE		MVE		DEN2	
MAb	Cross-reactivity	IFA	NT	IFA	NT	IFA	NT	IFA	NT
E-1c	**SLE**	<1.7	<1.0	**2.9**	**3.1**	<1.7	<1.0	<1.7	nd
E-1c	**MVE**	<1.7	<1.0	<1.7	<1.0	**2.9**	**3.0**	<1.7	nd
E-7	**JE/MVE**	**2.6**	<1.0	<1.7	nd	**2.9**	**3.3**	<1.7	nd
E-5a	**JE/MVE**	**2.3**	<1.0	<1.7	nd	**2.6**	**3.6**	<1.7	nd
E-2	**JE/SLE**	**2.3**	<1.0	**2.3**	<1.0	<1.7	nd	<1.7	nd
E-8	**JE/SLE/MVE**	**2.0**	<1.0	**2.6**	<1.0	**2.6**	**3.6**	<1.7	nd
E-3	**JE/SLE/MVE**	**2.0**	<1.0	**2.6**	<1.0	**2.3**	**2.1**	<1.7	nd
E-4b	**JE/SLE/MVE/DEN2**	**2.3**	**2.5**	**2.3**	**2.5**	**2.0**	**2.1**	**2.0**	**2.5**
VEE	**VEE**	<1.7	<1.0	<1.7	<1.0	<1.7	1.0	<1.7	<1.0

NOTE: MAbs were purified from murine ascitic fluids by ammonium sulfate precipitation and column chromatography on Sepharose 4B–protein A. Antibody concentrations were determined by BioRad protein assay and antibodies were standardized to 20 μg per mL. Virus from which MAb was derived is shown in bold. Serological cross-reactivity measured in IFA with virus-infected cells or ELISA with purified virus. Positive reactions are shown in bold.

ABBREVIATIONS: JE = Japanese encephalitis virus; SLE = St. Louis encephalitis virus; MVE = Murray Valley encephalitis virus; DEN2 = dengue 2 virus; VEE = Venezuelan equine encephalitis virus (negative control); IFA = end-point titer by indirect immunofluorescence on virus-infected Vero cells; NT = end-point plaque-reduction neutralization titer on PS cells; nd = not done.

TABLE 3. Relative virulence of challenge virus in mice

Challenge virus	PFU/100 i.p. LD$_{50}$	Median survival time (days)
JE	0.1	6.5
SLE	0.5	5.0
MVE	2.5	7.0

NOTE: The i.p. LD$_{50}$ was calculated by inoculating 3-week-old NIH-Swiss mice with 0.2 mL of the appropriate virus dilution containing 100 i.p. LD$_{50}$. Mice were observed daily for 15 days for clinical signs of viral encephalitis. Plaque-forming units (PFU) were determined by plaque assay on PS cells.

ABBREVIATIONS: JE = Japanese encephalitis virus; SLE = St. Louis encephalitis virus; MVE = Murray Valley encephalitis virus.

these MAbs are listed in TABLE 2. Included for comparison are virus-specific anti– E-1c MAbs for SLE and MVE viruses. Of particular interest was the variability in neutralizing capacity that some of these MAbs displayed. The MAbs reactive with epitopes E-5a, E-7, and E-8 neutralized MVE virus infectivity to high titer, but failed to neutralize JE or SLE viruses, even though virus binding in IFA could be detected.

TABLE 4. Cross-protection of mice from flavivirus challenge at 24 h after passive antibody transfer

MAb epitope	μg antibody transferred	% survival following virus challenge (MST in days)		
		JE	SLE	MVE
E-1c	0.2		100 (>15.0)	
E-1c	5			100 (>15.0)
	0.5			80 (>13.0)
E-7	100	40 (12.0)		30 (9.5)
	50	20 (10.5)		0 (7.0)
	5	0 (8.5)		0 (6.5)
E-5a	100	60 (>15.0)		100 (>15.0)
	50	20 (10.0)		40 (9.0)
	5	ND		0 (7.5)
E-5a + E-7	25 + 25	60 (>15.0)[a]		40 (9.5)
E-2	50	40 (13.5)	40 (13.0)	ND
E-8	100	50 (14.5)	30 (7.5)	50 (>15.0)
	50	10 (9.0)	0 (7.5)	50 (11.0)
	5	0 (10.0)		30 (8.0)
E-3	50	0 (13.5)	40 (8.0)	100 (>15.0)
PBS control	0	0 (6.5)	0 (5.0)	0 (7.0)

NOTE: Groups of 10 mice were used for each antibody dose. MAb not reactive with virus (blank areas): not tested.

ABBREVIATIONS: MST = median survival time; JE = Japanese encephalitis virus; SLE = St. Louis encephalitis virus; MVE = Murray Valley encephalitis virus; ND = not done.

[a]Corresponding PBS control for this challenge had a 10% survival rate.

Prior to performing antibody transfer–virus challenge studies, we first analyzed the relative virulence of each of our challenge viruses in two ways (TABLE 3). While the MST was shortest for SLE virus (5.0 days), JE virus was most virulent when comparing plaque-forming units (PFUs) to intraperitoneal (i.p.) LD_{50} (0.1 for JE, 0.5 for SLE, and 2.5 for MVE virus). All passively administered antibodies significantly increased the MST of JE virus–challenged mice in a dose-dependent manner (Mann-Whitney two-sample rank-sum test, $\alpha = 0.05$) (TABLE 4). No individual antibody or combination of cross-reactive antibodies produced a 100% protection level following JE virus challenge. Results were similar for SLE virus–challenged mice. Interestingly, for MVE virus–challenged mice, levels of protection with anti–E-5a MAb reached 100% when a dose of 100 μg was administered. While this level of protection was impressive, it was still not as good as protection mediated by type-specific anti–E-1c MAbs, which were able to protect 100% of the mice when as little as 5 μg was administered and 80% of mice when 0.5 μg was administered. On balance, these results show that cross-reactive neutralizing and nonneutralizing MAbs are indeed capable of protecting animals from peripheral challenge with a variety of closely related flaviviruses, provided they are present in sufficient quantities.

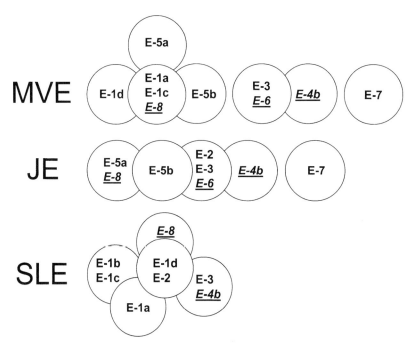

FIGURE 4. Competitive binding assay (CBA) maps of MVE, JE, and SLE virus E-glycoprotein. To determine spatial interrelationships between epitopes located in the glycoprotein of these related flaviviruses, CBAs were performed using MAbs with similar binding avidities as described previously.[50,54,55] Circles represent spatial identity for enclosed epitopes. Overlapping circles indicate spatial overlap of enclosed epitopes. Italicized and underlined epitopes are those that have been located to domain II of the E-glycoprotein in other studies.[48,53]

The interesting difference between protective efficacy and neutralization capacity of Mabs identifying the same epitope on two different viruses suggests that identical epitopes might have different topological arrangements in these viruses. To investigate further the topological arrangements of epitopes in these viruses, an enzyme-linked immunosorbent assay–based antibody competitive binding assay (CBA) was performed with JE virus and compared to previous results with SLE and MVE viruses (FIG. 4).[38,50,53–55] The results of this analysis revealed some variation in epitope topology from virus to virus, but did not readily explain the differences in MAb neutralization capacity with these viruses. For example, the E-3/E-6/E-4b epitope cluster is not linked to the type-specific neutralization domain in MVE virus, but they are linked in JE virus. This result could be explained, however, by the lack of MVE virus anti–E-2-reactive MAb. Because CBA maps do not reveal meaningful changes in spatial relationships of epitopes between viruses, it is likely that these differences in virus-neutralizing capacity are due to differences in epitope accessibility on the virion surface. It is clear that a more detailed structural analysis of both the JE and MVE virus E-glycoprotein will be necessary to fully explain these observations. Results from other studies have been able to localize some of these epitopes (italicized in FIG. 4) to domain II of the E-glycoprotein. The binding site of anti–E-6 and anti–E-4b MAbs have been localized to domain II on MVE virus E-glyco-protein.[46] The binding site of the anti–E-8 MAb on the MVE virus E-glycoprotein has been located between amino acids 200 and 327.[46] The binding site of anti–E-4b on dengue virus also has been localized to domain II.[53] However, virulence differ-ences between JE and MVE viruses could explain some of the observed differences in protective capacity (TABLE 3).

A recent study by Broom et al. determined that mice passively transferred with sera from other mice that had been either sublethally infected with Kunjin virus or vaccinated with JE virus were not protected from subsequent MVE virus chal-lenge.[26] In fact, mice passively transferred with the JE virus antiserum appeared to succumb more rapidly to MVE virus challenge than did untreated mice. Little is known about antibody-dependent enhancement (ADE) with encephalitic flaviviruses, but this mechanism could explain this result. While the ADE phenomenon is much better characterized for dengue viruses, it must be remembered that ADE was first observed with MVE virus.[56] The possibility of ADE functioning with encephalitic flaviviruses should be considered prior to administering JE vaccine to protect animals from challenge with a heterologous flavivirus (e.g., WN virus).

CONCLUSIONS

Experiments need to be done to investigate the efficiency of antibody passive pro-tection in primates. There have been anecdotal observations of murine MAbs being able to modulate JE virus infections in monkeys and humans; however, this work has never been officially published. It is clear from the work with animal models that the efficiency of passive antibody protection depends upon (1) the virulence of chal-lenge virus, (2) the dose of antibody transferred, and (3) the biological characteris-tics of transferred antibody (i.e., neutralizing activity, epitope specificity). It is also clear that cross-protection is not as efficient as specific protection. Furthermore, for an antibody to be effective therapeutically, it must be applied early in infection and prior to the time that the virus enters the central nervous system. Because of the low disease incidence of flaviviral encephalitis, antibody prophylaxis/therapy will require an artificial source of protective antibodies. Using murine MAbs in humans results in a human antimouse antibody (HAMA) response that eventually limits the effectiveness of subsequent murine antibody applications. To reduce the HAMA response and make these MAbs more generally useful for humans, murine MAbs can be "humanized" or human MAbs with analogous reactivities can be developed. Administration of antiflaviviral human or humanized MAbs might be a practical and cost-effective approach to prevent or modify flaviviral diseases.

REFERENCES

1. KANAMITSU, M., N. HASHIMOTO, S. URASAWA, et al. 1970. A field trial with an improved Japanese encephalitis vaccine in a nonendemic area of the disease. Biken J. **13:** 313–328.
2. KUNZ, C., F.X. HEINZ & H. HOFMANN. 1980. Immunogenicity and reactogenicity of a highly purified vaccine against tick-borne encephalitis. J. Med. Virol. **6:** 103–109.

3. SUSILOWATI, S., Y. OKUNO, T. FUKUNAGA, *et al.* 1981. Neutralization antibody responses induced by Japanese encephalitis virus vaccine. Biken J. **24:** 137–145.
4. POLAND, J.D., C.B. CROPP, R.B. CRAVEN & T.P. MONATH. 1990. Evaluation of the potency and safety of inactivated Japanese encephalitis vaccine in U.S. inhabitants. J. Infect. Dis. **161:** 878–882.
5. ROBINSON, P., T. RUFF & R. KASS. 1995. Australian case-control study of adverse reactions to Japanese encephalitis vaccine. J. Travel Med. **2:** 159–164.
6. DEFRAITES, R.F., J.M. GAMBEL, C.H. HOKE, *et al.* 1999. Japanese encephalitis vaccine (inactivated, BIKEN) in U.S. soldiers: immunogenicity and safety of vaccine administered in two dosing regimens. Am. J. Trop. Med. Hyg. **61:** 288–293.
7. ASHOK, M.S. & P.N. RANGARAJAN. 2000. Evaluation of the potency of BIKEN inactivated Japanese encephalitis vaccine and DNA vaccines in an intracerebral Japanese encephalitis virus challenge. Vaccine **19:** 155–157.
8. ZEITLIN, L., R.A. CONE & K.J. WHALEY. 1999. Using monoclonal antibodies to prevent mucosal transmission of epidemic infectious disease. Emerg. Infect. Dis. **5:** 54–64.
9. KELLER, M.A. & E.R. STIEHM. 2000. Passive immunity in prevention and treatment of infectious diseases. Clin. Microbiol. Res. **13:** 602–614.
10. SAWYER, L.A. 2000. Antibodies for the prevention and treatment of viral diseases. Antiviral Res. **47:** 57–77.
11. KUNZ, C., H. HOFMANN, M. KUNDI & K. MAYER. 1981. Efficacy of specific immuno-globulin against TBE [author's translation]. Wien. Klin. Wochenschr. **93:** 665–667.
12. KLUGER, G., A. SCHOTTLER, K. WALDVOGEL, *et al.* 1995. Tick-borne encephalitis despite specific immunoglobulin prophylaxis. Lancet **346:** 1502.
13. ARRAS, C., R. FESCHAREK & J.P. GREGERSEN. 1996. Do specific hyperimmunoglobulins aggravate clinical course of tick-borne encephalitis? Lancet **347:** 1331.
14. WALDVOGEL, K., W. BOSSART, T. HUISMAN, *et al.* 1996. Severe tick-borne encephalitis following passive immunization. Eur. J. Pediatr. **155:** 775–779.
15. MONATH, T.P., C.B. CROPP & A.K. HARRISON. 1983. Mode of entry of a neurotropic arbovirus into the central nervous system: reinvestigation of an old controversy. Lab. Invest. **48:** 399–410.
16. ELDADAH, A.H., N. NATHANSON & R. SARSITIS. 1967. Pathogenesis of West Nile virus encephalitis in mice and rats: 1. Influence of age and species on mortality and infection. Am. J. Epidemiol. **86:** 765–775.
17. ELDADAH, A.H. & N. NATHANSON. 1967. Pathogenesis of West Nile virus encephalitis in mice and rats: II. Virus multiplication, evolution of immunofluorescence, and development of histological lesions in the brain. Am. J. Epidemiol. **86:** 776–790.
18. WEINER, L.P., G.A. COLE & N. NATHANSON. 1970. Experimental encephalitis following peripheral inoculation of West Nile virus in mice of different ages. J. Hyg. (London) **68:** 435–446.
19. MONATH, T.P., C.B. CROPP, G.S. BOWEN, *et al.* 1980. Variation in virulence for mice and rhesus monkeys among St. Louis encephalitis virus strains of different origin. Am. J. Trop. Med. Hyg. **29:** 948–962.
20. TRENT, D.W., T.P. MONATH, G.S. BOWEN, *et al.* 1980. Variation among strains of St. Louis encephalitis virus: basis for a genetic, pathogenetic, and epidemiologic classification. Ann. N.Y. Acad. Sci. **354:** 219–237.
21. BRINTON, M.A. 1982. Characterization of West Nile virus persistent infections in genetically resistant and susceptible mouse cells. I. Generation of defective nonplaquing virus particles. Virology **116:** 84–98.
22. BRINTON, M.A., J. DAVIS & D. SCHAEFER. 1985. Characterization of West Nile virus persistent infections in genetically resistant and susceptible mouse cells. II. Generation of temperature-sensitive mutants. Virology **140:** 152–158.
23. MATHUR, A., K.L. ARORA & U.C. CHATURVEDI. 1983. Host defence mechanisms against Japanese encephalitis virus infection in mice. J. Gen. Virol. **64:** 805–811.
24. KIMURA-KURODA, J. & K. YASUI. 1988. Protection of mice against Japanese encephalitis virus by passive administration with monoclonal antibodies. J. Immunol. **141:** 3606–3610.
25. HAWKES, R.A., J.T. ROEHRIG, A.R. HUNT & G.A. MOORE. 1988. Antigenic structure of the Murray Valley encephalitis virus E glycoprotein. J. Gen. Virol. **69:** 1105–1109.

26. BROOM, A.K., M.J. WALLACE, J.S. MACKENZIE, et al. 2000. Immunisation with gamma globulin to Murray Valley encephalitis virus and with an inactivated Japanese encephalitis virus vaccine as prophylaxis against Australian encephalitis: evaluation in a mouse model. J. Med. Virol. **61:** 259–265.
27. MATHEWS, J.H. & J.T. ROEHRIG. 1984. Elucidation of the topography and determination of the protective epitopes on the E glycoprotein of Saint Louis encephalitis virus by passive transfer with monoclonal antibodies. J. Immunol. **132:** 1533–1537.
28. HEINZ, F.X., R. BERGER, W. TUMA & C. KUNZ. 1983. A topological and functional model of epitopes on the structural glycoprotein of tick-borne encephalitis virus defined by monoclonal antibodies. Virology **126:** 525–537.
29. PHILLPOTTS, R.J., J.R. STEPHENSON & J.S. PORTERFIELD. 1987. Passive immunization of mice with monoclonal antibodies raised against tick-borne encephalitis virus: brief report. Arch. Virol. **93:** 295–301.
30. NIEDRIG, M., U. KLOCKMANN, W. LANG, et al. 1994. Monoclonal antibodies directed against tick-borne encephalitis virus with neutralizing activity in vivo. Acta Virol. **38:** 141–149.
31. KREIL, T.R., I. BURGER, M. BACHMANN, et al. 1997. Antibodies protect mice against challenge with tick-borne encephalitis virus (TBEV)–infected macrophages. Clin. Exp. Immunol. **110:** 358–361.
32. KREIL, T.R. & M.M. EIBL. 1997. Pre- and postexposure protection by passive immunoglobulin, but no enhancement of infection with a flavivirus in a mouse model. J. Virol. **71:** 2921–2927.
33. KREIL, T.R., I. BURGER, E. ATTAKPAH, et al. 1998. Passive immunization reduces immunity that results from simultaneous active immunization against tick-borne encephalitis virus in a mouse model. Vaccine **16:** 955–959.
34. KREIL, T.R., E. MAIER, S. FRAISS & M.M. EIBL. 1998. Neutralizing antibodies protect against lethal flavivirus challenge, but allow for the development of active humoral immunity to a nonstructural virus protein. J. Virol. **72:** 3076–3081.
35. CHIBA, N., M. OSADA, K. KOMORO, et al. 1999. Protection against tick-borne encephalitis virus isolated in Japan by active and passive immunization. Vaccine **17:** 1532–1539.
36. SCHMALJOHN, C., D. CUSTER, L. VANDERZANDEN, et al. 1999. Evaluation of tick-borne encephalitis DNA vaccines in monkeys. Virology **263:** 166–174.
37. PEIRIS, J.S., J.S. PORTERFIELD & J.T. ROEHRIG. 1982. Monoclonal antibodies against the flavivirus West Nile. J. Gen. Virol. **58:** 283–289.
38. ROEHRIG, J.T., J.H. MATHEWS & D.W. TRENT. 1983. Identification of epitopes on the E glycoprotein of Saint Louis encephalitis virus using monoclonal antibodies. Virology **128:** 118–126.
39. HEINZ, F.X., W. TUMA, F. GUIRAKHOO, et al. 1984. Immunogenicity of tick-borne encephalitis virus glycoprotein fragments: epitope-specific analysis of the antibody response. J. Gen. Virol. **65:** 1921–1929.
40. HEINZ, F.X. 1986. Epitope mapping of flavivirus glycoproteins. Adv. Virus Res. **31:** 103–168.
41. HOLZMANN, H., C.W. MANDL, F. GUIRAKHOO, et al. 1989. Characterization of antigenic variants of tick-borne encephalitis virus selected with neutralizing monoclonal antibodies. J. Gen. Virol. **70:** 219–222.
42. MANDL, C.W., F. GUIRAKHOO, H. HOLZMANN, et al. 1989. Antigenic structure of the flavivirus envelope protein E at the molecular level, using tick-borne encephalitis virus as a model. J. Virol. **63:** 564–571.
43. HEINZ, F.X., G. AUER, K. STIASNY, et al. 1994. The interactions of the flavivirus envelope proteins: implications for virus entry and release. Arch. Virol. Suppl. **9:** 339–348.
44. HOLZMANN, H., K. STIASNY, M. ECKER, et al. 1997. Characterization of monoclonal antibody–escape mutants of tick-borne encephalitis virus with reduced neuro-invasiveness in mice. J. Gen. Virol. **78:** 31–37.
45. LOBIGS, M., L. DALGARNO, J.J. SCHLESINGER & R.C. WEIR. 1987. Location of a neutralization determinant in the E protein of yellow fever virus (17D vaccine strain). Virology **161:** 474–478.

46. GUIRAKHOO, F., F.X. HEINZ & C. KUNZ. 1989. Epitope model of tick-borne encephalitis virus envelope glycoprotein E: analysis of structural properties, role of carbohydrate side chain, and conformational changes occurring at acidic pH. Virology **169:** 90–99.

47. CECILIA, D. & E.A. GOULD. 1991. Nucleotide changes responsible for loss of neuro-invasiveness in Japanese encephalitis virus neutralization-resistant mutants. Virology **181:** 70–77.

48. GUIRAKHOO, F., R.A. BOLIN & J.T. ROEHRIG. 1992. The Murray Valley encephalitis virus prM protein confers acid resistance to virus particles and alters the expression of epitopes within the R2 domain of E glycoprotein. Virology **191:** 921–931.

49. HASEGAWA, H., M. YOSHIDA, T. SHIOSAKA, *et al.* 1992. Mutations in the envelope protein of Japanese encephalitis virus affect entry into cultured cells and virulence in mice. Virology **191:** 158–165.

50. MCMINN, P.C., E. LEE, S. HARTLEY, *et al.* 1995. Murray Valley encephalitis virus envelope protein antigenic variants with altered hemagglutination properties and reduced neuroinvasiveness in mice. Virology **211:** 10–20.

51. REY, F.A., F.X. HEINZ, C. MANDL, *et al.* 1995. The envelope glycoprotein from tick-borne encephalitis virus at 2 Å resolution. Nature **375:** 291–298.

52. RYMAN, K.D., T.N. LEDGER, R.C. WEIR, *et al.* 1997. Yellow fever virus envelope protein has two discrete type-specific neutralizing epitopes. J. Gen. Virol. **78:** 1353–1356.

53. ROEHRIG, J.T., R.A. BOLIN & R.G. KELLY. 1998. Monoclonal antibody mapping of the envelope glycoprotein of the dengue 2 virus, Jamaica. Virology **246:** 317–328.

54. ROEHRIG, J.T., J.W. DAY & R.M. KINNEY. 1982. Antigenic analysis of the surface glycoproteins of a Venezuelan equine encephalomyelitis virus (TC-83) using monoclonal antibodies. Virology **118:** 269–278.

55. ROEHRIG, J.T. & J.H. MATHEWS. 1985. The neutralization site on the E2 glycoprotein of Venezuelan equine encephalomyelitis (TC-83) virus is composed of multiple conformationally stable epitopes. Virology **142:** 347–356.

56. HAWKES, R.A. & K.J. LAFFERTY. 1967. The enhancement of virus infectivity by antibody. Virology **33:** 250–267.

Guidance for 2001

Panel Discussion

DUANE J. GUBLER, Moderator
Division of Vector-Borne Infectious Diseases,
Centers for Disease Control and Prevention, Fort Collins, Colorado 80522

DALE L. MORSE, Moderator
Office of Science and Public Health, New York State Department of Health,
Albany, New York 12237

DAVID A. DAME
American Mosquito Control Association, Gainesville, Florida 32605

JAMES L. HADLER
Infectious Diseases Division, Connecticut Department of Health,
Hartford, Connecticut 06134-0308

MARCELLE LAYTON
Communicable Disease, New York City Department of Health,
New York, New York 10013

STEPHEN M. OSTROFF
Associate Director for Epidemiologic Science,
Centers for Disease Control and Prevention, Atlanta, Georgia 30333

DUANE J. GUBLER: Good afternoon. We have come to our last panel discussion for this conference. I would like to introduce my co-moderator, Dale Morse, from the New York State Department of Health. Dale will introduce the panelists.

DALE L. MORSE: Thanks very much, Duane. We have a fine group of expert panelists here today. They are David Dame, from the American Mosquito Control Association; James Hadler, from the Connecticut Department of Health; Marcelle Layton, from the New York City Department of Health; and Stephen M. Ostroff, from the CDC in Atlanta. Thank you all for coming. We will begin with James Hadler.

JAMES L. HADLER: West Nile virus will likely re-emerge this season and be present in a much larger geographic area than last year. The virus became established here in New York City in 2000 and may spread northward in the spring and southward in the fall, following bird migration routes. In 2001, the mid-Atlantic area, the whole corridor between Washington, D.C., Philadelphia, and urban areas of New Jersey could be affected by West Nile virus. The cool, wet weather of 2000 may have been the critical factor in delaying the amplification of the virus. If we have a hot and dry summer this year, it is possible we could get an amplification of West Nile in many geographic areas. On the basis of experience in France and Spain in the

1960s and Romania in 1996, it would appear that the virus becomes established for a long time in local geographic areas with climates similar to ours.

Successful overwintering may become the rule, not the exception. Mosquitoes successfully overwintered in the area after 1999, and epizootic activity rapidly widened with intense levels of epizootic activity wherever the virus spread. In Europe they didn't have the high crow mortality marker of epizootic activity that we have here. I doubt we would have known the extent of West Nile infection in the United States in 2000 if we hadn't had the crow mortality marker. This past year we had fewer human cases; we were better prepared. Our early season mosquito control and awareness may have made a critical difference in the rate of amplification and the number of people at risk of exposure. Many took personal precautions. In addition, intense larviciding in May and June may have minimized the emerging mosquito population in areas affected by West Nile in 1999. Given the rates of severe human illness in sizable geographic areas of Bucharest and Volograd with high population densities, I am concerned that we may have a similar potential in some areas.

MORSE: Thanks Jim. Now we will hear from Stephen Ostroff.

STEPHEN M. OSTROFF: I have only a few comments. What I feel we need is to continue our public education efforts so that misinformation about West Nile virus is corrected. Education should start early and address the high level of public anxiety concerning efforts to control the virus. We need regional strategies to address all the diseases like West Nile, but we also need an exchange of information among states so that we can better learn new approaches to the problem. We can continue to learn to refine our information about interventions. As a result, the 2001 West Nile virus guidelines are more comprehensive and offer more scientific information.

MORSE: Thanks Steve. David Dame is next.

DAVID A. DAME: Our focus should be on continuing to build a strong scientific database and expanding our current resources for providing information to the states and local municipalities. Also we need to be proactive in sending out information, such as medical sources, to the public and media. Vectors and reservoirs where vectors may breed need to be identified. Focus needs to be put on the disease cycle phenomenon. We should remain alert to the increased virulence of the WNV strain and study the ecology of the disease. The role of direct transmission factors needs assessing. We need to increase funding to strengthen agencies and infrastructure, and we need to work with community leaders regarding potential disease transmission. The use of adulticides needs to be reviewed, as well as their health effects and mechanisms that result from their use. The CDC's training program for field observation and surveillance work needs to be expanded, and I recommend a consolidation of the public health agencies and mosquito control agencies.

MORSE: Thanks Dave. Now we will hear from Marci.

MARCELLE LAYTON: West Nile virus is certainly not a typical virus, and it's clear that the virus has broken all the rules. Given the experience of countries like Romania, where the virus has persisted for years, we must remain alert. Risks for human cases will be affected by how effective we are in source reduction. Risks also depend on how well the messages about personal protection measures get received by the public, especially the older population.

The people least likely to hear our message are the people most likely to be at high risk. As the virus spreads, it may be in areas where there may be some cross-protective immunity with SLE and other viruses. In New York City, we have mobilized a speaker's bureau that gives presentations to youth and community groups. Misinformation needs to be addressed through the use of solid scientific data to justify pesticide spraying.

In 1999, New York City had no mosquito control program and only a minimal surveillance program; as a result of inexperience with these programs, some residents have resisted, and may continue to resist, mosquito control efforts. We need to maintain and build our surveillance program. Surveillance tools, such as dead bird mortality rates, will remain a sensitive indicator of West Nile activity. I am concerned that as the story about West Nile virus becomes old news that it will be harder to get the message out. Our successes sometimes work against us; when there's no evidence of disease, the funding tends to disappear until there's another outbreak.

Fortunately, lab capacities have expanded to monitor infection rates in humans and other mammals. Funding from local, state, and federal agencies has led to additional staff. Within only one year, we have accumulated a wealth of information about the virus, and we will continue to analyze the data.

MORSE: Thanks Marci. Duane Gubler is next.

GUBLER: We need to be careful in predicting what will happen for the coming year. Perhaps is would be instructive to learn from Europe's experience with the virus. Response to this virus may be different depending on one's geographic area. For example, people in rural areas may not report dead birds the way residents of New York City do. One question that needs a solution is, How do we bring veterinary surveillance together with other agencies dealing with this problem? Finally, improving public outreach and education should be goals that we aim for.

Now we have some time for questions and comments. First, however, allow me to raise the topic of surveillance. You have to do not only surveillance for virus activity in the vertebrate host but also you've got to know what mosquitoes are there and what is transmitted.

ROBERT E. SHOPE (*University of Texas Medical Branch, Galveston, Texas*): If you had a vaccine, you could have a vaccination program.

GUBLER: We don't have a vaccine.

OSTROFF: I've become convinced by everything the mosquito control people tell me that source reduction is the way to go. And if the Canadians have some way of doing source reduction and can do the surveillance to show that there are no larval mosquitoes in certain bodies of water, then they can probably get away without doing larviciding.

DONNA REYNOLDS (*Durham Region Health Department, Whitby, Ontario, Canada*): I don't think we have any magic Canadian bullets for this. In fact, we have very few bullets in Canada due to very strong gun control. However, the reason I ask this is because we're having a follow-up meeting, which is organized by the local medical officers health organization in Ontario, asking our ministry to come. I think this is our major concern: What is the role of larviciding as a prevention mechanism? After this meeting we'll be going back to our colleagues and strongly advocating for us to build on the experience that you have here. I'm very concerned about our current state in Ontario, and particularly we have *no* mosquito control programs within our entire province. We'll be talking to you this season.

DAME: I'd like to make a comment based on the query. It goes back to the general principle that control is not applied until you can prove that there's a need to apply it. And both for adult and for larval control, surveillance is required. Wherever you have organized mosquito control, surveillance is a continuum, so they know where the mosquitoes are. If the mosquitoes are not there, they're not applying control to those particular habitats. With that in mind, I think the answer is obvious: if you're going to have a control program, you need to know where your targets are, and then you need to make a decision on whether you apply pesticides or not.

SHOPE: I have a comment regarding international representation. There's one international group that we don't have here and that's our neighbors to the south. It would be useful to me, Duane, and I think for the record also to hear your plans for inclusion of the Caribbean and Central and South America, and the plans for the future.

GUBLER: We all believe that this virus moves with migratory birds, so it's not unreasonable to think that if it hasn't already, it will move south into the Caribbean and into Central and South America. We are starting a program in Puerto Rico. We've already started a program to look at birds. If you look at the migration path, they go down to Florida, hit Cuba, and then island hop down through the Caribbean islands. Others fly right over and go to Brazil and Venezuela. Others go down into Texas and then into the Yucatan. Paul Reiter, who just left, and whose staff have been working with Nick Komar to collect birds—working with the fish and wildlife service down there—is collecting birds for testing. We're working with Barry Beatty who has a program in the Yucatan, and we're funded him to do bird surveillance in the Yucatan in collaboration with Jose Fartan at the university there. So that's in progress, and they've already collected several hundred birds for testing. We haven't found any positives yet. We will be funding Bob as well, in Galveston, to work with Ray Parsons in Texas, and also we would like to use that connection, since Bob has very close connections with Cuba, to start a program in Cuba to look at that, because that's one of the main places where birds go from Florida. So we'll be covering pretty much the Caribbean basin. We're also going to be working with the Pan American Health Organization to conduct a surveillance workshop at the Caribbean Epidemiology Center (CAREC) laboratory in Port of Spain, Trinidad. And that will probably be sometime in the fall and we would hope to bring in Venezuela, Brazil, and some of the Central American countries where the bird migrations go. So we haven't neglected this. It's just that we're a little bit slow, and we had to wait until we got our budget to get it off the ground, but we will be working with our partners to the south.

PETER JUPP (*Special Pathogens Unit, National Institute for Virology, Johannesburg, South Africa*): I'd like to make a few comments on the entomology side, if I may, as an outsider based on the experience we've had in South Africa. Perhaps my remarks follow quite nicely on Mike Turell's remarks yesterday. But he's gone away so he can't join me. Obviously, once you confirm the incriminated or principal vector or vectors of the virus, then you should be able to direct your pesticide measures better—if you like, more rationally. I realize that you have got some evidence to implicate vectors, but I think you need more. I think the key thing is what is actually transmitting the virus? And as Mike said, isolations on their own don't prove that. However, multiple isolations are usually very significant. I would suggest that there are two ways that you can demonstrate those vectors that transmit the most efficiently. One of them, of course, Mike Turell has already begun, and he's done some significant experiments. The use of birds—chickens of different ages, which have been inoculated—will give one different titers. Pigeons will also give different titers. And one can in that way do transmissions from bird to bird quantitatively, and you'll be able to get an assessment of transmission rates after infection at different titers. This is the best way, I think, of actually evaluating a vector in the laboratory.

In addition to that, you could also do natural transmissions, if you like, in the field in conjunction with your sentinel bird program. Now, I've advocated sentinel pigeons, and I've spoken to Nick Komar and it seems to me that pigeons would be very useful in this country. One could use a large number of cages, each containing pairs of pigeons. Then you can attach your traps, as I indicated the other day, at the bottom of the cage to actually collect from time to time what is feeding on the pigeons. This will give you an idea of which of the ornithophilic mosquitoes are present, but also you can then process those mosquitoes for virus and relate the results to your pigeons that are converting. If you really want to get sophisticated, you can change your birds as they convert and process a lot of samples, and you can actually get field transmission rates. This could be an interesting parallel to your laboratory work. Also, I think the design of the sentinel cage is important, and I can always explain in detail how we did it in South Africa, should anybody want to know.

The last comment I have is with regard to isolating virus from mosquitoes. We did some work the other day with Rift Valley fever that might apply to West Nile, and that is that the sensitivity of the baby mouse is considerably more sensitive than PCR for detecting virus. What we did recently with a large number of mosquitoes collected in Saudi Arabia was that we did PCR first, and anything that was suggested positive on PCR we put into mice the same day.

GUBLER: Peter, I'd like to follow-up. You know, I certainly agree. We need to get a better idea of what species of mosquitoes are transmitting to what animals, including humans, and that's going to be critical in our efforts for prevention and control. One of the things that hasn't come up in this meeting at all, and there haven't been any talks on it, is blood meal identification of mosquitoes. I know Dennis White is working on this. He's got a group that's going to be working this coming summer. We're funding Chuck Apperson to do a similar type of project. So, the other component of what you're saying is to get a good idea of which mosquitoes are feeding on which animals and put that together with the vector confidence that you're talking about. We certainly agree one hundred percent.

Just one comment on the virus isolation. We did a comparison in John Roehrig's lab, which compared baby mice, inoculation of baby mice, plaque assay in Vero cells, and fluid culture in Vero cells, and basically the Vero cells were more sensitive than the baby mice in our laboratory in the fall of 1999. So, probably it has something to do with the line of cells that you have and maybe the line of mice that you're working with as well.

MORSE: Tracey?

TRACY MCNAMARA (*Wildlife Conservation Society, The Bronx, NY*): My comments go to the lessons of West Nile, and clearly when we were faced with a zoonotic disease that involved wildlife, domestic animals, and humans, we were confronted with the fact that we had an utter lack of contingency planning as to how to deal with zoonotic disease. Since the discovery of West Nile, everything that's happened since then has been driven by funding and societal attitudes. Well, those were the problems that resulted in West Nile in the first place. The crows were telling us in late June and July in 1999 that there was a problem—*but* it was only a bunch of crows. All of the money goes to public health, food, animals, and agricultural veterinary species, and when you get down to the animals that were ruining us, they were the equivalent of the homeless, the uninsured. Who was going to pay for it; who cared about it. But, in fact, those crows turned out to be critical to public health.

The irony here is we are eighteen-plus months down the road and all the money that's been released is wonderful to see, but none of it has been going to the wildlife agencies, the veterinary agencies—it's still top-heavy up at public health. And so I'm concerned that if the next virus steps off a plane or comes in with a mosquito or a migratory bird, since that structural and societal issue has not been addressed, it won't be any different when Nipah virus hits our shores. I am very concerned that we have no BL-4 capabilities for veterinary diseases in the United States, and the fact that wildlife and captive wildlife still fall through the cracks. Clearly it's in everyone's best interest to address these issues—as you know, we're all part of one ecosystem.

The other thing I'm concerned about with the funding that's been released, as a person who does diagnostic testing, is the large number of epidemiologists hired. Someone needs to create the data that epidemiologists will later interpret. And I sleep better at night knowing that if I drop dead someone can stick a pin in a map eight months later. But where are the people actually running the PCR? Where are the lab technicians? I'm also concerned, again, with the way funding has been released—the lack of funding for research. Now, as a pathologist, I do what I do because I know you can't treat or prevent a disease unless you can recognize it and understand it. Some of the stuff that's come out at the meeting today could potentially go towards how we deal with this disease.

I would hope the next time we deal with a major infectious disease outbreak that the federal government—I mean, whoever pulls the strings—would fork over the money to do the necessary experimental trials. In our case, trials could have and should have been done eighteen months ago, because we knew there were things that needed to be looked at. But, in fact, many of those studies were being paid for by private funds. There's something fundamentally wrong with that. Again, just as a pathologist, I'd like to point out that we've been very reactive to all of this. Of course we're short-funded, understaffed, but I think we're taking a fatally shortsighted approach, in that tissues are not being banked for long-term pathology studies. What I showed raises the possibility that there may be long-term sequelae, and we are going to need to follow these cases. And so I would just emphasize perhaps the need for a national archive. Perhaps we need national serum banks. And even if we don't have the time, staff, or money to deal with it now, if it's banked somewhere maybe we can go back to it a year later and get the answers we need.

GUBLER: Comments?

HADLER: I'll take a small stab at one of your comments from a state perspective in terms of funding. Even though I'm certainly not one of the people in charge of funding at the federal level and how that gets distributed, I can say that at least in the second year, the funding has been very open. There's been the potential to use it to enhance all the different partners that play a role in the different forms of surveillance for West Nile virus, including all kinds of laboratory partners. And there's been the possibility to propose research type projects that anybody in your state can do for potential funding and then to get approval to use funds that are appropriated in that way. So I can say, at least in Connecticut, for example, that a substantial amount of money is going to the infrastructure at the Connecticut Agricultural Experiment Station, which does do a lot of wildlife work at the University of Connecticut Pathobiology Laboratory, which also does a lot of our veterinary work, as well as funding actually *one* epidemiologist and a number of laboratory people at the State Health Department. So the funding, I think, can be used in more diverse ways than you might have an impression of how it's being used.

GUBLER: Steve and I promised Jim a beer if he would say that (*general laughter*).

OSTROFF: My only comment is that if all the money is going to public health, I wasn't aware of it (*general laughter*).

ANDREW SPIELMAN (*Harvard School of Public Health, Boston, MA*): I'd like to make two dangerous remarks about the future. One of them is that a West Nile is not likely to lose a grip on public attention because it's an *urban* infection, and it affects older people. This group is extremely health conscious. It's a new fact of life in the United States that a high C in the middle of the night is dangerous. One would always imagine that the gun is loaded.

GUBLER: Explain what a high C is. Most people don't know what you're talking about.

SPIELMAN: The sound of a female's wings (*general laughter*). The other point is that I suspect that this infection is more likely to move north than it is south. That's a function of day length. If indeed it is *Culex pipiens* that is the vector, and if indeed fourteen and a quarter hours of light a day is the critical period, as one moves south, that window, that fourteen and a quarter hours of light, narrows. It disappears at about the level of Atlanta, Georgia. As you move north it widens so that Canada might very well anticipate more activity than Florida, if this reasoning is right.

GUBLER: Anybody want to comment about that?

DAME: The only comment I will make is that we really have no idea what the vectors will be, and *Culex pipiens* or *quinquefasciatus* may not be involved in the cycle when it gets here, but we don't know that.

SPIELMAN: The point, though, is that the situation that exists now in New York may very well *not* exist in the south. It would require some other kind of an adaptation, some additional point about which we have no idea at the moment. So the precise epidemiological circumstances that exist now, I argue, will be unlikely to go too much further south.

GUBLER: Andy, I would only say that if you look at this group of Japanese encephalitis serocomplex viruses, they're basically tropical viruses. They exist in enzootic cycles in tropical areas, periodically moving north causing epidemics in the north, and so I'm not sure what you're saying. Is it that the epidemics will likely be in the north and not in the south? I think that the rest of the complex bears that out, but it doesn't mean that it won't move south.

JULI TRTANJ (*NOAA Office of Global Programs, Silver Spring, MD*): I run a program on climate variability in human health. I came here in part to learn about what we know about the environmental and climatic variables that affect West Nile virus. Part of my job is to figure out how to better integrate climate environmental information into the decisions that U.S. public health officials have to make. Part of that is figuring out what decisions you have to make and what we know about the environmental components.

I have a couple of questions for the panel. I've heard a lot about the sequence of weather events—this dry and hot information. We actually sit on a task force, or a small part of a West Nile task force at the inner-agency level and provide them with—recently, as of last fall, actually—updates of climate information—climate forecasts. We're in the office that does the predictions related to *El Niño*, seasonal to inter-annual climate forecasting, but we also work very closely with the weather service, so we're trying to provide a continuum of information from weather on out to seasonal and interannual climate. I know when we sit on the task force there's a pretty easy mechanism for looking at the climate situation for the next month or the next three or six months. Is there a mechanism for doing so for a larger community? The media certainly do take some of that information. If you were to get something in the media, however, that said, we're going into another *El Niño*, that wouldn't necessarily mean the same thing as the last time you had an *El Niño*. Each one is a little different. So I'm not sure how the media message would actually be interpreted by the general public and that you would have all the information you would really need to make your decisions.

So, again, the question is, Is there a way to ensure that the people here who are interested in getting information that says the next three months are going to be hotter than normal, or they're not, or they're going to be normal will get it and know what that means? The second question is, To what extent do some of you have more specific data needs or information needs to either determine budget planning for spraying or just to prepare psychologically for public outreach. You do, I think, almost all have state climatologists. If you don't know them, we can help you find them. We can also help you find more specific and tailored information. There's somebody in my office who will help with that specifically.

The last inquiry is with regard to providing feedback to how the climate guys actually produce their stuff. What I'm hearing here is that the scale is a real issue. It's not a surprise. We need to get much more localized in the delivery of information, particularly rainfall predictions. So, one, how do we convey that information that we can get pretty readily? Two, we're willing to work with you in helping find resources in your own state, or more independently on specific projects if you have data needs.

Morse: Does anybody on the panel want the use of weather data—can that be helpful in managing the virus? I don't know if we have enough years of experience based on two years to be able to use weather to predict what's happening. It certainly would be helpful when people are spraying and adulticiding to know weather conditions.

Trtanj: If, for instance, we had a forecast coming out in a couple of weeks that said we're going into an *El Niño*, and for New York, New Jersey, Connecticut, and Massachusetts that means a couple degrees warmer than normal for the summer period, or between three and five degrees warmer than normal. How would you actually get that information? That's the nature of the question.

Gubler: I would urge all of you to get Julie's contact information. She is a tremendous resource for all of us in public health that we haven't really had access to before, and the types of data that you can get from NOAA I think will help us understand the influence of weather, temperature, and rainfall patterns on these diseases. So we're very happy to have NOAA and Julie as part of this group.

Hadler: How might we use that data? I think mostly we sort of keep it to ourselves and worry (*laughter*). So that if we started seeing West Nile virus emerge and emerge early enough, and if the prediction was for a considerably warmer season than usual, then that would certainly have us on edge and watching all our indices that we're planning on watching very closely and being prepared to come out with public warnings, if anything, even sooner.

Trtanj: If it's any consolation, we sit and worry too!

DANA FOCKS (*Gainesville, FL*): A lot of people like models. And models take a long time to develop. In light of the resource that Julie was just mentioning, it might be useful to make some kind of a minimal vectorial capacity model for *Culex pipiens*—just using the data that we have or using somebody else's data for another mosquito, if we don't have *Culex pipiens*, and then seeing how well that tracks 1999 and 2000. In the last two years the weather was quite different, and it might be that we will get lucky and find something that does have some relationship with the intensity of transmission—perhaps as measured by crows. And something as simple as that might then make the connect between Julie's forecast of two years—two degrees warmer the next three months. It might give us a way to connect that with risk.

DANIEL ARBEGAST (*DEP Field Operatons, Harrisburg, PA*): One of the things we haven't talked much about are the communications issues. We've kind of skirted around it, but we haven't talked a lot about it, and I guess that's probably because we're all technical types and technical types don't like the communication end. But we did see during the presentation notes that five to six percent of the public get their information from the internet. But we had the same results within a half a percent of that in Pennsylvania, and when we went back through the data we said, OK where did they get their information? They got their information from the media—print, radio, and television. So we did a survey of television and print media. Guess where they got their information? From the internet (*laughter*). We wasted two and a half days a week with one person's time every week getting stuff onto the internet, but in reality we got out the message. The message we delivered was linked—this technology stuff is just awesome, you know—by a hot button to all our county pages, which, in turn, got out exactly the same message, which was linked to our township and borough home pages, which got exactly the same message out. Forest County is one of our square counties in the north where there's five thousand people; 70 to 80% of the county is either state or fedcral forest land. When *The Forest Press* published an article, it had almost the exact wording that the *Philadelphia Inquirer* had in their article. So we were able to communicate.

My second comment is that we knew what happened in New York, and we knew what happened in New Jersey. I didn't have to call Bob Kent to find out what was happening in New Jersey. I could be in the field during the conference call on Wednesday because the stuff was on the net and we had the same information. I don't think we emphasize this much and realize how much communication affects us. This may be the first really major outbreak response kind of a situation where we've used that kind of technology to share that information with so many people.

West Nile Virus Serosurvey and Assessment of Personal Prevention Efforts in an Area with Intense Epizootic Activity: Connecticut, 2000

TARA A. MCCARTHY,[a] JAMES L. HADLER,[b] KATHLEEN JULIAN,[c]
STEPHEN J. WALSH,[d] BRAD J. BIGGERSTAFF,[e] STEVEN R. HINTEN,[c]
CAROLINE BAISLEY,[f] ANTHONY ITON,[g] TIMOTHY BRENNAN,[b]
RANDALL S. NELSON,[b] GARY ACHAMBAULT,[b] ANTHONY A. MARFIN,[e]
AND LYLE R. PETERSEN[e]

[a]*Epidemic Intelligence Service, assigned to the Connecticut Department of Public Health, Epidemiology Program Office, Centers for Disease Control and Prevention, Atlanta, Georgia 30333, USA*

[b]*Connecticut Department of Public Health, Epidemiology Program, Hartford, Connecticut 06134-0308, USA*

[c]*Epidemic Intelligence Service, assigned to the National Center for Infectious Disease, Vector-Borne Infectious Diseases, Centers for Disease Control and Prevention, Fort Collins, Colorado 80522, USA*

[d]*University of Connecticut, Farmington, Connecticut 06030, USA*

[e]*National Center for Infectious Disease, Vector-Borne Infectious Diseases, Centers for Disease Control and Prevention, Fort Collins, Colorado 80522, USA*

[f]*Greenwich Department of Health, Greenwich, Connecticut 06830, USA*

[g]*Stamford Health Department, Stamford, Connecticut 06901, USA*

ABSTRACT: West Nile virus (WNV) can cause large outbreaks of febrile illness and severe neurologic disease. This study estimates the seroprevalence of WNV infection and assesses risk perception and practices regarding potential exposures to mosquitoes of persons in an area with intense epizootics in 1999 and 2000. A serosurvey of persons aged ≥12 years was conducted in southwestern Connecticut during October 10–15, 2000, using household-based stratified cluster sampling. Participants completed a questionnaire regarding concern for and personal measures taken with respect to WNV and provided a blood sample for WNV testing. Seven hundred thirty persons from 645 households participated. No person tested positive for WNV (95% CI: 0–0.5%). Overall, 44% of persons used mosquito repellent, 56% practiced ≥ two personal precautions to avoid mosquitoes, and 61% of households did ≥ two mosquito-source reduction activities. In multivariate analyses, using mosquito repellent was associated with age <50 years, using English as the primary language in the home, being worried about WNV, being a little worried about pesticides, and finding mosquitoes frequently in the home (P<0.05). Females (OR = 2.0; CI = 1.2–2.9) and persons very worried about WNV (OR = 3.8; CI = 2.2–6.5)

Address for correspondence: James L. Hadler, M.D., M.P.H., Infectious Disease Division, Connecticut Department of Public Health, 410 Capitol Avenue, MS #11 EPI, Hartford, CT 06134-0308. Voice: 860-509-7995; fax: 860-509-7910.
James.hadler@po.state.ct.us

were more likely to practice ≥ two personal precautions. Taking ≥ two mosquito source reductions was associated with persons with English as the primary language (OR = 2.0; CI = 1.1–3.5) and finding a dead bird on the property (OR = 1.8; CI = 1.1–2.8).

An intense epizootic can occur in an area without having a high risk for infection to humans. A better understanding of why certain people do not take personal protective measures, especially among those aged ≥50 years and those whose primary language is not English, might be needed if educational campaigns are to prevent future WNV outbreaks.

KEYWORDS: West Nile virus; flavivirus; arbovirus; encephalitis; seroprevalence; cluster sampling

INTRODUCTION

West Nile virus (WNV) was first identified in the Western Hemisphere in the greater New York City area in September 1999.[1] In 1999 and 2000, WNV caused outbreaks of severe human neurologic disease in the greater New York City area.[1,2] Each of the outbreaks of human disease was preceded by an epizootic of WNV among birds.[3,4] In October 1999, a seroprevalence survey in northern Queens, the epicenter of the 1999 outbreak, estimated that 2.6% (95% confidence interval [CI]: 1.2–4.1%) of persons in the study area were infected with WNV.[5]

Connecticut, especially towns in coastal Fairfield County, experienced substantial bird mortality due to WNV in 1999 and 2000, yet no human cases of severe neurologic disease were diagnosed. In 2000, one mildly symptomatic person tested positive for WNV in Fairfield County. Epizootic activity in 2000 was particularly intense in an 18 square mile area of southern Stamford and neighboring southeastern Greenwich, the two Fairfield County towns closest to New York City.[6] Between July 5 and October 31, 2000, 96 (9%) of the 1093 WNV-infected crows collected in Connecticut and 5 (36%) of the 14 WNV-positive mosquito pools statewide were found in this area. In addition, this area had a higher peak density of dead crow sightings than any single town in Connecticut, peaking at 2.3 dead crows per square mile during the week of August 13–19.

The primary prevention activities that occurred in this area and throughout Connecticut were late spring larviciding of catch basins, public education aimed at eliminating peridomestic and municipal *Culex* mosquito breeding sites, and encouraging personal protective measures. Adulticiding to kill adult mosquitoes was negligible.

Little is known about human infection rates in areas with intense epizootic activity, active efforts at public education, large preseason larviciding programs, and no documented severe human illness. The purpose of this study was to estimate the seroprevalence of recent WNV infection and to assess the knowledge, attitudes, and practices of the population concerning WNV, as well as the prevention of exposures to mosquitoes in such an area.

METHODS

During October 10–15, 2000, a serosurvey was conducted in an 18 square mile area of southeastern Greenwich and southern Stamford, Connecticut (population approximately 99,000 persons), where WNV epizootic activity in Connecticut was most intense. A stratified cluster sampling design was used to obtain a representative number of households. The area was stratified into three strata on the basis of predominant vegetation cover and urbanization as determined by satellite imagery (Lee DeCola, USGS, Reston, VA). Within each of these strata, census blocks were grouped into clusters so that each cluster contained a minimum of 50 households. Clusters were then selected within strata approximately proportional to the number of households in each cluster. A total of 71 clusters were sampled. Within each cluster, start points were chosen randomly and successive households were approached until at least seven households were enlisted.

Eligibility included all persons at home at the time of the survey who were at least 12 years of age and had lived in the household since the summer of 2000. Translators were available for those who spoke Spanish or Creole. After informed consent was obtained, each participant submitted a serum sample and completed an on-site interview that used a standardized questionnaire regarding knowledge, attitudes, and behaviors to prevent WNV infections and potential exposures to mosquitoes. One person in each household completed a second questionnaire regarding selected household characteristics, and peridomestic mosquito reduction measures taken. All participants were offered the results of their blood tests. Institutional Review Board approval at both the Centers for Disease Control and Prevention (CDC) and the Connecticut Department of Public Health (DPH) were obtained prior to initiation of the survey.

Serum samples were initially tested at the DPH Laboratory for WNV antibody using an immunogloblin (Ig) M-capture enzyme-linked immunosorbent assay (ELISA).[7] Any positive or equivocal result was sent to the CDC for confirmation by a plaque-reduction neutralization test (PRNT).

Statistical analyses were done using Epi Info version 6 and STATA.[8,9] Sampling weights were used to estimate population parameters and reflected a person's probability of inclusion in the study. Statistical tests were performed incorporating these weights and the stratified cluster sampling design. Stratified analyses were used to examine possible interactions between exposure variables found to be associated with outcome variables. Confidence intervals for the human seroprevalence study were calculated using the exact binomial interval.[10] Various self-reported personal protective measures were the primary outcome variables of interest. Multivariate analyses were performed by using backwards stepwise logistic regression in STATA. Basic demographic variables were retained in the model. In all statistical tests, $P < 0.05$ was considered to be significant.

RESULTS

A total of 3007 households were approached. In 1653, no one was home or the household was ineligible. Of the remaining 1354 households, 645 (48%) agreed to participate. A total of 730 persons from participating households were enrolled in the study. All percentages in these analyses are weighted and are estimates of the population parameters.

TABLE 1. Demographic, exposure, and behavioral characteristics of serosurvey participants

Characteristics	Percent[a]	Confidence Interval (percent)
Age (years)		
12–49	63	59–68
50–64	21	17–24
≥65	16	13–19
Mean age 45.7 years (CI = 43.9–47.4)		
Sex		
Female	57	53–60
Male	43	40–47
Race/Ethnicity		
White	68	61–76
Black	5	2–9
Hispanic	16	11–21
Other/Unknown	10	7–13
Language		
English	81	76–87
Spanish	11	6–15
Creole	2	0–3
Other	6	4–8
Educational level		
0–11 years	11	7–15
12–15 years	45	39–50
≥16 years	44	38–50
Insurance		
Private	80	76–85
Medicaid/Husky/Medicare	6	5–8
No health insurance	12	7–15
Do not know	2	0–4
Dwelling		
Single family	64	56–72
Multifamily	31	24–38
Other	5	2–9
Screens on all windows		
Yes	91	89–94
No/Do not know	9	6–12
Air conditioning		
Yes	86	83–90
No	14	10–17
How often did you see mosquitoes inside your house?		
Daily	8	5–10
More than once a week	10	7–13
Once a week	15	29–38
Once or twice a month	34	12–18
Never	33	30–39

TABLE 1. Demographic, exposure, and behavioral characteristics of serosurvey participants (Continued)

Characteristics	Percent[a]	Confidence Interval (percent)
Found dead birds(s) on property		
Yes	17	14–21
No	83	79–86
≥2 hours outside at dusk or dawn		
Yes	13	10–15
No	87	85–90
How worried were you about getting WNV?		
Very worried	14	11–18
A little worried	44	39–48
Not worried at all	40	36–45
Never heard about WNV/Do not know	2	0–4
How worried were you about getting sick from pesticides used to kill mosquitoes?		
Very worried	17	13–20
A little worried	31	27–35
Not worried at all	51	46–56
Never heard of using pesticides to kill mosquitoes/Do not know	1	0–3
What worried you more?		
Getting WNV	37	33–42
Getting sick from pesticides	19	16–23
Equally worried about WNV and pesticides	17	14–20
Not worried about WNV or pesticides	27	23–31
During this past July and August, how often did you do any of the following to protect yourself from mosquitoes?		
Avoid areas where mosquitoes are likely to be a problem		
Always	22	18–25
Sometimes	33	29–37
Never	45	41–49
Avoid going outdoors		
Always	3	2–5
Sometimes	26	23–29
Never	71	67–74
Wear long sleeves, long pants when outside		
Always	13	10–15
Sometimes	30	26–35
Never	57	53–62
Wear mosquito repellent when outside for 30 minutes or more		
Always	12	9–15
Sometimes	32	28–36
Never	56	52–60
Did at least one personal precaution		
Yes	79	76–82
No	21	18–24
Took all four personal precautions		
Yes	7	5–9
No	93	91–95

TABLE 1. Demographic, exposure, and behavioral characteristics of serosurvey participants (Continued)

Characteristics	Percent[a]	Confidence Interval (percent)
Mosquito-Source Reductions		
During the past summer did you or anyone ... remove objects that might collect water from around the outside of your home or apartment building?		
Yes	55	49–60
No/Do not know	45	40–51
check all screens and repair if necessary?		
Yes	63	59–67
No/Do not know	37	33–41
check and clean all rain gutters if necessary?		
Yes	55	49–60
No	45	40–51
did one of these mosquito source reductions?		
Yes	86	83–89
No	14	11–17
did all three mosquito source reductions?		
Yes	25	21–29
No	75	71–79

[a]Weighted percentages.

Seroprevalence Results

None of the 730 persons who provided a blood sample had a positive WNV IgM and neutralizing antibody test indicating recent infection. The upper 95% confidence limit for seroprevalence was 0.5% (seroprevalence = 0%; 95% CI = 0–0.5%).

Description of the Sample Population and Exposure to Mosquitoes

Population estimates of demographic, exposure, attitudinal, and behavioral characteristics are shown in TABLE 1. Mean age was 45.7 years (range: 12–88 years). Fifty-seven percent were female; 32% were racial-ethnic minorities; 19% spoke a language other than English in the home; and 89% had completed ≥12 years of schooling.

Most households (64%) were single-family homes; 95% had a yard and 14% had a swimming pool. Nearly all dwellings had screens (91%) and air-conditioning (86%). Only 18% of persons noticed indoor mosquitoes more than once per week, and 13% spent ≥ two hours outside at dusk or dawn. Seventeen percent of households reported finding a dead bird on their property.

Concern about WNV and Prevention

Nearly all participants (99%) had heard of WNV. Overall, 58% were a little or very worried about getting WNV. Because there was substantial media coverage regarding the risks for exposure to pesticides that might be used to control exposure to WNV, we also asked about concern regarding pesticide exposure. Forty-eight percent were a little or very worried about getting sick from the pesticides that were used to kill the mosquitoes. However, when given a choice, people were more worried about getting WNV (37%) than about getting sick from pesticides (19%).

Most persons (79%) practiced ≥ one personal precaution to avoid WNV exposure. A total of 55% reported avoiding areas with mosquitoes; 44% used mosquito repellent; 43% wore long-sleeved shirts and long pants; and 29% avoided the outdoors at least sometimes. Although practicing some personal precautions was common, only 7% reported practicing all four personal precautions.

Similarly, most (86%) households did ≥ one mosquito-source reduction activity. Sixty-three percent of households reported that they checked their screens; 55% cleaned their gutters; and 55% removed objects from around their property that contained water. However, only 25% did all three mosquito-source reductions.

People were also asked where they had received their most useful information concerning WNV and how to avoid mosquito bites. The media (*i.e.*, television, newspaper, or radio) was the most common response (79%).

Multivariate Analyses

Using multivariate logistic regression, we examined three different outcome variables: mosquito repellent use, practicing ≥ two personal precautions, and doing ≥ two larval source reductions (TABLE 2). Among other variables, significant associations were found between self-reported behavior of at least some mosquito repellent use and speaking English as the primary language in the home, being worried about WNV, age <50 years, and finding mosquitoes in the home at least twice a week.

Practicing ≥ two personal precautions was associated with higher perceived risk for WNV and being female. Doing ≥ two larval source reductions was associated with speaking English as the primary language in the home (Odds ratio [OR] 2.0; CI =1.1–3.5) and finding a dead bird on the property (OR 1.8; CI = 1.1–2.8).

TABLE 2. Multivariate logistic regression of predictors of taking personal protective measures and efforts to reduce mosquito populations

Mosquito repellent use (sometimes or always vs. never)		
English as the primary language spoken in the home vs. another language primarily spoken in the home	2.0	1.2–3.3
Being very worried about WNV vs. not worried about WNV	1.9	0.95–3.6
Being a little worried about WNV vs. not worried about WNV	1.9	1.3–2.6
Having private insurance vs. not having private insurance	1.9	1.1–3.1
Being a little worried about pesticides vs. not worried about pesticides	1.7	1.1–2.6
Age <50 years vs. age ≥65 years		
Finding mosquitoes in the home at least twice a week vs. once a week	1.6	1.03–2.5
or less	1.6	1.02–2.5
Practicing two or more personal precautions (sometimes or always vs. never)		
Being very worried about WNV vs. not worried about WNV	3.8	2.2–6.5
Females vs. males	2.0	1.2–2.9
Doing two or more mosquito-source reductions		
English as the primary language spoken in the home vs. another language primarily spoken in the home	2.0	1.1–3.5
Finding a dead bird on the property	1.8	1.1–2.8

DISCUSSION

In 2000, WNV reemerged in a wide geographic area, affecting 12 states and the District of Columbia.[4] Although Connecticut experienced intense epizootic activity, no severe human disease was documented. Because most WNV infections are expected to be asymptomatic or mild,[11] population-based serosurveys are important tools that can be used to estimate the proportion of persons who are infected. This serosurvey showed that despite a prolonged epizootic among birds, there was little evidence of transmission to humans. The reasons for this are unclear. Although WNV can be focal in nature, prevention measures implemented in 2000 might have contributed to the low incidence of disease among humans and the lack of apparent infection in the study area. Because preventive measures taken by individuals and households to reduce the number of mosquitoes and mosquito bites is a major means of limiting the human health impact of WNV, understanding what levels of prevention were achieved and whether this might have contributed to the apparent low human risk for WNV infection is critical. Results from the serosurvey in northern Queens, New York, in 1999 demonstrated that the highest infection rates occurred among people who spent substantial time outdoors between dusk and dawn and did not use mosquito repellent.[12] In that survey, only 9% of individuals routinely used mosquito repellent and 70% never used it.

People in the Connecticut study area were highly aware of WNV. Most took at least some personal protective measures and almost 50% used mosquito repellent sometimes or always. This suggests that public education and awareness might have contributed substantially to the lower human risk in 2000.

Nonetheless, not all Connecticut serosurvey participants were concerned about WNV or took personal protective measures. Substantial improvements could be made. Despite two seasons with intensive media coverage, 42% of persons were not particularly concerned about WNV. This is important because persons who perceive themselves as being at risk were more likely to take personal protective measures. Of particular concern, those persons who were at highest risk for severe WNV disease, namely, people over 50 years of age, were, if anything, less likely to take personal protective measures. In addition, cultural and language issues involved in educating groups about the use of personal protective measures to reduce one's exposure to mosquito bites might have an impact on prevention actions taken. In our study, 74% of those whose primary language in the home was not English reported that they were a little or very worried about WNV, but only 34% used mosquito repellent; 53% practiced ≥ two personal precautions; and 47% of households did ≥ two source reductions. Although providing literature in appropriate languages is an important first step, more information is needed to assess why people from homes where English is not the primary language were less likely to take personal protective measures. Cultural issues and prior experience with mosquito-borne diseases might play a role in beliefs regarding the utility of protective measures.

Our findings also demonstrate that the media play an important role in educating the public. Local and state public health officials were routinely interviewed by the media, which tried to convey accurate information regarding WNV and the personal protective measures the public could do to reduce their risk of exposure to mosquitoes. Heightened media interest in WNV might have enhanced public awareness of

WNV and protective measures that were taken. As media interest wanes, working with local media to define appropriate public health education messages and disseminate information in a timely fashion is critical.

This study was limited in several ways. First, the self-reporting nature of the interview does not allow for independent validation of respondents' answers. Visual household surveys could validate certain responses and should be considered in future surveys. Second, translators were routinely available only for those who spoke Spanish or Creole. Potential participants who only spoke other languages were considered refusals; however, the percent of persons only speaking other languages in this area is thought to be low, and thus the potential for selection bias was thought to be small. Last, the response rate was approximately 50%. Nonrespondents could differ in important and relevant ways from respondents, and no systematic attempt was made to follow up with those who refused to participate. Consequently, the extent and direction of this possible source of bias is unknown.

Persons living or traveling to areas in which WNV is known to occur should be aware of the need to avoid mosquito bites and understand how to reduce their exposure. Further study is needed to determine why some people do not take protective measures and how they can be motivated to change their behavior to reduce their risk of mosquito-borne diseases.

ACKNOWLEDGMENTS

We thank the Greenwich and Stamford health departments for their assistance and support which made the serosurvey possible; Marcy Gray from the National Center for Infectious Disease, Vector-Borne Infectious Diseases, Centers for Disease Control and Prevention, Fort Collins, Colorado, for her time and patience in coordinating the logistics of the study; the numerous persons at the local and state health departments, the public health prevention specialists, and the phlebotomists and translators who walked the streets and collected the data.

REFERENCES

1. CENTERS FOR DISEASE CONTROL AND PREVENTION. 1999. Outbreak of West Nile-like viral encephalitis—New York, 1999. Morb. Mortal. Wkly. Rep. **48:** 845–849.
2. CENTERS FOR DISEASE CONTROL AND PREVENTION. 2000. Update: West Nile virus activity—northeastern United States, January–August 7, 2000. Morb. Mortal. Wkly. Rep. **49:** 714–717.
3. LANCIOTTI, R.S., J.T. ROEHIG, V. DEUBEL, *et al.* 1999. Origin of the West Nile virus responsible for an outbreak of encephalitis in the northeastern United States. Science **286:** 2333–2337.
4. CENTERS FOR DISEASE CONTROL AND PREVENTION. 2000. Update: West Nile Virus activity—eastern United States, 2000. Morb. Mortal. Wkly. Rep. **49:** 1044–1047.
5. CENTERS FOR DISEASE CONTROL AND PREVENTION. 2001. Serosurveys for West Nile virus infection—New York and Connecticut counties–2000. Morb. Mortal. Wkly. Rep. **50:** 37–39.
6. HADLER, J., R. NELSON, T. MCCARTHY, *et al.* 2001. West Nile Virus surveillance in Connecticut 2000: Evidence that an intense epizootic can occur without humans being at high risk for severe disease. Emerg. Infect. Dis. **7:** 646–642.

7. MARTIN, D.A., D.A. MUTH, T. BROWN, *et al.* 2000. Standardization of immunoglobulin M capture enzyme-linked immunosorbent assays for routine diagnosis of arboviral infections. J. Clin. Microbiol. **38:** 1823–1826.
8. DEAN, A.G., A.J. DEAN, D. COULOUMBIER, *et al.* 1994. Epi Info, version 6: a word processing, database, and statistical program for epidemiology on microcomputers. U.S. Department of Health and Human Services, Centers for Disease Control and Prevention. Atlanta, GA.
9. STATA, version 5. 1997. Stata Corporation. College Station, TX.
10. KORN, E. & B.I. GRAUBARD. 1998. Confidence intervals for proportions with small expected number of positive count estimated from survey data. Surv. Methodol. **24**(2): 193–201.
11. MCINTOSH, B.M., P.G. JUPP, I. DOS SANTOS & G.M. MEENEHAN. 1976. Epidemics of West Nile and Sindbis viruses in South Africa with *Culex* (Culex) *univittatus* Theobold as vector. South Afr. J. Sci. **72:** 295–300.
12. MOSTASHARI, F., M.L. BUNNING, P.T. KITSUTANI, *et al.* 2001. Epidemic West Nile encephalitis, New York, 1999: results of a household-based seroepidemiologic survey. Lancet **358:** 261–264.

Potential North American Vectors of West Nile Virus

MICHAEL J. TURELL, MICHAEL R. SARDELIS, DAVID J. DOHM,
AND MONICA L. O'GUINN

*Virology Division, U.S. Army Medical Research Institute of Infectious Diseases,
1425 Porter Street, Fort Detrick, Maryland 21702-5011, USA*

ABSTRACT: The outbreak of disease in the New York area in 1999 due to West
Nile (WN) virus was the first evidence of the occurrence of this virus in the
Americas. To determine potential vectors, more than 15 mosquito species (including *Culex pipiens, Cx. nigripalpus, Cx. quinquefasciatus, Cx. salinarius,
Aedes albopictus, Ae. vexans, Ochlerotatus japonicus, Oc. sollicitans, Oc. taeniorhynchus,* and *Oc. triseriatus*) from the eastern United States were evaluated for
their ability to serve as vectors for the virus isolated from birds collected during the 1999 outbreak in New York. Mosquitoes were allowed to feed on one- to
four-day old chickens that had been inoculated with WN virus 1–3 days previously. The mosquitoes were incubated for 12–15 days at 26°C and then allowed
to refeed on susceptible chickens and assayed to determine transmission and
infection rates. Several container-breeding species (e.g., *Ae. albopictus,
Oc. atropalpus,* and *Oc. japonicus*) were highly efficient laboratory vectors of
WN virus. The *Culex* species were intermediate in their susceptibility. However, if a disseminated infection developed, all species were able to transmit WN
virus by bite. Factors such as population density, feeding preference, longevity,
and season of activity also need to be considered in determining the role these
species could play in the transmission of WN virus.

KEYWORDS: West Nile virus; North American vectors; temperature

INTRODUCTION

The recent outbreak of illness due to infection with West Nile (WN) virus in the
New York City metropolitan area[1–3] represents the first documented introduction of
WN virus into the New World. Previous studies in Africa, Asia, and southern Europe, where WN virus is enzootic, isolated WN virus from numerous species of mosquitoes, as well as from several species of both hard (Ixodid) and soft (Argasid)
ticks.[4,5] However, most WN virus isolations have been made from *Culex* (*Culex*)
spp. mosquitoes.

As part of the surveillance program for WN virus in the eastern United States, extensive efforts were made to collect mosquitoes to determine which species were responsible for this outbreak. In both 1999 and 2000, most WN virus-positive pools

Address for correspondence: Michael J. Turell, Department of Vector Assessment, Virology
Division, USAMRIID, 1425 Porter Street, Fort Detrick, Maryland 21702-5011. Voice: 301-619-
4921; fax: 301-619-2290.
michael.turell@det.amedd.army.mil

contained *Culex* (*Culex*) species, principally *Cx. pipiens, Cx. restuans,* and *Cx. salinarius.*[6] In addition, WN virus was also detected in at least nine pools each of *Aedes vexans, Ochlerotatus j. japonicus,* and *Oc. triseriatus,* indicating that they might also be involved in viral transmission. Other species, including *Anopheles punctipennis, Ae. albopictus, Oc. trivittatus, Culiseta melanura, Oc. cantator,* and *Psorophora ferox,* yielded between one and three WN virus-positive pools.[6] These isolation studies provide preliminary evidence of involvement in the transmission cycle. However, there are potential problems associated with virus isolation studies that might cause a mosquito species to be erroneously implicated as a vector. These include misidentification of mosquitoes, contamination of a pool either in the laboratory or with a leg of an infected mosquito, or detection of virus in the remnant of a partially digested infected blood meal in an otherwise uninfected mosquito. Also, some mosquito species may be susceptible to infection but are unable to transmit the virus by bite. In addition, the type of trap used to capture the mosquitoes will determine, in large part, which mosquito species are captured. Gravid traps are more likely to capture *Culex* mosquitoes, while dry ice–baited miniature light traps are more likely to collect host-seeking *Aedes* or *Ochlerotatus* species. Other species, such as *Ae. albopictus* or *Oc. j. japonicus* may be common as larvae, but be difficult to capture as adults. This may result in a significant underestimation of their involvement based on trap collection data. Thus, depending on the trapping method used, certain species might be over- or underrepresented in the pools tested for the virus.

Vector Incrimination

To be incriminated as a vector, several criteria need to be met.[7] These include repeated isolation of virus from field-caught individuals of the species and demonstration in the laboratory that the species is able to become infected and transmit the virus by bite after it ingests a viremic blood meal (i.e., vector competence). In addition, there needs to be data demonstrating that the mosquito species feeds, in nature, on a host that develops an appropriate viremia, and that it is active at the time of year that viral transmission is occurring. However, the relative role that the species will play in viral transmission is determined not only by how efficient a vector it is in the laboratory, but also by factors such as its relative abundance, feeding patterns, longevity relative to the extrinsic incubation period, and environmental factors such as temperature and rainfall. All of these need to be taken into account when trying to determine the importance of a particular species as a potential vector.

Vector Competence Tests

Mosquitoes were selected for evaluation either because evidence of WN virus infection was detected in that species or because that species is known to be involved with another arbovirus with a similar epidemiology (i.e., enzootic transmission cycle involving birds and disease occurring in humans or equines). The species evaluated are listed in TABLE 1.

We allowed mosquitoes to feed on two- to four-day-old leghorn chickens that had been inoculated with 10^{2-3} plaque-forming units (PFU) of WN virus one to three days earlier. We used a strain of WN virus isolated from the brain of a crow that died in the Bronx in 1999. The virus was used either unpassed or passaged one time in

TABLE 1. Potential for selected North American mosquitoes to transmit West Nile (WN) virus based on distribution, bionomics, vector competence, virus isolations, and involvement with other arboviruses

Species	Field isolations of WN virus[a]	Other viruses[b]	Host preference	Vector competence for WN virus[c]	Potential to serve as a Enzootic vector[d]	Bridge vector[e]
Aedes albopictus	+	EEE	Opportunistic	++++	+	++++
Ae. vexans	+++	EEE	Mammals	+	0	++
Culex nigripalpus	0	EEE/SLE	Opportunistic	++	++	++
Cx. pipiens	+++++	SLE	Birds	+++	+++++	++
Cx. quinquefasciatus	0	SLE	Birds	+++	++++	++
Cx. restuans	+++	SLE	Birds	–+++	+++++	++
Cx. salinarius	+++	EEE/SLE	Opportunistic	–+++	+++	++++
Ochlerotatus atropalpus	0	—	Mammals	–+++	+	++
Oc. canadensis	0	EEE	Mammals	+	0	+
Oc. cantator	+	—	Mammals	+	0	+
Oc. j. japonicus	+++	—	Opportunistic	–+++	+	++++
Oc. sollicitans	0	EEE	Large mammals	++	0	+
Oc. taeniorhynchus	0	EEE	Large mammals	+	0	+
Oc. triseriatus	+++	—	Mammals	+++	0	+++

[a]Relative number of WN virus-positive pools detected. 0 = none; + = one; +++++ = many.

[b]EEE = eastern equine encephalomyelitis virus; SLE = St. Louis encephalitis virus.

[c]Efficiency with which this species is able to transmit WN virus in the laboratory. 0 = incompetent; + = inefficient; ++++ = extremely efficient vector (Turell *et al.*,[9,20], Sardelis &Turell[22], Dohm, O'Guinn, Sardelis, Turell unpublished data).

[d]Potential for this species to be an enzootic or maintenance vector based on virus isolations from the field, vector competence, feeding behavior, etc. 0 = little to no risk; +++++ = this species may play a major role.

[e]Potential for this species to be an epizootic or bridge vector based on virus isolations from the field, vector competence, feeding behavior, etc. 0 = little to no risk; +++++ = this species may play a major role.

African green monkey kidney (Vero) cells. Engorged mosquitoes were placed in 3.8-liter cardboard cages with netting across the open end and held at 26°C for 12–15 days until tested for virus infection, dissemination, and transmission. After incubation for 12–15 days, mosquitoes were allowed to refeed either individually or in small groups on susceptible young chickens and were then killed by freezing at −20°C. They were then examined for the presence of blood, and their legs and bodies triturated separately in 1 mL of diluent (10% heat-inactivated fetal bovine serum in Medium 199 with Earle's salts, $NaHCO_3$, and antibiotics). Both the leg and body suspensions were tested for infectious virus by a plaque assay on Vero cell monolayers. Detecting virus in the body suspension indicated an infected mosquito, while detecting virus in the leg suspension indicated that virus had disseminated from the midgut to the hemocoel in that individual.[8] Each of the chickens fed upon in the transmission trial was bled 24 or 48 h later, and the presence of virus in their blood indicated transmission.

Examination of blood from the WN virus–inoculated chickens indicated that viremia titers were related to both the age of the chicken and the time interval between WN virus inoculation and bleeding.[9] We determined infection, dissemination, and transmission rates for mosquitoes that fed on chickens with viremia levels that were approximately 10^7 PFU of WN virus/mL of blood at the time the mosquitoes fed on these chickens. Although infection rates varied from >80% to <5%, at least some of the individual mosquitoes in all of the species tested were susceptible to infection with WN virus. Similarly, transmission rates for the various species varied greatly. In some species, >50% of the orally exposed mosquitoes transmitted WN virus by bite, while in others <5% were able to transmit WN virus (TABLE 1).

Transmission Cycles

West Nile virus, like many other arboviruses, has two distinct transmission cycles: a primary enzootic or amplification cycle involving one set of vectors and avian hosts and secondary cycles involving potentially different arthropods and transmission to other hosts such as humans and horses. To predict and control the occurrence of WN virus, it is necessary to understand how these cycles are related and how the vertebrate hosts, strain of virus, vector species, and environmental factors affect them. In the primary cycle of WN virus, ornithophagic mosquitoes, such as *Cx. pipiens*, feed on viremic birds (amplification hosts), become infected, and transmit WN virus to other amplification hosts. If the proper conditions exist (i.e., temperature, mosquito species, mosquito population density, number of susceptible hosts, etc.) an epizootic will occur in the avian population.

Although numerous avian hosts might become infected, this will not necessarily result in human or equine disease. In addition to being competent transmitters of virus, the most efficient primary vectors are those that feed exclusively on avian hosts, particularly those species that develop high-level viremias. Because they feed almost exclusively on avian hosts, these primary vectors pose little risk of transmitting WN virus to humans or equines. On the other hand, mosquitoes that are more general feeders would not be efficient amplification vectors. However, they could pose a much greater threat to humans and equines. These species, known as bridge vectors, could become infected when feeding on an infected bird and then transmit WN virus to a susceptible vertebrate host. The greater the number of infected birds at a given period of time, the more likely that a bridge vector would feed on an infected bird, become infected, and transmit WN virus to other vertebrate hosts (e.g., humans or equines).

Effect of Environmental Temperature

Environmental factors, particularly temperature and rainfall, have long been known to influence the transmission cycles of arboviruses.[10–14] Several laboratory studies indicate that mosquitoes are more efficient vectors of flaviviruses when they are held at higher, rather than lower, environmental temperatures.[12,14–16] Studies at the United States Army Medical Research Institute of Infectious Diseases[23] indicated that *Cx. pipiens* was a significantly more efficient vector of WN virus when maintained at 30°C rather than at 18, 20, or 26°C. To complement these laboratory studies, Hess[11] found that outbreaks of the closely related St. Louis encephalitis (SLE) virus in North America were more likely to occur in years with above-average temperatures from April to June. These observations are consistent with the outbreak in New York in 1999 in which 62 cases of encephalitis were documented over a relatively small geographic area, indicative of intense WN virus transmission, during one of the warmest summers on record. By contrast, the summer of 2000 was much cooler, and although there was WN viral activity over a much larger geographical area in the United States, there were only 22 diagnosed cases of WN encephalitis. Similarly, the recent outbreaks of WN viral activity in Bucharest, Romania, in 1996[17–18] and in Volgograd, Russia, in 1999[19] were also associated with above-average temperatures. As with other flaviviruses such as dengue[15] and SLE,[11] transmission of WN virus might be more efficient at warmer temperatures, and this might have serious implications as WN virus extends its range south.

Although cooler temperatures probably played a role in the reduced intensity of WN transmission during 2000 as compared to 1999, other factors also need to be considered. In 1999, mosquito control was not initiated until nearly all of the human cases had already been infected. However, in 2000 extensive mosquito control efforts, including larval control of *Culex* mosquitoes, were initiated early in the spring. This may have reduced the population density of primary amplification vectors, principally *Cx. pipiens*, sufficiently that the amplification cycle in birds was not as explosive as it had been in 1999. This, in turn, may have reduced the chance that bridge vectors, such as *Cx. salinarius, Oc. j. japonicus,* and *Ae. vexans,* would have fed on an infectious bird, become infected, and transmitted WN virus to humans and equines.

Potential North American Vectors

Primary (Amplification) Cycle

Based on the criteria mentioned above, several species have the potential to be involved in the primary amplification cycle of WN virus in North America. *Culex pipiens* and *Cx. restuans* have both been implicated as enzootic maintenance vectors. WN virus has been detected in numerous pools of each of these species. Both are competent laboratory vectors (Sardelis, unpublished data),[9,20] feed readily on avian hosts,[21] and are active in areas where and when WN activity has been reported. In addition, because of the involvement of *Cx. nigripalpus* and *Cx. quinquefasciatus* with the closely related SLE virus and their ability to transmit WN virus in the laboratory,[24] these two species should also be considered as potential vectors in the amplification cycle of WN virus.

Secondary (Bridge Vectors) Cycle

Several species, including *Ae. vexans, Cx. salinarius, Oc. j. japonicus,* and *Oc. triseriatus,* have already been implicated as bridge vectors. There have been repeated WN virus-positive pools of each of these species, and they are all competent laboratory vectors of WN virus (Sardelis, unpublished data).[9,20,22] In addition, as the range of WN viral activity extends further south, species such as *Ae. albopictus* and *Cx. nigripalpus* may become involved as bridge vectors. Both species are opportunistic feeders and are competent laboratory vectors of WN virus (Sardelis, unpublished data).[9] A number of groundwater-breeding *Aedes* and *Ochlerotatus* species, including *Oc. canadensis, Oc. cantator, Oc. sollicitans,* and *Oc. taeniorhynchus,* were competent but inefficient vectors of WN virus (O'Guinn, unpublished data).[9]

SUMMARY

The outbreak of disease in the New York area due to West Nile (WN) virus in 1999 was the first evidence of the occurrence of this virus in the Americas. Because little is known about the ability of North American mosquitoes to transmit this virus, we conducted laboratory studies to evaluate several mosquito species epidemiologically linked to WN virus in North America. These included *Culex pipiens, Cx. nigripalpus, Cx. quinquefasciatus, Cx. salinarius, Aedes albopictus, Ae. vexans, Ochlerotatus j. japonicus, Oc. sollicitans, Oc. taeniorhynchus,* and *Oc. triseriatus* from the eastern United States. Mosquitoes were allowed to feed on one- to four-day-old chickens inoculated previously with a strain of WN virus isolated from a crow collected during the New York outbreak in 1999. The mosquitoes were incubated for 12–15 days at 26° C and then allowed to refeed on susceptible chickens and assayed to determine infection and transmission rates. Several container-breeding species (e.g., *Ae. albopictus, Oc. atropalpus,* and *Oc. j. japonicus*) were highly efficient laboratory vectors of WN virus. By contrast, most of the floodwater *Aedes/ Ochlerotatus* species tested were relatively refractory to infection with WN virus. The *Culex* species were intermediate in their susceptibility. However, if a disseminated infection developed, all species were able to transmit WN virus by bite. Factors such as population density, feeding preference, environmental temperature, longevity, and seasonal activity also need to be considered in determining the role these species could play in WN transmission.

ACKNOWLEDGMENTS

We thank T. McNamara (Wildlife Conservation Society) for providing the Crow 397-99 strain of WN virus used in this study, and D. Schachner and M. Delgado for their assistance in rearing mosquitoes. We also thank J. Blow, C. Bosio, and K. Kenyon for critically reading the manuscript.

In conducting research using animals, the investigators adhered to the "Guide for the Care and Use of Laboratory Animals," as prepared by the Committee on Care and Use of Laboratory Animals of the Institute of Laboratory Animal Resources, National Research Council (NIH Publication No. 86-23, Revised 1996). The facilities are fully accredited by the Association for Assessment and Accreditation of Laboratory Animal Care, International.

REFERENCES

1. CENTERS FOR DISEASE CONTROL. 1999. Outbreak of West Nile-like viral encephalitis— New York, 1999. Morb. Mortal. Wkly. Rep. **48:** 845–849.
2. CENTERS FOR DISEASE CONTROL. 1999. Update: West Nile virus encephalitis—New York, 1999. Morb. Mortal. Wkly. Rep. **48:** 944–946.
3. LANCIOTTI, R.S., J.T. ROEHRIG, V. DEUBEL, et al. 1999. Origin of the West Nile virus responsible for an outbreak of encephalitis in the northeastern United States. Science **286:** 2333–2337.
4. HAYES, C. 1989. West Nile fever. In Arboviruses: Epidemiology and Ecology. Vol. V. T. Monath, Ed.: 59–88. CRC Press. Boca Raton, FL.
5. HUBALEK, Z. & J. HALOUZKA. 1999. West Nile virus—a reemerging mosquito-borne viral disease in Europe. Emerg. Infect. Dis. **5:** 643–650.
6. CENTERS FOR DISEASE CONTROL. 2000. Update: West Nile virus activity–eastern United States, 2000. Morb. Mortal. Wkly. Rep. **49:** 1044–1047.
7. REEVES, W.C. 1957. Arthropods as vectors and reservoirs of animal pathogenic viruses. In Handbuch de Virusforschung. Vol. 4 (Suppl. Vol. 3). C. Hallauer & K.F. Meyer, Eds.: 177–202. Springer-Verlag. Vienna. Vol. 4 (Suppl. Vol. 3).
8. TURELL, M.J., T.P. GARGAN II & C.L. BAILEY. 1984. Replication and dissemination of Rift Valley fever virus in Culex pipiens. Am. J. Trop. Med. Hyg. **33:** 176–181.
9. TURELL, M.J., M.L. O'GUINN, D.J. DOHM & J.W. JONES. 2001. Vector competence of North American mosquitoes (Diptera: Culicidae) for West Nile virus. J. Med. Entomol. **38:** 130–134.
10. DAVIS, N.C. 1932. The effect of various temperatures in modifying the extrinsic incubation period of yellow fever virus in Aedes aegypti. Am. J. Hyg. **16:** 163–176.
11. HESS, A.D., C.E. CHURUBIN & L.C. LAMOTTE. 1963. Relationship of temperature to activity of western and St. Louis encephalitis viruses. Am. J. Trop. Med. Hyg. **12:** 657–667.
12. LAMOTTE, L.C., JR. 1963. Effect of low environmental temperature upon Japanese B encephalitis virus multiplication in the mosquito. Mosq. News **23:** 330–335.
13. HURLBUT, H.S. 1973. The effect of environmental temperature upon the transmission of St. Louis encephalitis virus by Culex pipiens quinquefasciatus. J. Med. Entomol. **10:** 1–12.
14. CORNEL, A.J., P.G. JUPP & N.K. BLACKBURN. 1993. Environmental temperature on the vector competence of Culex univittatus (Diptera: Culicidae) for West Nile virus. J. Med. Entomol. **30:** 449–456.
15. WATTS, D.M, D.S. BURKE, B.A. HARRISON, et al. 1987. Effect of temperature on the vector efficiency of Aedes aegypti for dengue 2 virus. Am. J. Trop. Med. Hyg. **36:** 143–152.
16. JUPP, P.G. 1974. Laboratory studies on the transmission of West Nile virus by Culex (Culex) univittatus Theobald; factors influencing the transmission rate. J. Med. Entomol. **11:** 455–458.
17. HAN, L.L., F. POPOVICI, J.P. ALEXANDER, JR., et al. 1999. Risk factors for West Nile virus infection and meningoencephalitis, Romania, 1996. J. Infect. Dis. **179:** 230–233.
18. SAVAGE, H.M., C. CEIANU, G. NICOLESCU, et al. 1999. Entomologic and avian investigations of an epidemic of West Nile fever in Romania in 1996, with serologic and molecular characterization of a virus isolate from mosquitoes. Am. J. Trop. Med. Hyg. **61:** 600–611.

19. PLATONOV, A.E., G.A. SHIPULIN, O.Y. SHIPULINA, *et al.* 2001. Outbreak of West Nile virus infection, Volgograd Region, Russia, 1999. Emerg. Infect. Dis. **7:** 128–132.
20. TURELL, M.J., M. O'GUINN & J. OLIVER. 2000. Potential for New York mosquitoes to transmit West Nile virus. Am. J. Trop. Med. Hyg. **62:** 413–414.
21. TEMPELIS, C.H. 1975. Host-feeding patterns of mosquitoes, with a review of advances in analysis of blood meals by serology. J. Med. Entomol. **11:** 635–653.
22. SARDELIS, M.R. & M.J. TURELL. 2001. *Ochlerotatus j. japonicus* in Frederick County, Maryland: discovery, distribution, and vector competence for West Nile virus. J. Am. Mosq. Cont. Assoc. **17:** 137–141.
23. DOHM, D.J., M.L. O'GUINN & M.J. TURELL. 2002. Effect of environmental temperature on the ability of *Culex pipiens* (Diptera: Culicidae) to transmit West Nile virus. J. Med. Entomol. In press.
24. SARDELIS, M.R., M.J. TURELL, D.J. DOHM & M.L. O'GUINN. 2001. Vector competence of selected North American *Culex* and *Coquillettidia* mosquitoes for West Nile virus. Emerg. Infect. Dis. **7:** 1006–1010.

West Nile Virus Envelope Protein

Role in Diagnosis and Immunity

TIAN WANG,[a] JOHN F. ANDERSON,[b] LOUIS A. MAGNARELLI,[b]
SANDRA BUSHMICH,[c] SUSAN WONG,[d] RAYMOND A. KOSKI,[e]
AND EROL FIKRIG[a]

[a]Section of Rheumatology, Department of Internal Medicine,
Yale University School of Medicine, New Haven, Connecticut, 06520, USA

[b]Department of Entomology, Connecticut Agricultural Experiment Station,
New Haven, Connecticut 06504, USA

[c]Department of Pathobiology, University of Connecticut, Storrs, Connecticut 06269, USA

[d]Wadsworth Center, New York State Department of Health,
Albany, New York 12201, USA

[e]L[2] Diagnostics, New Haven, Connecticut 06530, USA

ABSTRACT: The role of antibodies to the West Nile virus envelope (E) protein in serodiagnosis and protection was examined. The E protein was expressed and purified in recombinant form. Antibodies to the E protein were detected in patients with West Nile virus infection. Passive immunization with rabbit anti-E protein sera also partially protected mice from challenge with West Nile virus. The humoral response to the West Nile virus E protein is therefore useful as an aid in the diagnosis and may also play a role in immunity to infection.

KEYWORDS: West Nile virus; E protein; serologic tests

West Nile (WN) virus is a flavivirus that is closely related to Japanese encephalitis virus, St. Louis encephalitis virus, and Murray Valley encephalitis virus. Approximately half of the flaviviruses cause human disease, with symptoms such as fever, hemorrhage, vascular collapse, and encephalitis.[1] Epidemics of WN virus infection have been reported in Africa, Asia, and Eastern Europe.[1–4] WN virus had not been documented in North America until an outbreak occurred in the New York City area in 1999.[5,6] WN virus has now been identified in mosquitoes, birds, and other animals in the United States, has survived seasonal changes, and has been responsible for sporadic cases of lethal human and equine infection.[5–9]

New serologic tests to aid in the diagnosis of WN virus infection are necessary. Present methods of diagnosis include an IgM capture ELISA,[10] detection of neutralizing antibody in cerebrospinal fluid or serum using a plaque assay, virus isolation

Address for correspondence: Erol Fikrig, M.D., 608 Laboratory of Clinical Investigation, Section of Rheumatology, Department of Internal Medicine, Yale University School of Medicine, 333 Cedar Street, New Haven, CT 06520-8031. Voice: 203-785-2453; fax: 203-785-7053.
erol.fikrig@yale.edu

TABLE 1. The antibody response to the recombinant WN virus E proteins is important in diagnosis and immunity[a]

Human antibodies to E protein during infection
Patients with WN virus infection
5/5
Normal individuals (controls)
0/4
E protein antibodies are protective in mice
Delay in time to death
4/5 mice given 10^3 PFU of WN virus
Prevention of death
3/5 mice given 10^1 PFU of WN virus

[a]Recombinant E protein was probed in immunoblot with sera from patients with WN virus infection and sera from normal individuals (controls). Groups of 5 C3H/HeN mice were administered E protein antisera, then challenged with either 10^3 or 10^1 plaque-forming units (PFU) of WN virus (isolate 2741), and examined daily for 14 days. Control mice usually died at 7–8 days. Mice that had a delay in mortality of at least 24 hours compared with controls were considered to have an alteration in the course of disease. Mice that lived to day 14 were considered to have survived WN virus infection.

from fluid or tissues, and RT-PCR.[7,11] We have focused on identifying WN virus antigens that may be used in assays to help diagnose infection. The viral genome is processed to eight proteins—the envelope (E) protein, the matrix protein, the nucleocapsid protein, and five nonstructural proteins.[5,6] The E proteins of several flaviviruses elicit neutralizing antibodies and may be important in the protective immune response.[12–14]

We cloned the gene encoding the WN virus E protein. RNA was isolated from WN virus (2741) from *Culex pipiens* during the recent outbreak.[5] The gene encoding the WN virus E protein was amplified by RT-PCR and expressed in *Escherichia coli* as a fusion protein.[15] The recombinant E protein was then purified and used as an antigen in an IgG Western blot analysis. Sera from persons with well-documented WN virus infection from the New York State Department of Health had antibodies that reacted with the E protein (TABLE 1).[15] Sera from normal individuals served as controls (TABLE 1).

WN virus infection causes death in various strains of laboratory mice, including C3H/HeN mice.[14,16,17] To investigate the role of the antibody response to the WN virus E protein in immunity, E protein–specific antisera was generated. Rabbits were immunized with 50 μg of E protein in Freund's adjuvant, boosted twice, and then phlebotomized. The rabbit antisera contained antibodies to the recombinant E protein, detectable in ELISA. Naive mice were then passively immunized with 200 μL of rabbit E protein antisera and challenged one day later with WN virus (either 10^3 or 10^1 plaque-forming units). Depending on the viral doses, the E protein antisera either delayed the time to death or protected the animals from infection (TABLE 1). These data demonstrate that recombinant E protein can be used as antigen in serologic assays to aid in the diagnosis for WN viral infection and that E protein antibodies may be important in immunity.

REFERENCES

1. HUBALEK, Z. *et al.* 2000. West Nile virus investigations in South Moravia, Czechland. Viral Immunol. **13**(4): 427–433.
2. HUBALEK, Z. 2000. European experience with the West Nile virus ecology and epidemiology: could it be relevant for the New World? Viral Immunol. **13**(4): 415–426.
3. HUBALEK, Z. & J. HALOUZKA. 1999. West Nile fever—a reemerging mosquito-borne viral disease in Europe. Emerg. Infect. Dis. **5**(5): 64.
4. CEAUSU, E. *et al.* 1997. Clinical manifestations in the West Nile virus outbreak. Rom. J. Virol. **48**(1–4): 3–11.
5. ANDERSON, J.F. *et al.* 1999. Isolation of West Nile virus from mosquitoes, crows, and a Cooper's hawk in Connecticut. Science **286**(5448): 2331–2333.
6. LANCIOTTI, R.S. *et al.* 1999. Origin of the West Nile virus responsible for an outbreak of encephalitis in the northeastern United States. Science **286**(5448): 2333–2337.
7. LANCIOTTI, R.S. *et al.* 2000. Rapid detection of West Nile virus from human clinical specimens, field-collected mosquitoes, and avian samples by a TaqMan reverse transcriptase-PCR assay. J. Clin. Microbiol. **38**(11): 4066–4071.
8. CDC. 2000. Surveillance for West Nile virus in over-wintering mosquitoes—New York, J. Am. Med. Assoc. **283**(18): 2380–2381.
9. CDC. 2000. Guidelines for surveillance, prevention, and control of West Nile virus infection—United States. J. Am. Med. Assoc. **283**(8): 997–998.
10. TARDEI, G. *et al.* 2000. Evaluation of immunoglobulin M (IgM) and IgG enzyme immunoassays in serologic diagnosis of West Nile virus infection J. Clin. Microbiol. **38**(6): 2232–2239.
11. BRIESE, T. *et al.* 1999. Identification of a Kunjin/West Nile-like flavivirus in brains of patients with New York encephalitis. Lancet **354**(9186): 1261–1262.
12. GOVERDHAN, M.K. *et al.* 1992. Two-way cross-protection between West Nile and Japanese encephalitis viruses in bonnet macaques. Acta Virol. **36**(3): 277–283.
13. PRICE, W.H. & I.S. THIND. 1971. Protection against West Nile virus induced by a previous injection with dengue virus. Am. J. Epidemiol. **94**(6): 596–607.
14. LUSTIG, S. *et al.* 2000. A live attenuated West Nile virus strain as a potential veterinary vaccine. Viral Immunol. **13**(4): 401–410.
15. WANG, T. *et al.* 2001 Immunization of mice against West Nile virus with recombinant envelope protein. J. Immunol. **167:** 5273–5277.
16. LUSTIG, S. *et al.* 1992. Viral neuroinvasion and encephalitis induced by lipopolysaccharide and its mediators. J. Exp. Med. **176**(3): 707–712.
17. HALEVY, M. *et al.* 1994. Loss of active neuroinvasiveness in attenuated strains of West Nile virus: pathogenicity in immunocompetent and SCID mice. Arch. Virol. **137**(3–4): 355–370.

Characterization of West Nile Virus from Five Species of Mosquitoes, Nine Species of Birds, and One Mammal

JOHN F. ANDERSON,[a] CHARLES R. VOSSBRINCK,[b] THEODORE G. ANDREADIS,[b] ANTHONY ITON,[c] WILLIAM H. BECKWITH III,[d] AND DONALD R. MAYO[d]

[a]*Department of Entomology, The Connecticut Agricultural Experiment Station, New Haven, Connecticut 06504, USA*

[b]*Department of Soil and Water, The Connecticut Agricultural Experiment Station, New Haven, Connecticut 06504, USA*

[c]*Stamford Department of Health and Social Services, 888 Washington Boulevard, Stamford, Connecticut 06904, USA*

[d]*Arbovirus/Molecular Diagnostics, Connecticut Department of Public Health, Hartford, Connecticut 06144, USA*

KEYWORDS: West Nile virus; nucleotide sequences; amino acid substitutions

INTRODUCTION

An outbreak of West Nile (WN) virus occurred in New York City and surrounding environs in 1999, infecting and killing humans, birds, and horses.[1,2] We compared nucleotide sequences of 82 independent Connecticut WN virus isolates to WN-NY99 from a Chilean flamingo that died in 1999 in New York City. Isolates were obtained from nine species of birds, five species of mosquitoes, and one striped skunk.

MATERIAL AND METHODS

A 921 nucleotide sequence of 82 Connecticut WN virus isolates from 1999 and 2000 was compared to the homologous sequence region of the WN-NY99 isolate from a Chilean flamingo that died at the Bronx Zoo in New York City in 1999. This sequence begins at nucleotide 205 and ends at 1125. It includes a 261-nucleotide region of the nucleocapsid gene, the entire 501 nucleotide premembrane and membrane regions, and a 159 nucleotide fragment of the envelope gene. Four of the isolates were made in 1999, and 78 were cultured in 2000.

Address for correspondence: John F. Anderson, The Connecticut Agricultural Experiment Station, P. O. Box 1106, New Haven, CT 06504.Voice: 203-974-8440; fax: 203-974-8502.
John.F.Anderson@po.state.ct.us

TABLE 1. Nucleotide regions exhibiting variability

Nucleotide Position	Nucleotide Change	Number of Isolates with Mutation	Hosts
381	C to T	2	*Cx. restuans*; crow
400	C to G	1	*Cx. salinarius*
456	C to T	2	Crow (2)
516	T to C	2	Crow (2)
527	A to G	1	Crow
528	T to C	1	Crow
543	A to G	1	Crow
588	G to A	1	Crow
615	T to C	1	Crow
673	A to G	1	Crow
711	C to T	1	Crow
721	C to T	1	Crow
726	A to G	3	Crow, *Cs. melanura*; *Cx. restuans*
735	T to C	1	Crow
775	C to T	1	Crow
795	T to C	1	Skunk
812	A to G	1	Skunk
825	T to C	3	Crow, *Ae. vexans*; *Cx. pipiens*
826	T to C	1	*Cx. salinarius*
858	C to T	26	Crow (13); Canada goose; Mourning dove; blue jay (3); robin (2); skunk; *Cx. pipiens* (2); *Cs. melanura; Cx. restuans*; house sparrow
867	T to C	1	Cooper's hawk
885	C to T	1	Crow
905	G to A	1	Crow
933	C to T	1	Crow
940	T to C	1	Crow
951	G to A	1	*Cs. melanura*
1000	T to C	1	Crow
1032	T to C	1	Crow
1041	C to T	1	Crow
1047	C to T	1	*Cx. pipiens*

WN virus was cultured in Vero cells[1] from tissues of brain, heart, or kidney from avian specimens. Isolates were also made from triturated pools of mosquitoes[1,3] and from kidney and spleen of one striped skunk. Purification, amplification, and analysis of the DNA segments of each isolate were done according to methods previously described.[1]

RESULTS

WN virus was isolated from nine species of birds (American crow, American robin, blue jay, brown-headed cowbird, Canada goose, house sparrow, mourning dove, red-shouldered hawk, and Cooper's hawk). WN virus also was isolated from a striped skunk and from five species of mosquitoes (*Culex pipiens, Culex restuans, Culex salinarius, Culiseta melanura, and Aedes vexans*).[1,3]

Thirty of the 921 nucleotide positions showed variability, and six nucleotide positions showed identical changes in two or more isolates (TABLE 1). Thirty-four WN virus isolates had sequences identical to the WN-NY99 isolate, 37 had a single nucleotide change, eight had two nucleotide changes, and three isolates had three nucleotide changes. For example, the same mutation at nucleotide position 381 occurred in isolates from *Culex restuans* and a crow. The most common change occurred at nucleotide 858. Twenty-six isolates, primarily from Stamford in southwestern Connecticut, showed a mutation at this position of C to T.

Amino acid changes occurred at seven loci within six isolates. Five of the isolates had one amino acid substitution. One isolate from an American crow had changes in two amino acids. Changes occurred in the nucleocapsid (n=1), premembrane (n=4), and membrane (n=2) coding regions.

DISCUSSION

Our WN virus sequence data suggest that we are seeing microevolutionary events unfold and that we can, by sequence analysis, observe temporal and geographical genetic variation. Although the majority of the 30 mutations were silent, seven of the mutations, or 23%, resulted in amino acid substitutions.

The clustering of isolates from Stamford, CT with the mutation C to T at position 858 likely represents a single event and is not a repeated example of convergence among unrelated isolates. This C to T change was recovered from six bird species, a striped skunk, and three mosquito species in Stamford, further indicating this variant WN virus is widespread within vertebrate and mosquito populations.

The introduction of WN virus into the United States is a unique opportunity for studying the causes, dissemination, and control of a virus in nonimmune host and vector populations. The comparative phylogenetic approach using RNA sequences may be an important method for understanding these processes.

ACKNOWLEDGMENTS

We thank Jodie Correia, Melanie Baron, Michael Vasil, Bonnie Hamid, John Shepard, Michael Thomas, Ira Kettle, and Shirley Tirrell for technical help. We also thank Skip Sirpenski, Dr. Randall Nelson, and Lynn Wilcox for their efforts in coordinating the avian surveillance program in Connecticut and Dr. Richard A. French and Meghan Tucker for necropsy work.

This work was supported in part by Hatch Grant 763, Epidemiology and Laboratory Capacity for Infectious Diseases Cooperative Agreement number U50/CCU116806-

01-1 from the Centers for Disease Control and Prevention, and United States Department of Agriculture Specific Cooperative Agreement number 58-6615-1-218.

REFERENCES

1. ANDERSON, J.F., T.G. ANDREADIS, C.R. VOSSBRINCK, *et al.* 1999. Isolation of West Nile virus from mosquitoes, crows, and a Cooper's Hawk in Connecticut. Science **286:** 2331–2333.
2. LANCIOTTI, R.S., J.T. ROEHRIG, V. DEUBEL, *et al.* 1999. Origin of the West Nile virus responsible for an outbreak of encephalitis in the northeastern United States. Science **286:** 2333–2337.
3. ANDREADIS, T.G., J.F. ANDERSON & C.R. VOSSBRINCK. 2001. Mosquito surveillance for West Nile virus in Connecticut, 2000: Isolation from *Culex pipiens, Culex restuans, Culex salinarius* and *Culiseta melanura*. Emerg. Infect. Dis. **7:** 670–674.

West Nile Virus Strains Differ in Mouse Neurovirulence and Binding to Mouse or Human Brain Membrane Receptor Preparations

DAVID W. C. BEASLEY, LI LI, MIGUEL T. SUDERMAN,
AND ALAN D. T. BARRETT

*WHO Collaborating Center for Tropical Diseases and Department of Pathology,
University of Texas Medical Branch, Galveston, Texas 77555-0609, USA*

KEYWORDS: West Nile virus; mouse neurovirulence; membrane receptor preparations

The recent introduction of West Nile (WN) virus into the Western Hemisphere has focused considerable attention on this virus as a public health problem. As a result, there have been considerable advances in our knowledge of the molecular biology and phylogeny of WN virus strains from different geographical origins. However, relatively little is known about the virulence phenotypes of these viruses. Human infections with WN virus generally result in a mild, self-limiting, undifferentiated fever. However, recent outbreaks in North America and eastern Europe have been associated with a relatively high percentage (up to 10%) of cases involving potentially fatal neurological manifestations.[1]

The aim of this study was to systematically compare 19 strains of WN virus (TABLE 1) to determine whether biological differences exist between them that can be correlated with genotype. To facilitate this, we undertook a series of mouse neurovirulence experiments, and compared the ability of these viruses to bind to mouse and human brain tissue membrane receptor preparations (MRPs). In addition, we sequenced a ~500 bp region of the NS5 gene/3′-noncoding region (NCR) junction for comparison with other phylogenetic analyses that used segments of the E protein gene. Viruses were chosen to represent each of the known WN virus lineages: lineage I (primarily European and Middle Eastern isolates, but also isolates from the 1999 New York outbreak and some African isolates); lineage II (which comprises African isolates only); Kunjin (KUN) viruses; and Indian WN virus isolates (antigenically distinct from both lineages I and II).[2,3]

As has been reported previously with a smaller group of WN viruses,[3] considerable variation was observed in the region of the 3′-NCR immediately following the

Address for correspondence: David W. C. Beasley, Department of Pathology, University of Texas Medical Branch, Galveston, TX 777555-0609. Voice: 409-772- 2547; fax: 409-747-2415. dwbeasle@utmb.edu

TABLE 1. Characteristics of West Nile and Kunjin virus strains used in this study

Designation	Strain	Origin/Year	Line-age[a]	LD$_{50}$ (ip) (pfu)	MRP binding index (log$_{10}$)
CAR67	Arb-310/67	Central African Republic/1967	I	13	1.2
NIG65	IbAn7019	Nigeria/1965	I	3	1.2
SEN79	ArD-27875	Senegal/1979	I	<1	2.1
USA99a	31A	United States/1999	I	<1	1.0
USA99b	385-99	United States/1999	I	3	1.0
IND68	68856	India/1968	I	3	≥3.8
EGY50	Egypt101	Egypt/1950	I	50	2.2
ETH	EthAn4766	Ethiopia/n.k.[b]	I	n/a[c]	3.0
AUS60	MRM16 (Kunjin)	Australia/1960	KUN	≥ 10,000	1.2
AUS91	K6453 (Kunjin)	Australia/1991	KUN	≥ 10,000	0.2
IND57	IG-15578	India/1957	IND	n/a	2.4
IND80	804994	India/1980	IND	n/a	1.3
SEN90	ArD-76104	Senegal/1990	II	50	1.2
CAR82	ArB3573/82	Central African Republic/1982	II	<1	1.0
SA58	SAH-442	South Africa/1958	II	3	3.3
SA89	SPU116-89	South Africa/1989	II	5	1.2
MAD-88	ArMg-979	Madagascar/1988	II	n/a	2.7
CYP68	Q3574-5	Cyprus/1968	II	n/a	3.5
MAD78	DakAnMg798	Madagascar/1978	II	≥ 10,000	0.9

[a]Determined by sequencing of NS5/3-NCR junction and comparison with lineages defined by Lanciotti et al.[2] and Jia et al.[3]
[b]n.k., not known.
[c]n/a indicates LD$_{50}$ values could not be determined for these viruses.

NS5 stop codon (FIG. 1). In general, lineage I viruses contained a shorter 3′-NCR sequence than did viruses of lineage II. Both the Kunjin viruses and the Indian viruses IND57 and IND80 could be readily distinguished from the lineage I and II viruses.

Considerable variation was observed in the neuroinvasive phenotype of the strains examined (TABLE 1). Groups of five three- to four-week old female NIH Swiss mice were injected intraperitoneally with 10-fold dilutions of WN virus strains [10^4 to 10^{-1} plaque forming units (pfu) per animal]. Lineage I viruses as a group were most virulent, with LD$_{50}$ values ranging between ~0.2 and 50 pfu. Several lineage II strains (SA58, SA89, CAR82, SEN90) had similar neuroinvasive characteristics. By contrast, the KUN viruses (AUS60 and AUS91) and the lineage II virus MAD78 were non-neuroinvasive. Other viruses of lineage II and the Indian WN viruses were poorly neuroinvasive and caused sporadic deaths at some dilutions, but LD$_{50}$ values could not be determined for these viruses (data not shown).

The ability of WN viruses to bind to mouse or human brain tissue MRPs was also investigated (TABLE 1). MRPs were prepared and binding experiments performed as

```
                  1                                                                                              100
CAR67     (I)     CTTTGGTTGAGGACACAGTACTGTAAATACTT----------------C-AT-CAATTGTA-------------------AATAGACAATATAAGCATGT
NIG65     (I)     ....................T.........----------------T-..-........-------------------....................
SEN79     (I)     ....................T.........----------------T-..-........-------------------......A.............
USA99a    (I)     .........................G...T..----------------A-..-........-------------------..............T....C
USA99b    (I)     .........................G...T..----------------A-..-........-------------------..............T....C
IND68     (I)     ................................----------------T-..-T.......-------------------..........G.........
EGY50     (I)     ................................----------------T-..-T.......-------------------..........G.........
ETH       (I)     ....................T......C....----------------T-..-T.......-------------------..........G.........
AUS60     (KUN)   .A..................T........G..----------------T-G.-T.......-------------------...AG..T.G.C.TT.....
AUS91     (KUN)   .A...........T......T...........----------------T-G.-T.......-------------------....A.T.T.G.T.TT....
IND80     (IND)   .A..A..G......T.....GT.......G.AA--CAGT---------TA.GGT.TG.......-------------------.....T..GTGTTG.AA
IND57     (IND)   .A..A..G......T.....GT.......G.AA--CAGT---------TA.GGT.TGT......-------------------.....T..GTGTTG.AA
SEN90     (II)    T.G.A..G.......T..TT.....A.A.AAAGCTGTATTGAGTAGTTG.AT.G.....GTGT-------------TC....CA.T.TG..TT...A
CAR82     (II)    T.G.A..G.......T..TT........A.AAAGCTGTATTGAGTAGTTGCAT.G.....GC---------------TT....CA.T.TG..TT...A
SA58      (II)    T.G.A..G.......T..TT........A.AAAGCTGTATTGAGTAGTTGCAT.G.....GC---------------TT....CA.T.TG..TT...A
SA89      (II)    T.G.A..G.......T..TT........A.AAAGCTGTATTGAGTAGTTG.AT.G.....GTGT-------------TT....CA.T.TG..TT...A
MAD88     (II)    .CG.A..G.......T..TT........A.AAAGTTGTATTGAATAGTTG.A..G...C.GTGT-------------TT....CA.T.TG..TT...A
CYP68     (II)    T.A.A..G..A..T..T..TT.....G...A.GAAGTTGAGATGAATAGTT-.GTG......GTTTAGTTAATTTTATAAT.....T..T.TGG.TT...A
MAD78     (II)    .AG.T..A.......T..TT........G.GAAGTCAC---------------------------------------------------------------

                  101                                                                                            200
CAR67     (I)     ACAAAATTATAGGTTTATAGTAGCATTT-AGTGATGTTAGTGTAAATAGTTAAGAAAATTTTAAGGA-GGAAGTCAGGCCGGGAAGTTTCCGCCACCGGA
NIG65     (I)     .TG...G.....T...............-......................................-................................
SEN79     (I)     .TG...G.....T..-............-..............G.......................-................G...............
USA99a    (I)     .T....G.G...T.........T.....-....G............................G....-A...................C..........
USA99b    (I)     .T....G.G...T.........T.....-....G............................G....-A...................C..........
IND68     (I)     GT....G.....T...............-......................................-..............A...............
EGY50     (I)     GT....G.....T...............-......................................-..............A...............
ETH       (I)     GT....G.....C..C............-......................................-..............A....C..........
AUS60     (KUN)   GT.G..GCT...C......A...TG...T....TGT..AGAGT------..G.........GT..-..............A..A.............
AUS91     (KUN)   GT.G..G.T...C...G..A...TG...-....TGT..AGAGT-------..G.........GT..-..............A..A..C..........
IND80     (IND)   .T.GG.--T...C--..A....----GC.TGT.G...AGTGTT---------..G......GTTAGA..............AGCA.............
IND57     (IND)   .T.GG.--T...C--..A....----GC.TGT.G...AGTGTT---------..G......GTTAGA..............AGCA.............
SEN90     (II)    TT..TTA.T....C...AGA...T.C.AT...T.GT..AGTGTAAA----..G..TTT-A..G..A.T...........A.ATTAA.G.T.........
CAR82     (II)    TT..TTA.T....C...AGA...T...AA...T.GT..AGTGTAAA----TAGGATTT-A..G..A.T...........A.ATTAA.G.T.........
SA58      (II)    TT..TCA.T....C...AGA...T...AT...T.GT..AGTGTAAA----TGGGATTT-A..G..A.T...........A.ATTAA.G.T.........
SA89      (II)    TT..TTA.T....C...AGA...T...AT...T.GC..AGTGTAAA----TAGGATTT-A..G..A.T...........A.ATTAA.G.T.........
MAD88     (II)    TT..TTA.T.......GAGA...T...AT...T.GTG.AGTGTTAA----TAGGATTTTA..G..A.T.............CTTAACG.T.........
CYP68     (II)    TT.G.CA.G.....G..GGA...TG..AT...T.GTG.AGTGTATA----TAAAATTA-A.....A.T...........A.AC.AA.G.T.........
MAD78     (II)    ---------------------------------------------ATT...TTTGTTAA..T....A.AG.........A.ACTAGAG.T.........
```

FIGURE 1. Alignment of ~200 bp of NS5/3′-NCR junction sequences of 19 WN virus strains. Stop codons shown underlined in bold text. Dots (.) indicate conserved residues; dashes (—) indicate deletions. Virus genotypes shown in brackets: I, lineage I; II, lineage II; KUN, Kunjin; IND,

described previously.[4] The majority of viruses tested had mouse brain MRP binding indices around 1 (indicating a 10-fold reduction in virus titer following binding to MRP). However, several strains from both lineage I and II underwent approximately 100-fold (EGY50, IND57, SEN79) or 1000-fold (ETH, IND68, CYP68, MAD88, SA58) reductions in titer. A small quantity of human brain MRP was also available, and this was used with representative high- (SA58) and low-binding index (AUS91 and USA99b) strains for comparison. Strain SA58 bound to human brain MRP to a greater degree than did either AUS91 or USA99b (binding indices of 1.3, 0.8 and 0.6, respectively). Mice were inoculated intracerebrally with serial 10-fold dilutions (10^4 to 10^{-1} pfu; 20 µL volumes) of representative high- and low-binding index strains (SA58, EGY50, SEN79, SEN90; see TABLE 1). No significant differences were observed in neurovirulence in terms of either LD_{50} values or average survival times for the viruses tested (data not shown).

On the basis of these results, we conclude that differences exist in the neuroinvasiveness of WN virus strains that can be correlated with genotype. Of interest is that viruses of lineage I, which have been associated with human encephalitic disease, were highly virulent in mice while many other viruses lacked this neuroinvasive phenotype. We also observed differences in the ability of WN virus strains to bind to human and/or mouse brain tissue MRPs, although these differences were not correlated with genotype or neuroinvasiveness/neurovirulence of the viruses.

ACKNOWLEDGMENTS

This work was funded in part by a grant from the Clayton Foundation for Research. The authors thank Dr. Robert Tesh and Hilda Guzman for providing virus strains used in this study.

REFERENCES

1. GARMENDIA, A.E., H.J. VAN KRUININGEN & R.A. FRENCH. 2001. The West Nile virus: its recent emergence in North America. Microbes Infect. **3:** 223–229.
2. LANCIOTTI, R.S., J.T. ROEHRIG, V. DEUBEL, *et al.* 1999. Origin of the West Nile virus responsible for an outbreak of encephalitis in the northeastern United States. Science **286:** 2333–2337.
3. JIA, X.-Y., T. BRIESE, I. JORDAN, *et al.* 1999. Genetic analysis of West Nile New York 1999 encephalitis virus. Lancet **354:** 1971–1972.
4. NI, H. & A.D.T. BARRETT. 1998. Attenuation of Japanese encephalitis virus by selection of its mouse brain membrane receptor preparation escape variants. Virology **241:** 30–36.

Surveillance for Avian-borne Arboviruses in Connecticut, 2000

WILLIAM BECKWITH, SKIP SIRPENSKI, AND DONALD MAYO

Connecticut Department of Public Health Laboratory, 10 Clinton Street, Hartford, Connecticut 06144, USA

KEYWORDS: avian, bird, West Nile virus, eastern equine encephalitis virus, WNV, EEEV, arbovirus

The emergence of the West Nile virus (WNV) in the northeastern United States has drawn emphasis to the need of expanded arbovirus surveillance in Connecticut (CT). Although the state of CT began a comprehensive mosquito-screening program in 1997, only since the emergence of WNV have efforts been made to determine the prevalence of arboviruses in CT's bird populations. Herein, we report on our arbovirus survey of 1704 dead birds that were submitted for WNV testing during the year 2000 arbovirus transmission season from May to October.

In total, our surveillance identified 1095 isolations of WNV and 9 isolations of eastern equine encephalitis (EEE) virus in the year 2000.[1] All of the WNV isolates were obtained from crow species including the American crow (*Corvus brachyrhynchos*) and the fish crow (*Corvus ossifragus*). Our findings indicate a statewide distribution of WNV, with infected crows submitted from each of CT's eight counties. Most striking are the high rates of WNV isolation (66%) from the two densely populated CT counties (Fairfield and New Haven counties) located along the shore of Long Island Sound in the greater New York City metropolitan area. Significant percentages of WNV-infected crows were also detected in the New London (71%), Hartford (60%), Middlesex (57%), Tolland (54%), Litchfield (25%), and Windham (19%) counties. Interestingly, the highest rates of isolation occurred in the human population centers and along the waterways of CT. Taken together, our findings indicate a statewide distribution of WNV, with the highest rates of isolation made during the peak arbovirus transmission season in September and October.

In addition to WNV, we also detected and isolated EEE virus from nine birds (eight crows and one wild turkey) that tested negative for WNV. Unlike WNV, however, the EEE virus isolates were collected exclusively from New Haven, Fairfield, and Hartford counties in the southwest and central regions of CT.[1] Not surprisingly, the collection dates of the nine EEE virus–infected birds also coincided with peak WNV activity in late summer and early fall. Furthermore, our findings suggest a prevalence of EEE virus in a region of the state where the virus is not commonly found.

Address for correspondence: William Beckwith, Connecticut Department of Public Health Laboratory, 10 Clinton Street, P.O. Box 1689, Hartford, CT 06144. Voice: 860-509-8553; fax: 860-509-8699.

william.beckwith@po.state.ct.us

In addition to presenting data on the geographical and temporal distribution of our arbovirus isolations, we also presented a summary of the changes made to our protocol that collectively allowed us to streamline our diagnostics for avian-borne arboviruses. Beginning with the implementation of standard reverse transcriptase polymerase chain reaction (RT-PCR) in August, we made a gradual transition to molecular diagnostics after testing 534 specimens using Vero cell culture alone for virus isolation. Following an initial validation study, we determined that both RT-PCR and our cell culture diagnostics were equally able to detect WNV in crow brains. All 59 specimens tested by RT-PCR and cell culture were positive using both techniques. Following this validation study, we went on to test 1096 specimens using both methods at different times of the week to take advantage of the inherent qualities of each technique. For example, specimens received early in the week (i.e., Monday through Wednesday) were tested by RT-PCR and confirmed test results reported by the end of the week. Specimens received later in the week (i.e., Thursday through Saturday) were routinely inoculated into cell culture. Given the longer turnaround time of culture diagnostics (3–5 days for a positive), positive cultures exhibited a cytopathic effect within 3 to 5 days and could be confirmed via immunofluoresent assay (IFA) early the following week. Using this algorithm, we screened 564 specimens by RT-PCR (432 WNV positives) and 532 by cell culture (431 WNV positives). All WNV RT-PCR negative specimens were routinely inoculated into cell culture. Of the 132 WNV RT-PCR negatives, 16 yielded viable WNV in culture.

Aside from the implementation of RT-PCR, we also made a number of other changes to our protocol that had considerable effects on cost and turnaround time. Some examples of these cost- and timesaving cutbacks include: glass-bead vortexing for tissue preparation (instead of a mortar and pestle), using a 1% (w/v) suspension of brain for direct inoculation (instead of multiple dilutions), and using 25 µl RT-PCR reactions (instead of 50 µL). In total, these changes had a profound effect on our throughput, turnaround times, and specimen costs. For example, in August, 49% of WNV confirmed positive tests were reported out in five days or less; in October, that percentage jumped to 81. Similarly, whereas the cost of a confirmed positive specimen in July was $15, the cost in October was reduced to $4. Similar savings are also evident in our culture diagnostics ($10 initial cost vs. $3 for a confirmed positive cell culture).

Based on our experiences in 2000, we enter this season in a state of preparedness for the high-throughput screening of avian tissues. With the addition of real-time RT-PCR as a diagnostic tool, we look to screen avian brains for the presence of WNV, while still relying on virus isolation in times of low positivity, as well as additional follow-up studies. Together with limitations on the numbers of birds tested from any given town, we aim to employ these methodologies to gain a better understanding of the avian-borne distribution of WNV in CT, especially in the regions of the state where WNV was not as common.

REFERENCE

1. BECKWITH, W., S. SIRPENSKI, R.A. FRENCH, *et al.* Isolation of eastern equine encephalitis virus and West Nile virus from cows during increased arbovirus surveillance in Connecticut, 2000. Am. J. Trop. Med. Hyg. In press.

Experimental Infection of Horses with West Nile Virus and Their Potential to Infect Mosquitoes and Serve as Amplifying Hosts

M. L. BUNNING,[a,b] R. A. BOWEN,[c] B. CROPP,[b] K. SULLIVAN,[b] B. DAVIS,[b] N. KOMAR,[b] M. GODSEY,[b] D. BAKER,[c] D. HETTLER,[b] D. HOLMES,[b] AND C. J. MITCHELL[b]

[a]*Epidemiology Program Office, Centers for Disease Control and Prevention (CDC), Public Health Service (PHS), United States Department of Health and Human Services (DHHS), Atlanta, Georgia 30333, USA*

[b]*Division of Vector-Borne Infectious Diseases, National Center for Infectious Diseases (NCID), Centers for Disease Control and Prevention (CDC), Fort Collins, Colorado 80522-2089, USA*

[c]*Department of Physiology, Colorado State University, Fort Collins, Colorado 80522, USA*

KEYWORDS: West Nile virus; horses

West Nile virus (WNV) was responsible for outbreaks of encephalomyelitis in humans and horses in southeastern New York during 1999. Continuing widespread virus activity in the northeastern United States during 2000 suggests that WNV has become endemic. Historically, infections were thought to result in mild clinical disease or inapparent infections in equids, with only occasional cases resulting in severe disease. Unusually high morbidity and mortality rates in a cluster of equine cases in eastern Suffolk County, New York, during the 1999 epizootic indicated otherwise. These observations raised the question of whether horses might be serving as amplifying hosts for WNV, thereby exacerbating public health and veterinary problems. A total of 12 random-bred, varying aged horses were infected with WNV. Horses were infected via the bites of infected *Aedes albopictus* mosquitoes. Half of the horses were infected with a viral isolate from the brain of a horse (BC787) and the remaining animals were infected with an isolate from a crow brain (NY99-6625), both NY99 isolates. On days 3, 4, and 5 postinfection, uninfected female *Ae. albopictus* were fed on eight of the infected horses. All 12 horses became infected with WNV after being bitten by infected mosquitoes and there was 1 case of clinical encephalomyelitis; all survivors developed neutralizing (Nt) antibody. In the first trial, Nt anti-

Address for correspondence: M.L. Bunning, Division of Vector-Borne Infectious Diseases, Centers for Disease Control and Prevention, P.O. Box 2087, Fort Collins, CO 80522.Voice: 970-266-3565; fax: 970-221-6476.
zyd7@cdc.gov

body titers reached ≥1:320, 1:20, 1:160, and 1:80 for horses 1 to 4, respectively. In the second trial, the seven horses with subclinical infections developed Nt antibody titers that were ≥1:10 between days 7 and 11 postinfection. Peak titers in six horses were reached between days 9 and 13 following infection. The highest viremia in horses fed upon by the recipient mosquitoes was approximately 460 Vero cell PFUs/mL. All mosquitoes that fed upon viremic horses were tested and all were negative for the presence of virus. This work supports the conclusions that horses infected with the NY99 strain of WNV develop viremias of low magnitude and short duration and that infected horses are unlikely to serve as important amplifying hosts for WNV in nature.

Department of Defense West Nile Virus Surveillance

C. E. CANNON,[a] J. A. PAVLIN,[b] M. F. VAETH,[c] G. V. LUDWIG,[d] J. V. WRITER,[b] B. B. PAGAC,[a] M. B. GOLDENBAUM,[e] AND P. W. KELLEY[b]

[a]U.S. Army Center for Health Promotion and Preventive Medicine–North (CHPPM–N), Fort Meade, Maryland 20755, USA

[b]Department of Defence Global Emerging Infections System (DoD–GEIS), Silver Spring, Maryland 20910, USA

[c]Walter Reed Army Medical Center (WRAMC), Washington, D.C. 20307, USA

[d]U.S. Army Medical Research Institute of Infectious Diseases (USAMRIID), Fort Detrick, Maryland 21702, USA

[e]Walter Reed Army Institute of Research (WRAIR), Silver Spring, Maryland 20910, USA

After the 1999 West Nile encephalitis outbreak in the New York City metropolitan area it was recognized that spread beyond this region was likely and that surveillance efforts to track and characterize the emerging infection were needed. The Department of Defense (DoD) has many military installations in areas potentially at high risk for the emergence of the West Nile virus. As part of the broad national response to the potential spread of West Nile virus in 2000, the DoD performed surveillance of humans, mosquitoes, and birds and other animals during the transmission season. Forty-one military installations participated in the surveillance effort.

It was recognized that military installations could play a key role in regional surveillance. The DoD's larger installations have abundant mosquito, avian, and mammalian populations. Many of these large installations do routine mosquito trapping and identification. The DoD also has the laboratory capabilities to identify mosquito species; to collect and process avian, mammalian, and human specimens; and to determine the presence of WNV in specimens, including humans. The military health care system has a large active-duty, beneficiary and retiree population on the East and Gulf Coasts. Information collected from these medical facilities could play a role in defining the epidemiology in the active force and across the full spectrum of beneficiaries (i.e., spouses, children, and retirees).

The military's public health infrastructure can be analogous to a state's. Each installation could be considered to operate as a city or county. The regional Preventive Medicine Service acts as a de facto state health department. Supporting entomological, veterinary, and laboratory activities are available.

In response to the WNV threat, Department of Defense (DoD) Health Affairs and the U.S. Army's North Atlantic Regional Medical Command (NARMC) instituted a

Address for correspondence: James V. Writer, USDA-APHIS, 4700 River Rd., Unit 150, Riverdale, MD 20737. Voice: 301-734-7121; fax: 301-734-5992.
jwriter@aphis.usda.gov

TABLE 1. Results of the U.S. Department of Defense's West Nile virus mosquito, dead bird and mammal, and human surveillance activities in 2000

Species	Collection Dates	No. Tested	No. Positives	Remarks
Mosquitoes	5 Jun–7 Nov	2806 pools	1 pool	Ft. Hamilton, NY[a]
Birds/mammals	Jun–Nov	Unknown	5 (birds)	West Point, NY (4)[b] Ft. Hamilton, NY (1)[c]
Humans	Jun–Oct	18	0[d]	See note[e]

[a]1 pool of 3 *Culex pipiens* collected in a gravid trap on 23 August.
[b]1 house sparrow (submitted on 31 August), 2 cedar waxwings (submitted on 28 August), and 1 ruby-throated hummingbird (submitted on 8 September).
[c]1 crow (submitted on 25 September)
[d]All IgG-negative; 1 IgM-borderline-positive, but was negative on WNV neutralizing antibody assay.
[e]IgG and IgM antibodies; 4 from West Point, 10 from Washington, D.C., and 2 from Virginia.

surveillance program on 5 June 2000. The NARMC plan laid out specific surveillance, response and reporting functions for subordinate activities in the region.

Overall program management, development of clinical and practice guidelines, and coordination of human surveillance were performed by NARMC at the Walter Reed Army Medical Center (WRAMC), Washington, D.C. The Chief of the Preventive Medicine Service at WRAMC received weekly human surveillance reports that included the number of patients suspected of or confirmed as having WNV encephalitis and the test results received. The Naval Environmental Health Center reported on human surveillance of Navy beneficiaries weekly. If there had been confirmed positive test results they were would have been telephonically reported to the appropriate military, state, and federal agencies immediately.

The U.S. Army Medical Research Institute of Infectious Diseases (USAMRIID) tested human samples (using IgM and IgG ELISA and plaque-reduction neutralization test). Testing was also available from state public health laboratories.

The U.S. Army Center for Health Promotion and Preventive Medicine (CHPPM) through its subordinate command, the CHPPM–North (CHPPM–N) at Fort Meade, Maryland, provided mosquito surveillance program management and guidance. Mosquito pools were collected by the Preventive Medicine Services at installations in the NARMC and submitted to CHPPM–N for speciation and testing. The pools were tested for WNV by standard ELISA and PCR assays. Seventeen Army and three Air Force installations submitted pools. CHPPM–N reported results of NARMC mosquito trapping activities and WNV test results weekly to the senior Environmental Science Officer (ESO) at each post, to NARMC, and to the DoD's Global Emerging Infections System (DoD–GEIS). Positive results were to be reported to the submitting installation's Preventive Medicine Service, to the NARMC senior ESO, and to the appropriate state health department within 24 hours of confirmation. CHPPM–N also provided on-site technical support and assistance to installations in the North Atlantic region.

The U.S. Air Force activity at Brooks Air Force Base, Texas, collected and speciated mosquitoes, but did not test for WNV. The U.S. Navy coordinated activities with local and state health departments.

Animal and bird specimens collected at installations were processed through the U.S. Army North Atlantic Regional Veterinary Command (NARVC). WNV testing could be performed by the New York State, New York City, New Jersey, and U.S. Geological Survey laboratories. Veterinary Services in NARVC reported results of all analyses to the NARVC Commander, who provided a report of bird and animal surveillance to the Chief, Preventive Medicine Service and to WRAMC and DoD–GEIS monthly. Positive results were reported by the local veterinary clinics to the installation's Preventive Medicine Service.

These military agencies reported their test results to DoD–GEIS. The DoD–GEIS compiled a weekly report of surveillance efforts at all installations. The report was faxed to the CDC.

The results of the DoD's surveillance efforts are presented in TABLE 1.

Although costs were not tallied, the DoD, especially with regard to activities in the Army's North Atlantic region, expended significant resources to implement the program. There was no apparent human health impact on the military installations surveilled. Only installations in southern New York State reported WNV-positive tests (mosquitoes and birds). The reporting system for 2000 was cumbersome. In 2001 a more streamlined system is likely to be implemented. The DoD's WNV efforts did increase awareness and surveillance of all arthropod-borne encephalitides and led to increased surveillance and control of potential disease vectors.

[NOTE: The authors are solely responsible for the contents of this article. The contents do not necessarily reflect the policy of the Department of the Army, Department of Defense, or the United States Government.]

Sentinel Chickens as a Surveillance Tool for West Nile Virus in New York City, 2000

BRYAN CHERRY,[a] SUSAN C. TROCK,[b,c] AMY GLASER,[b] LAURA KRAMER,[d] GREGORY D. EBEL,[d] CARLA GLASER,[a] AND JAMES R. MILLER[a]

[a]New York City Department of Health, New York, New York 10013, USA

[b]Cornell University, Ithaca, New York, USA

[c]New York State Department of Agriculture and Markets, Albany, New York, USA

[d]Arboviral Research Laboratory, New York State Department of Health, Albany, New York, USA

KEYWORDS: West Nile virus; sentinel chicken; arboviral surveillance

INTRODUCTION

West Nile (WN) virus was first identified in the Western Hemisphere during an outbreak of encephalitis in New York City (NYC) in 1999. Prior to 1999, NYC had not had a locally acquired human arboviral infection since the 1800s (yellow fever), although eastern equine and St. Louis encephalitis have occurred in surrounding areas. There was also no existing surveillance system for arthropod-borne viruses and no citywide mosquito control program in NYC prior to 1999. The identification of this new agent prompted the NYC Department of Health to develop surveillance and control programs to prevent future outbreaks of WN and other arboviral diseases. Among the systems implemented for the 2000 mosquito season were sentinel chicken flocks. Experimental evidence has shown that domestic chickens are readily infected with isolates of NY-99 WN virus, shed virus for only a brief period of time, and experience a viremia high enough to infect mosquitoes for only about two days.[1,2] The Centers for Disease Control and Prevention supported the use of sentinel chickens as a surveillance tool for the local presence and transmission of WN virus during the 2000 mosquito season.[1]

METHODS

Chicken coops were established at a convenience sample of live poultry markets in four boroughs of New York City (flocks 1–13, FIG. 1). An existing chicken flock in a Staten Island (SI) park was also used for this surveillance program (flock 14). Chickens were placed at sites 1–13 on 5/3/00. Flocks 1–13 were established and maintained with an average of seven birds per flock (range: 1–16). Additional chick-

Address for correspondence: Bryan Cherry, NYC Department of Health, 125 Worth Street, Box 22-A, New York, NY 10013. Voice: 212-295-5673; fax: 212-295-5421.
bcherry@health.nyc.gov

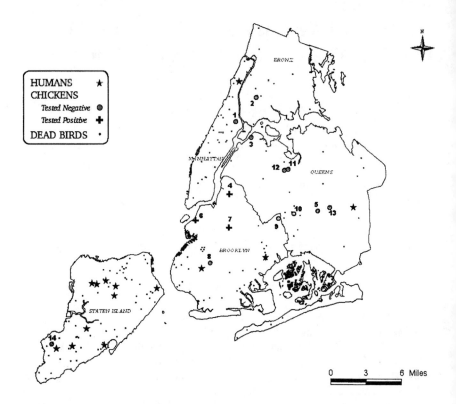

FIGURE 1. NYC map showing placement of sentinel chicken flocks relative to human WN cases and WN-positive dead birds.

ens were added to replace any that died. Flock 14 contained 23 chickens, of which 8 were used for this study.

Blood serum samples from flocks 1–13 were tested at the Veterinary Diagnostic Laboratory at Cornell University via indirect immunofluorescent antibody (IFA) tests for IgM and IgG. Confirmatory testing of positive or suspect samples was done using serum neutralization tests at the National Veterinary Services Laboratory. Blood samples from flock 14 were collected using a "finger prick" method on the comb. Samples were collected on filter paper strips and air-dried prior to shipment to the Arboviral Research Laboratory of the New York State Department of Health. Screening tests there were done using indirect ELISA followed by confirmatory indirect IFA. Positive results were reported directly to staff of the NYC Department of Health.

RESULTS

Blood samples were collected weekly from flocks 1–13 between 5/3/00 and 11/3/00. Birds from flock 14 were tested weekly from 6/20/00 through 8/16/00.

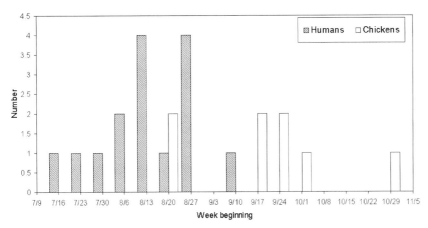

FIGURE 2. Epidemic curve of WN human cases and infected sentinel chickens in 2000.

FIGURE 1 shows the location of each flock on a map of NYC, with the dates that WN infection was first recognized in each flock that seroconverted. Overall, 8 chickens developed detectable antibody to WN virus at three sites in Brooklyn. FIGURE 2 shows the epidemic curve of human cases and seropositive chickens. The first birds seroconverted on 8/23/00 in flock 6, although final confirmation of these results was obtained on 9/23/00. One bird in each of flocks 4 and 7 seroconverted on 9/20/00. Two more birds from flock 7 seroconverted on 9/29/00, and two more birds from flock 4 seroconverted on 10/6/00 and 11/3/00. The nearest human case to a WN-positive sentinel flock was in southwestern Brooklyn, approximately 3 miles from flock 6, with an onset date of 8/15/00. Only five human WN cases occurred anywhere in NYC after infection was first identified in sentinel chickens. All 14 human cases had onset dates prior to our first confirmation of infection in chickens (9/23/00). Six of the 8 chickens became infected after the onset date of the last human WN case.

DISCUSSION

As used by NYC in 2000, sentinel chicken flocks did not provide an early warning for the presence or local transmission of WN virus. Dead bird and mosquito surveillance for WN virus provided a much more sensitive system for detection of virus before the occurrence of human infection. Sentinel chicken infection with WN virus occurred too late to prompt any adult mosquito control activities (adulticide spraying).

Curiously, the three WN virus–positive chicken flocks were located in an area where very few positive dead birds were found, yet nearly all of the other sentinel flocks were surrounded by WN viral activity in birds (FIG. 1). Flock 14, in particular, was surrounded by virus in birds and humans, as well as in mosquito pools (data not shown). All 23 chickens in flock 14 were retested on 4/10/01, and 1 was positive for

WN antibody. This positive chicken was one that had been tested during the 2000 WN season and was negative for WN antibody at its last testing on 8/16/00.

In order to determine the usefulness of sentinel bird surveillance programs for WN virus, further research is warranted. Field studies that integrate sentinel flock, mosquito, and dead bird testing with evaluation of flock location and sentinel species selection are necessary to define the most effective means of implementing sentinel surveillance for WN virus.

ACKNOWLEDGMENTS

We would like to thank Annette Gonzalez and Michelle Gaeta from the New York State Department of Agriculture and Markets for their tremendous assistance in collecting blood samples from sentinel chickens and maintaining the flocks, and Chris Cuschieri and his staff at Clay Pit Ponds State Park Preserve for their assistance with the sentinel chickens on Staten Island. We extend special thanks to Susan Resnick at the NYC Department of Health for her mapping expertise.

REFERENCES

1. CDC. 1999 (November 8). Epidemic/epizootic West Nile virus in the United States: guidelines for surveillance, prevention, and control. Fort Collins, CO.
2. SCHMITT, B., B. PANIGRAHY, J.C. PEDERSEN, et al. 2000 (January 19–21). Pathogenicity of West Nile virus in chickens. Presented at the WN Virus Action Workshop, Tarrytown, NY.

West Nile Virus Human Surveillance in Nassau County, New York: 1999–2000

ABBY J. GREENBERG AND MARGARET SHERMAN

Nassau County Department of Health, 240 Old Country Road, Mineola, New York 11501, USA

KEYWORDS: West Nile virus; disease surveillance; meningitis; encephalitis; meningoencephalitis; Nassau County, NY, 1999–2000; human disease; suspect disease; case investigation; disease reporting; public health; epidemiology

In September 1999, following initial notification by the New York City Department of Health of a cluster of meningoencephalitis cases in Queens, NY, the Nassau County Department of Health initiated heightened surveillance for potential cases of viral encephalitis and viral meningitis, in order to identify cases of what ultimately would be identified as West Nile virus encephalitis.[1–4] Components of the system included sending periodic informational letters by mailings and fax alerts to key personnel in all 13 Nassau County hospitals (to the chief executive officers, emergency room directors, infection control practitioners, and chairpersons of the Departments of Medicine, Pediatrics, Infectious Diseases, and Neurology) and to local medical societies; contacting hospital infection control practitioners on a weekly basis to identify potential cases; providing formal professional education at various professional meetings; and providing information on all aspects of human surveillance, disease transmission, and prevention to health-care providers through telephone and in-person consultations. In 1999, department staff collected all acute and convalescent laboratory specimens from hospitals and physicians' offices and mailed the specimens to the New York State Department of Health Laboratory. When necessary, department staff obtained convalescent specimens directly from patients. In 2000, hospitals and health-care providers were instructed to send laboratory specimens directly to the New York State Department of Health Laboratory.

The contents of the surveillance information provided periodically to health-care professionals included the following components: the most current information about the West Nile virus (WNV) outbreak; a request for physicians to report suspect cases of aseptic meningitis, encephalitis, meningoencephalitis; the clinical case definition of WNV meningoencephalitis; clinical case reporting forms; the availability of laboratory testing; instructions regarding specimen submission; and the availability of 24-h public health medical consultation. The clinical case definition used for public health surveillance for WNV disease was any adult or pediatric patient with aseptic meningitis or encephalitis characterized by at least two of four criteria: fever >100°F; cerebrospinal fluid pleocytosis; altered mental status; muscle weakness.[3]

Address for correspondence: Margaret Sherman, Nassau County Department of Health, 240 Old Country Road, Mineola, NY 11501. Voice: 516-571-3436; fax: 516-571-1537. msherman@health.co.nassau.ny.us

WNV meningoencephalitis human surveillance in Nassau County for the two-year period 1999–2000 resulted in 173 suspect reports. Information obtained for suspect WNV case reports consisted of patient demographics, clinical symptoms, laboratory tests, antiviral treatment, and risk factors such as travel information and animal or arthropod exposure. The majority (97%) of suspect reports were not confirmed cases (167/173). In 1999, there were 70 suspect case reports (incidence of 5.2/100,000 residents) and 6 confirmed cases with one death (17% mortality); the incidence of confirmed cases was 0.4/100,000. In 2000, there were 103 reports of suspect cases for an incidence of 7.7/100,000 and no confirmed cases (FIG. 1).

Confirmed cases and non-cases for the two-year period 1999–2000 were analyzed and compared with respect to the presence or absence of the four specific criteria for the case definition of WNV meningoencephalitis (fever, cerebrospinal fluid pleocytosis, altered mental status, and muscle weakness) and for the number of criteria present in each case report. Cases and non-cases were compared with respect to age range, median age, age ≥60 years, gender, and the results of initial serum antibody tests obtained soon after the onset of clinical symptoms of disease. Three of 6 confirmed cases and 7 of 167 non-cases met all four case criteria (odds ratio [OR] 14.2); 4 of 6 cases and 47 of 167 non-cases met at least three case criteria (OR 5.1). Four of the 6 confirmed cases and 63 of the 167 non-cases had altered mental status (OR 2.7); 3 of the 6 cases and 53 of the non-cases had muscle weakness (OR 2.2). The confirmed cases ranged in age from 58 to 83 years while the non-cases ranged in age from ≤1 to 94 years; the median age for confirmed cases was 70.5 and for non-cases was 47.0; 83% (5/6) confirmed cases were ≥60 years while 29% (48/167) non-cases were ≥60 years old (OR 12.4); 4 of 6 confirmed cases were females and 78 of 167 non-cases were females (OR 2.3). The factors most likely to predict a confirmed case were the presence of all four clinical criteria and age ≥60 years.

All three confirmed cases that had serum antibody tests obtained during the acute phase had positive test results. The remaining three confirmed cases had laboratory testing obtained only during the convalescent phase. Convalescent serum antibody test results were available for only 63% (109) of the 173 suspect cases reported in the two-year surveillance period; 3% (6) were confirmed cases of West Nile virus meningoencephalitis; 2% (2) had confirmed nonspecific antibody test results; 58% (101) were confirmed negative by convalescent serum antibody testing; 3% (5) of the suspect cases were not tested; 27% (46) with negative initial tests were not available for final testing despite extensive outreach efforts; and 9% (15) were diagnosed with other meningoencephalitic diseases (TABLE 1).

The intensive surveillance for WNV meningoencephalitis was conducted for a two-year period to determine the incidence of this newly emerging infection and to measure the effects of an intensive public health program directed at eliminating the vectors of WNV disease and preventing human illness. This intensive surveillance is appropriate and important for identifying the incidence and epidemiology of a new disease. However, WNV disease clinical criteria lack sufficient specificity and the ratio of confirmed to suspect cases is very low so that surveillance becomes very laborious, time consuming, and unproductive. Continued intensive surveillance for suspect WNV disease deflects from the surveillance and control of other communicable diseases. After a baseline incidence for WNV disease has been established and effective prevention and control programs have been implemented, then on-going surveillance and reporting for WNV disease should be initiated only following re-

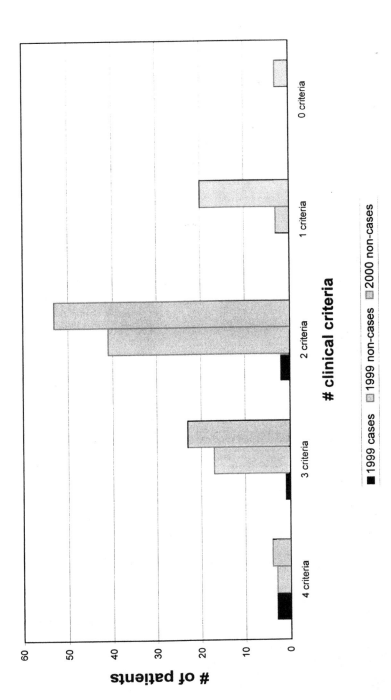

FIGURE 1.

TABLE 1. 1999–2000 Cohort of suspect cases (N=173)

Factor	Cases (N)	Non-cases (N)	Odds ratio for disease
WNV chacteristics			
Fever	6	139	
(+) Cerebrospinal fluid	6	113	
Altered mental state	4	63	2.7
Muscle weakness	3	53	2.2
WNV disease criteria met			
All four	3	7	14.2
At least three	4	47	5.1
At least two	6	141	
At least one	6	164	
None		3	
Females	4	78	2.3
Males	2	89	0.4
Age ≥ 60 years	5	48	12.4
Age range (years)	58–83	<1–94	
Median age	70.5	47	
Results			
Acute test positive	3	0	
nonspecific	0	2	
convalescent test positive	6	0	
negative	0	101	
nonspecific	0	2	
Not tested	0	5	
Lost to follow-up	0	46	
Other diagnosis	0	15	

ports of laboratory-confirmed cases. In order to obtain an accurate incidence of WNV, health-care providers will need to consider WNV in their differential diagnosis of aseptic meningitis and encephalitis and order the appropriate diagnostic tests.

REFERENCES

1. CENTERS FOR DISEASE CONTROL AND PREVENTION. 1999. Outbreak of West Nile–like viral encephalitis—New York, 1999. Morb. Mortal. Wkly. Rep. **48:** 845–849.
2. ASNIS, D.S. *et al.* 2000. The West Nile virus outbreak of 1999 in New York: the Flushing Hospital experience. Clin. Infect. Dis. **30:** 413–418.
3. CENTERS FOR DISEASE CONTROL AND PREVENTION. 1999. Update: West Nile–like viral encephalitis—New York, 1999. Morb. Mortal. Wkly. Rep. **48:** 890–892.
4. CENTERS FOR DISEASE CONTROL AND PREVENTION. 1999. Update: West Nile–like viral encephalitis—New York, 1999. Morb. Mortal. Wkly. Rep. **48:** 944–946, 955.

West Nile Virus Laboratory Surveillance Program

Cost and Time Analysis

ELIZABETH B. KAUFFMAN, KRISTEN A. BERNARD, SUSAN A. JONES,
JOSEPH MAFFEI, KIET NGO, AND LAURA D. KRAMER

Arbovirus Research Laboratory, Wadsworth Center,
New York State Department of Health, Albany, New York 12159, USA

KEYWORDS: West Nile virus; cost analysis; time analysis

The expense and time commitment involved in establishing and maintaining a West Nile virus (WNV) laboratory testing program has been reviewed. The information is based on the experience of the Arbovirus Laboratory of Wadsworth Center, where testing of more than 10,000 mosquito pools and 6000 bird and mammal specimens took place during the 2000 surveillance season.

The backbone of the mosquito testing program was the initial screening of all specimens by real-time RT-PCR using the ABI Prism 7700 Sequence Detector (Taq-Man, Applied Biosystems) with a sensitive WNV-specific primer/probe set.[1,2] Pools of 10–50 mosquitoes were homogenized using a Spex Mill (Spex Certiprep, Rahway, NJ, $4208), after which RNA was extracted using Rneasy kits (Qiagen) at a cost of $3.60 per sample. The cost of each real-time RT-PCR assay, after the initial investment of $100,000 for the instrument, was $3.60 per sample. If the initial test was negative, that sample was declared negative, and no further testing was done. Confirmatory TaqMan assays ($3.60 per sample), using a second WNV primer/probe set, were performed on samples that tested positive or borderline positive.[2] Those samples that were positive with both primer/probe sets were considered confirmed positives. Samples with ambiguous results (e.g., positive with one TaqMan primer/probe set and negative or borderline with the other primer/probe set) were tested further by standard RT-PCR with primers defining other regions of the WNV genome. If one TaqMan assay and one standard RT-PCR were positive, the sample was declared a confirmed positive. Virus isolation was attempted for select speci-

Address for correspondence: Elizabeth Kauffman, New York State Department of Health, Arbovirus Laboratory, Griffin Lab, 5688 State Farm Road, Slingerlands, NY 12159. Voice: 518-869-4525; fax: 518-869-4530.

ebk01@health.state,ny.us

TABLE 1. Assay costs and time commitment

	Description	Cost per sample[a]	Person Hours
Database	Accession Record results Reports		2.5 h per 50 samples
Preparation of RNA	Excise tissue (birds and mammals) Homogenize tissue Extract RNA	$3.75 (mosquitoes) $4.00 (birds, mam- mals)	6 h per 50 samples
Real-time RT-PCR (TaqMan)	Assay 84 samples + 12 controls per plate	$3.60	4 h per 84 samples
Virus Isolation	Plate on Vero or C6- 36 Observe for CPE Identify virus by IFA	$7.50	5 h per 10 samples
NASBA	Amplify RNA Detect RNA	$17.60	6 h per 45 samples

[a]These costs are for specific supplies only and do not reflect costs for personnel or general laboratory supplies and services, such as gloves, Kimwipes, underpads, disinfectant, and autoclaving.

mens (2900 in year 2000) at a cost of $1.50 per assay. Cost and time commitment estimates for each phase of testing is summarized in TABLE 1. TABLE 2 summarizes the cost and time required for testing by the arbovirus lab during the 2000 surveillance season. During 2000 a total of 10,571 mosquito pools were tested at a cost of more than $87,000. Testing required at least 3417 person hours, which amounted to 171 person hours per week for the 20-week testing period (TABLE 2). Most of the samples (9737) required only one TaqMan assay, but 383 samples, required two TaqMan assays, and 451 specimens required three or more assays.

The testing program for birds and mammals was similar to mosquitoes. TaqMan assays were used to screen one tissue (usually kidney) for each bird and four tissues per mammal, at a cost of $4.00 per tissue for tissue excision, homogenization, and RNA purification and $3.60 for each TaqMan assay. TaqMan confirmatory tests were performed as for mosquitoes. In addition, immunofluorescent assays on frozen sections were used as confirmatory tests for selected bird tissues, at a cost of $7.50 per specimen. During the 2000 surveillance season 3711 birds and 78 mammals were tested for a cost of more than $54,000 (TABLE 2). The time commitment for bird and mammal testing amounted to more than 247 person hours per week for the 20-week period.

For the 2001 surveillance season, our lab will continue to use TaqMan for screening and confirmatory tests. For specimens with equivocal TaqMan results, further tests will be performed using NASBA (Nucleic Acid Sequence-Based Amplification).[3] The cost of the instrument used for this assay (NucliSens Reader System, Organon Teknika, Durham, NC) is $20,000, and the cost of the assay using NASBA amplification and detection reagents from Organon Teknika is approximately $13.50 per sample.

TABLE 2. Cost and time estimates for 2000 season (20 weeks)

	Number of specimens	Cost per specimen	Total cost	Total person hours
Mosquitoes: 10,571 Pools				
One TaqMan assay (negatives)	9737	$7.35	$71,567	1655
Two TaqMan assays	383	$10.95	$4194	84
Three or more Taq-Man assays	451	≥$14.55	≥ $6562	≥122
Standard RT-PCR	212	$1.50	$318	106
Virus isolation	2900	$1.50	$4350	1450
			≥$86,991	≥3417
				Person hours per week ≥171
Birds: 3711 specimens				
One TaqMan assay (negatives)	1104	$7.60	$8390	188
Two TaqMan assays	2323	$11.20	$26,017	511
Three or more TaqMan assays	284	≥$14.80	≥$4203	≥77
Standard RT-PCR	691	$1.50	$1037	3455
Virus isolation	825	$5.00	$4125	413
IFA	100	$7.50	$750	50
			≥$44,522	≥4694
				Person hours per week ≥235
Mammals: 78 specimens (tested 4 tissues each)				
One TaqMan assay (negatives)	45	$30.40	$1368	30
Two TaqMan assays	70	$44.80	$3136	66
Three or more Taq-Man assays	38	≥$59.20	≥$2250	≥41
Standard RT-PCR	16	$1.50	$24	32
Virus isolation	80	$5.00	$400	40
IFA	41	$7.50	$3075	21
			≥$9953	≥230
				Person hours per week ≥12

[a]These costs are for specific supplies only and do not reflect costs for personnel or general laboratory supplies and services, such as gloves, Kimwipes, underpads, disinfectant, and autoclaving.

REFERENCES

1. LANCIOTTI, R.S., A.J. KERST, R.S. NASCI, *et al.* 2000. Rapid detection of West Nile virus from human clinical specimens, field-collected mosquitoes, and avian samples by a TaqMan reverse transcriptase-PCR assay. J. Clin. Microbiol. **38:** 4066–4071.
2. SHI, P.Y., E.B. KAUFFMAN, P. RENA, *et al.* 2001. High throughput detection of West Nile virus RNA. J. Clin. Microbiol. **39:** 1264–1271.
3. LANCIOTTI, R.S., A.J. KERST & B.C. ALLEN. 2000. Development of NASBA based assay for the rapid detection of West Nile virus. Am. J. Trop. Med. Hyg. (Suppl.) **62:** 340.

Sumithrin®: From Inception to Integration within West Nile Virus Programs

F. KRENICK, W. JANY, AND J. L. CLARKE III

Clarke Mosquito Control, Roselle, Illinois 60172, USA

KEYWORDS: West Nile virus; Sumithrin; Anvil

BACKGROUND

Synthetic pyrethroids were developed in the 1950s. This class of insecticide is derived from pyrethrins, naturally occurring chemicals found in the chrysanthemum flower. Pyrethroids act on the peripheral and central nervous systems of insects by interfering with sodium channels in nerve axons. D-Phenothrin (Sumithrin®) was first synthesized in 1969 and has been in use for mosquito control since 1977. Sumithrin is the active ingredient in Anvil®. Sumithrin is metabolized in mammals and has no tendency to accumulate in tissues; it does not bioaccumulate in the environment.[1]

Animal studies of Sumithrin indicate that the chemical is not a carcinogen or teratogen; it does not cause gene mutation, chromosomal aberration, or unscheduled DNA synthesis.[1] The EPA has noted the following with respect to the approved uses of Sumithrin: "Pyrethroids used in mosquito-control programs do not pose unreasonable risk to wildlife or the environment."[2]

Anvil has been used to control mosquitoes since 1996. Forty-three caged and natural population studies were performed against many species of mosquitoes under diverse operational conditions. These trials proved Anvil to be effective against over 25 species including the following potential West Nile virus vectors at 95–100% effectiveness: *Culex pipiens, Culex restuans, Culex salinarius, Aedes vexans, Ochlerotatus albopictus, Ochlerotatus canadensis,* and *Psorophora ferox.*

In the aftermath of Hurricane Floyd in 1999, Anvil was applied aerially to over 2.5 million acres in North and South Carolina, which included 20 counties in North Carolina. Results revealed an average 80% reduction in mosquito populations in treated areas. Species most affected were *Ochlerotatus atlanticus, Ochlerotatus canadensis,* and *Psorophora ferox.*[3]

METHODS

In response to signs of West Nile virus, Staten Island, New York underwent spraying with Anvil 10+10 at a rate of 0.0036 lbs active ingredient/acre. Operational

Address for correspondence: Fran Krenick, Clarke Mosquito Control, 159 N. Garden Avenue, Roselle, IL 60172. Voice: 1-800-323-5727; fax: 630-894-1774.
frankrenick@clarkemosquito.com

caged trials and a natural population study were conducted. Weather parameters were recorded during all trials by an on-site weather station. Particle size (MMD), temperature, and wind were noted.

The caged trials were conducted in operational settings during normal applications. A standard protocol was applied. All equipment was calibrated and characterized prior to application. Either aerial or ground spraying was performed and mosquito knockdown/mortality was recorded at 2, 12, and 24 hours. Test mosquitoes were collected via CO_2-baited light traps from treatment areas in addition to *Culex pipiens* that were laboratory reared. Control (untreated) mosquitoes were collected and handled identically to treated mosquitoes.

The natural population study was conducted over a period of four days. Three test sites and two control sites were selected on Staten Island and at the Flushing airport, respectively. The total number of mosquitoes collected pre- and posttreatment were recorded. Aerial spraying (treatment) was performed on day 3 at dusk.

RESULTS

These trials were conducted during aerial and ground adult mosquito control activities in an attempt to control West Nile virus on Staten Island, NY. Results from aerial caged trials reveal a 97–99% mortality 24 h posttreatment (FIG. 1). Results from the ground caged trial recorded up to 99% knockdown/mortality in cages placed 150′ and 300′ from the spray truck (FIG. 2). Results from the aerial natural population study indicate significant reductions in mosquito populations at the three treatment sites, while the two control sites experienced increases in mosquito populations.

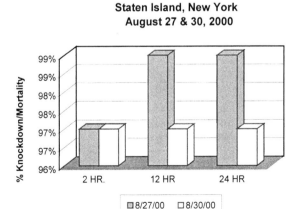

**Aerial Anvil 10+10 Caged Trials
Staten Island, New York
August 27 & 30, 2000**

FIGURE 1. Aerial caged trials.

Anvil 10+10 Ground ULV Operational Field Trial
September 17,2000
Staten Island, New York

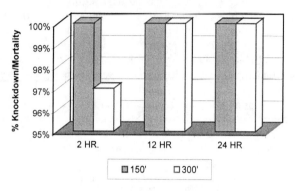

FIGURE 2. Ground caged field trial.

CONCLUSIONS

Sumithrin is a pyrethroid insecticide determined to be of negligible mammalian toxicity. Trials performed with Anvil since its introduction to mosquito control use in 1996 proved Sumithrin's effectiveness against over 25 mosquito species. The trials summarized in this study substantiate Sumithrin's significant effectiveness toward mosquito control. Anvil is another important weapon in the control of West Nile virus vectors.

REFERENCES

1. WHO. 1990. Environmental Health Criteria 96. Geneva.
2. EPA periodical. Synthetic Pyrethroids for Mosquito Control. Doc. #735-F-00-004. May 2000. p. 3.
3. FLORIDA MOSQUITO CONTROL ASSOCIATION. Wing beats. Vol. **11**(2). Aug. 2000. p. 4.

Use of an Arboviral Immunofluorescent Assay in Screening for West Nile Virus

KAREN E. KULAS, VALERIE L. DEMAREST, CAROL S. FRANCHELL, AND SUSAN J. WONG

New York State Department of Health, Wadsworth Center, David Axelrod Institute for Public Health, Diagnostic Immunology Laboratory, Albany, New York 12208, USA

KEYWORDS: arbovirus; West Nile virus; immunofluorescent assay; 1999 West Nile outbreak, metropolitan New York City region; St. Louis encephalitis

In 1999, the New York State Department of Health, Wadsworth Center, Diagnostic Immunology Laboratory responded to the public health outbreak of possible viral encephalitis in Queens, New York. Specimens were submitted from the metropolitan New York City region and neighboring counties, including those in the mid-Hudson region.

The laboratory provided arboviral antibody testing from the symptomatic population. Specimens ($n = 191$) from 147 patients were submitted for serological testing during the outbreak period. Of those specimens submitted, 160 specimens were tested from 135 patients (TABLE 1, section 4). The testing protocol used a commercially manufactured immunofluorescent assay (MRL Diagnostics, Cypress, CA), which included St. Louis, western equine, eastern equine, and California group (LaCrosse strain) encephalitis virus in tissue culture.

METHODS

The MRL Diagnostics ARBOVIRUS IFA IgG®, Catalog No. IF0300G, Cypress, CA uses Vero cells virally infected with EEE, New Jersey 60 strain; WEE, Fleming strain; SLE, TBH-28 strain; and CE, LaCrosse strain, group viruses. The indirect-immunofluorescent antibody (IFA) assay is a two-stage (sandwich) procedure. Diluted patient sera is added to slide wells in contact with the substrate and incubated. Following incubation, the slide is washed in phosphate-buffered saline, which removes unbound serum antibodies. Each well is overlaid with fluorescein-labeled antibody to IgG. The slide is incubated, allowing antigen-antibody complexes to react with the fluorescein-labeled anti-IgG. After the slide is washed, dried, and mounted, it is examined using fluorescent microscopy. Positive reactions appear as cells ex-

Address for correspondence: Karen E. Kulas, NYS Department of Health, Wadsworth Center, David Axelrod Institute for Public Health, Diagnostic Immunology Laboratory, Room 3001, 120 New Scotland Ave., Albany, NY 12208. Voice: 518-474-8566; fax: 518-486-7971.
kek01@health.state.ny.us

TABLE 1. Analysis of SLE IFA results from New York State Department of Health, Wadsworth Center, Diagnostic Immunology

Section 1	$(n = 32^a)$
SLE IgG positive = 28/32	SLE IgM positive = 8/32
negative = 2/32	negative = 17/32
nonspecific = 2/32	nonspecific = 2/32
Section 2	$(n = 3^b)$
SLE IgG positive = 3/3	SLE IgM positive = 1/3
negative = 0/3	negative = 2/3
nonspecific = 0/3	nonspecific = 0/3
Section 3	$(n = 100^c)$
SLE IgG positive = 16/100	SLE IgM positive = 1/100
negative = 82/100	negative = 99/100
Section 4	$(n = 135^d)$
SLE IgG positive = 47/135	SLE IgM positive = 10/135
negative = 86/135	negative = 118/135
nonspecific = 2/135	nonspecific = 2/13

[a]Subjects selected as those determined to be cases at CDC/VBDD. 5/32 specimens were not tested for SLE IgM.
[b]Subjects selected as probable cases at CDC/VBDD.
[c]Subjects selected as those determined to be noncases by either NYSDOH or CDC/VBDD.
[d]Subjects selected to represent the patient population submitted to the NYSDOH Diagnostic Immunology Laboratory for serological testing in response to the 1999 outbreak.

hibiting bright apple-green cytoplasmic fluorescence in 5–25% of the cells against a background of red negative control cells. Negative sera should exhibit negligible reactivity. Semiquantitative end-point titers are obtained by testing serial dilutions of positive specimens. Fluorescence is graded on a negative to 4+ scale. Nonspecific reactions are those in which all or a percentage of cells exhibit a weak cytoplasmic staining. If this staining is too intense to permit a confident reading, the test must be run by an alternate method or referred for further testing.

RESULTS AND CONCLUSION

The Center for Disease Control and Prevention, Division of Vector-Borne Infectious Diseases, Fort Collins, Colorado determined that 55 patients from the outbreak population were confirmed as cases of West Nile virus (WNV) infection, and that another six patients were probable WNV infected.[1] Our laboratory received specimens from 32 (TABLE 1, section 1) of the 55 confirmed cases and 3 (TABLE 1, section 2) of the 6 probable cases of WNV infection. Onset of symptoms of the confirmed cases occurred in late summer through early fall (FIG. 1). The analysis of our data regarding antibody reactivity to SLE virus indicates that the use of this surrogate

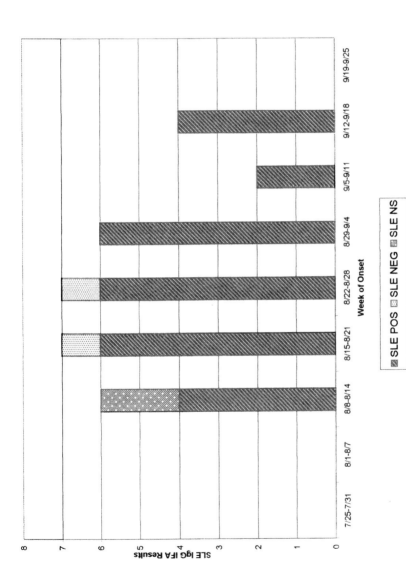

FIGURE 1. NYSDOH Diagnostic Immunology subset of SLE IgG results (*n* = 32).

marker led to the early detection of flavivirus involvement within the outbreak population. The SLE IFA findings presented on the 35 confirmed and probable WNV cases indicate the potential for use of the IFA test as preliminary evidence of flavivirus exposure. The presence of SLE IgG by IFA was noted in 87.5% of the selected population, whereas SLE IgM by IFA appeared in 25% (TABLE 1, sections 1 and 2). The CDC identified the causative agent as WNV.[2] The SLE virus, a group B flavivirus, shares structural homology and immunoreactivity with WNV.[3] Once the virus was identified as WNV, the CDC recommended IgM-capture ELISA and it was implemented in the laboratory. The specimens that reacted with SLE were retested using the MAC-ELISA and confirmed by CDC using plaque reduction neutralization testing (PRNT). In retrospect, the SLE IgM by IFA was less sensitive than the MAC-ELISA results.

Prior to the implementation of the MAC-ELISA, the IFA was the standard procedure in our laboratory for arboviral antibody testing. Immunofluorescent techniques are common to most clinical laboratory settings. Commercially prepared IFA procedures are cost effective, require minimal time, and technical training. The MRL Arbovirus IgG IFA that uses infected tissue culture cells, specifically, SLE, has proven to be a good preliminary surrogate antigen for the detection of WNV. This assay may be well suited for laboratories in which cost, time, and technical expertise may be prohibitory when considering incorporating an ELISA for arboviral detection.

ACKNOWLEDGMENTS

We thank Lance Kingsley and Reg Taylor, Diagnostic Immunology Laboratory, Wadsworth Center, New York State Department of Health, Albany, NY. Denise Martin, Robert Lanciotti, and John Roehrig, Division of Vector-Borne Infectious Diseases, Centers for Disease Control and Prevention, Fort Collins, CO. Iqbal Poshni, Bureau of Laboratories, New York City Department of Health, New York, NY. Marcelle Layton, Communicable Disease Program, New York City Department of Health, New York, NY.

REFERENCES

1. CDC. Update: Guidelines for surveillance, prevention, and control of West Nile virus infection—United States. 2000. Morb. Mortal. Wkly. Rep. **49**(2): 25P–28.
2. CDC. Update: West Nile virus Encephalitis—New York, 1999. 1999. Morb. Mortal. Wkly. Rep. **48**(41): 944–946, 955.
3. LANCIOTTI, R.S. et al. 1999. Origin of the West Nile virus responsible for an outbreak of encephalitis in the northeastern United States. Science **286**(5448): 2333–2337.

Biological Significance of Glycosylation of the Envelope Protein of Kunjin Virus

J. H. SCHERRET,[a,b] J. S. MACKENZIE,[a] A. A. KHROMYKH,[c] AND R. A. HALL[a]

[a]Department of Microbiology and Parasitology,
University of Queensland, St Lucia, QLD, 4072, Australia

[b]WHO Collaborating Center for Tropical Diseases and Department of Pathology,
University of Texas Medical Branch, Galveston, Texas 77555-0609, USA

[c]Sir Albert Sakzewski Virus Research Centre, Royal Children's Hospital,
Brisbane, QLD, 4029, Australia

KEYWORDS: West Nile virus; Kunjin virus; Australia

INTRODUCTION

Kunjin (KUN) virus, a subtype of West Nile (WN) virus, belongs to the Japanese encephalitis antigenic complex of the *Flavivirus* genus in the family Flaviviridae.[1] Kunjin virus is enzootic in northern Australia and possibly Papua New Guinea and is associated with occasional spread into southeastern Australia. *Culex annulirostris* mosquitoes are the major vector of KUN virus, while birds appear to act as the primary vertebrate host.[2]

The envelope (E) protein of most flaviviruses is glycosylated at a conserved site (residues 154–156) in the protein. A high proportion of KUN[3] and WN[4] virus isolates, however, lack glycosylation at this site. While several studies have shown that neuroinvasiveness and neurovirulence of the encephalitic flaviviruses are effected by specific amino acid substitutions within the E protein, the biological significance of glycosylation of the E protein remains unclear.

METHODS

Site-directed mutagenesis was performed on an infectious clone of KUN (FLSD),[5] which lacks the glycosylation motif (N-Y-T/S) in the E protein. By mutating the N-Y-F at position 154–156 in the E protein to N-Y-S, glycosylated mutant virus (156ser) was produced. To establish whether cell passage influenced the glycosylation status of these viruses, KUN virus was serially passaged 10 times through either Vero or C6/36 cells, digested with N-glycosidase F and analyzed by Western blot.

Address for correspondence: Jacqueline H. Scherret, Ph.D., WHO Collaborating Center for Tropical Diseases, Department of Pathology, University of Texas Medical Branch, 301 University Blvd., Galveston, TX 77555-0609. Voice: 409-772-2547; fax: 409-747-2415.
jhscherr@utmb.edu

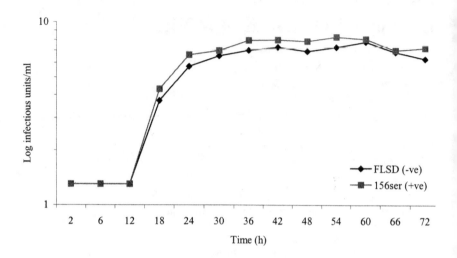

FIGURE 1. Growth kinetics of viral replication in FLSD-infected cultures. Vero cultures were inoculated with 156ser (glycosylated) and FLSD (nonglycosylated) viruses at a multiplicity of infection of 0.1. Culture fluids were collected at regular intervals between 2 and 72 h postinfection and analyzed for infectious viral titer by TCID$_{50}$ assay.

Growth kinetics were performed in Vero and C6/36 cell lines to assess the effect of glycosylation of the E protein on viral replication. Likewise, to determine the effect of the mutation in the E protein on the neuroinvasiveness of 156ser, weanling mice were inoculated intraperitoneally with 10-fold dilutions of low passage stocks of FLSD and 156ser viruses.

RESULTS

Growth kinetics of the glycosylated clone versus its nonglycosylated parent revealed the former to grow more successfully and produce 10- to 100-fold more virus in Vero cells (FIG. 1). Similar results were observed in C6/36 cells. This indicates that glycosylation of the E protein of KUN virus provides some advantage for virus growth *in vitro* and is positively selected during cell culture. Indeed, when nonglycosylated field isolates of KUN virus were serially passaged through Vero cell passage, the viruses generally (with one exception) gained glycosylation by passage 3-4 and in most cases remained glycosylated during subsequent passages (TABLE 1). This effect was less consistent for viruses grown in C6/36 cells. Although glycosylated virus was more effective in producing a productive infection in mice after intraperitoneal inoculation, as determined by a detectable antibody response, there was no clear correlation between neuroinvasiveness and glycosylation status.

TABLE 1. Glycosylation status of KUN and WN isolates following passage through Vero cells

Virus	P0	P1	P2	P3	P4	P5	P6	P7	P8	P9	P10
FLSD	−	−	±	±	±	±	±	±	±	±	±
156ser	+	+	+	+	+	+	+	+	+	+	+
OR4	+	+	+	+	+	+	+	+	+	+	+
35911	−	−	±	+	+	+	+	+	+	+	+
CX255	+	+	+	+	+	+	+	+	+	+	+
MRM16	−	±	+	+	+	+	+	+	+	+	+
Hu6774	+	±	+	±	+	+					
OR205	−	−	−	±	±	±					
MRM61C^a	−	−	±	±	±	±					
WN Sarafend	+										
MP502-66^b	−	−	−	−	−						

± Mixed population of glycosylated and nonglycosylated progeny.
^{a}FLSD parental strain.
^{b}KUN isolate from Malaysia.

CONCLUSIONS

Kunjin 156ser virus displayed more efficient replication in peripheral tissues, indicated by higher seroconversion rates and growth kinetics in Vero and C6/36 cells, than the nonglycosylated counterpart, FLSD virus. Therefore, at higher intraperitoneal doses, 156ser virus may induce a more rapid and intense immune response to clear the virus before neuroinvasion can take place. At lower doses of 156ser virus, there may be time during initial replication for a nonglycosylated revertant to occur. This would result in a neuroinvasive variant within the population, which is polymorphic at position 156, allowing invasion of the central nervous system before the immune system can eliminate virus from the host.

REFERENCES

1. HEINZ, F.X. *et al.* 2000. Family Flaviviridae. *In* Virus Taxonomy: Classification and Nomenclature of Viruses. M.H.V. Regenmortel *et al.*, Eds.: 859–878. Academic Press. San Diego, CA.
2. RUSSELL, R.C. 1995. Arboviruses and their vectors in Australia: an update on the ecology and epidemiology of some mosquito-borne arboviruses. Rev. Med. Vet. Ent. **83:** 141–158.
3. ADAMS, S.C. *et al.* 1995. Glycosylation and antigenic variation among Kunjin virus isolates. Virology **206:** 49–56.
4. WENGLER, G. *et al.* 1985. Sequence analysis of the membrane protein V3 of the flavivirus West Nile virus and of its gene. Virology **147:** 264–274.
5. KHROMYKH, A.A. & E.G. WESTAWAY. 1994. Completion of Kunjin virus RNA sequence and recovery of an infectious RNA transcribed from stably cloned full-length cDNA. J. Virol. **68:** 4580–4588.

Analysis of Mosquito Vector Species Abundances in Maryland using Geographic Information Systems

SCOTT M. SHONE,[a] PATRICIA N. FERRAO,[b] CYRUS R. LESSER,[b]
DOUGLAS E. NORRIS,[a] AND GREGORY E. GLASS[a]

[a]The W. Harry Feinstone Department of Molecular Microbiology and Immunology,
The Johns Hopkins Bloomberg School of Public Health,
Baltimore, Maryland 21205, USA

[b]Mosquito Control Section, Maryland Department of Agriculture,
Annapolis, Maryland 21401, USA

KEYWORDS: West Nile virus; mosquitoes; geographic information system
(GIS); *Culex*; *Ochlerotatus*; *Aedes*; *Culiseta*; *Psorophora*; *Anopheles*

INTRODUCTION

Following the outbreak of West Nile virus (WNV) in 1999, *Culex pipiens* was considered to be the primary vector of the disease in the United States.[1] Field collections from the 2000 WNV surveillance campaign indicate that the virus infects at least 14 species in six genera of mosquitoes, including *Culex*, *Ochlerotatus*, *Aedes*, *Culiseta*, *Psorophora*, and *Anopheles*.[2] The goal of the present study was to use a geographic information system (GIS) to graph or map indices of both weekly and seasonal abundances for each vector species using the 2000 WNV surveillance data from Maryland so that we could locate areas where certain species were prevalent.

METHODS

Collection

Mosquitoes were collected weekly from May 19 through October 31, 2000 at 184 sites throughout 11 counties in Maryland using unbaited or dry ice–baited CDC light traps (John W. Hock, Co., Gainesville, FL). For each trap site, either an address or GPS coordinates were obtained. Mosquitoes were killed on dry ice and sorted by sex and species using a series of dichotomous keys.[3–5] Only female *Ae. albopictus*, *Ae. vexans*, *An. punctipennis*, *Cs. melanura*, *Cx. pipiens*, *Cx. restuans*, *Cx. salinarius*,

Address for correspondence: Scott M. Shone, The W. Harry Feinstone Department of Molecular Microbiology and Immunology, The Johns Hopkins Bloomberg School of Public Health, 615 N. Wolfe St., Baltimore, MD 21205. Voice: 410-955-8898; fax: 410-955-0105.
sshone@jhsph.edu

A

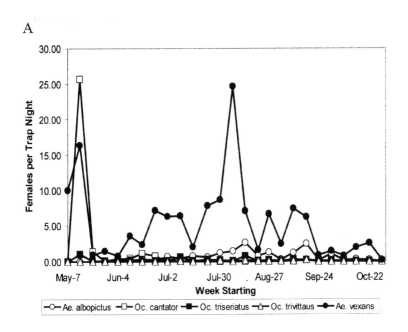

B

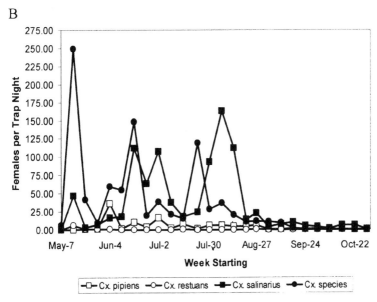

FIGURE 1. Abundance of *Aedes* and *Ochlerotatus* (**A**) and *Culex* (**B**) mosquitoes in females per trap night plotted as a function of weeks during 2000.

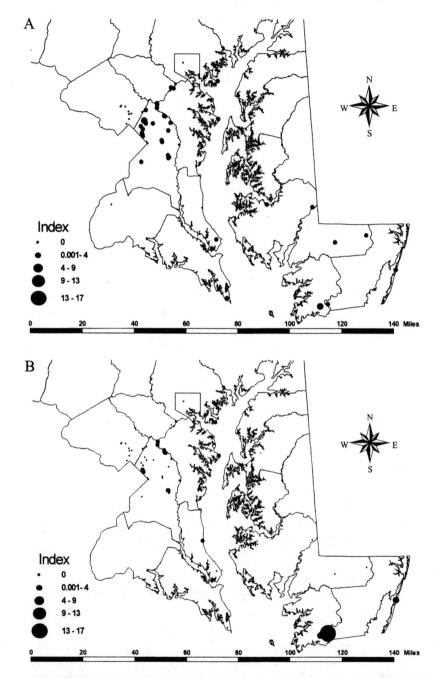

FIGURE 2. Maps of seasonal abundance index for *Ae. vexans* (**A**) and *Cx. salinarius* (**B**). *Ae. vexans* had a uniform spatial distribution over all trap sites in Maryland, whereas *Cx. salinarius* is an example of a species that exhibited geographical clustering.

Cx. species, Oc. cantator, Oc. japonicus, Oc. triseriatus, Oc. trivittatus, and *Ps. ferox* were analyzed because these were the species that tested positive for WNV in 2000.[2] *Oc. japonicus* was not caught in any of our surveillance traps and was not included in the analyses. *Cx. species* includes all *Culex* mosquitoes for which a specific identity could not be determined because of loss of differential characteristics.

Calculations

Weekly abundances of each species were determined using the following equation: (Total # female species s caught in week w)/(# trap nights in week w). Seasonal abundance indices at each trap site for each species were determined using the following equation: [(Total # female species s caught at site t for the season)/(Total # female species s caught at all sites for the season)]/(# trap nights for site t).

Graphs and GIS

The weekly abundance of each species was graphed as a function of week. Using the GIS software package ArcView GIS® (ESRI, Redlands, CA) and the GPS coordinates or geocoded addresses for each trap site, the seasonal abundance indices were plotted on a map of Maryland.

RESULTS

The weekly abundance graphs revealed that *Ae. albopictus, Oc. triseriatus, Oc. trivittatus* (FIG. 1A), *Cx. pipiens,* and *Cx. restuans* (FIG. 1B) were found at low abundance throughout the season. Although *Oc. cantator* was abundant in May, it was found at low levels during the rest of the season (FIG. 1A). *Ae. vexans* abundance peaked in mid-May (16.3 females/trap night) and at the end of June (24.6 females/ trap night), and was moderately abundant for the rest of season (FIG. 1A). In contrast, for *Cx. salinarius, Cx. species* (FIG. 1B), *An. punctipennis, Cs. melanura,* and *Ps. ferox* (data not shown) abundance peaked several times throughout the season. In addition to variable temporal abundances, all of the species were geographically clustered (FIG. 2B) throughout the state, except for *Ae. vexans* (FIG. 2A), which was uniformly distributed over all of the trap sites.

DISCUSSION

Both temporal and spatial abundances for several mosquito species potentially important in the transmission of WNV were identified using GIS. This analysis is the first step in determining environmental and climatic factors important in the distribution of vectors and the transmission of WNV. Once these factors are elucidated, we will be able to model and predict vector abundances and target surveillance and control resources to areas where disease transmission is most likely to occur.

ACKNOWLEDGMENTS

We thank the employees of the Mosquito Control Section at the Maryland Department of Agriculture for collecting and supplying the 2000 WNV surveillance data from Maryland. We also acknowledge NIH training grant AI07417-01 for providing support for S.M.S.

REFERENCES

1. CENTERS FOR DISEASE CONTROL. 1999. Update: West Nile virus encephalitis—New York, 1999. Morb. Mortal. Wkly. Rep. **48:** 944–9456.
2. CENTERS FOR DISEASE CONTROL. 2000. Update: West Nile Virus Activity—Eastern United States, 2000. Morb. Mortal. Wkly. Rep. **49:** 1044–1047.
3. CARPENTER, S. J. & W. J. LA CASSE. 1955. Mosquitoes of North America (North of Mexico). University of California Press. Berkeley, CA.
4. DARSIE, R. F., JR. & R. A. WARD. 1981. Identification and geographical distribution of mosquitoes of North America, North of Mexico. Mosq. Syst. (Suppl. 1): 1–313.
5. SLAFF, M. & C. S. APPERSON. 1989. A Key to the Mosquitoes of North Carolina and the Mid-Atlantic States. The North Carolina Agricultural Extension Service. Raleigh, NC.

Long-term Stability of West Nile Virus IgM and IgG Antibodies in Diluted Sera Stored at 4°C

SUSAN J. WONG[a] AND STEPHEN J. SELIGMAN[b]

[a]*Diagnostic Immunology Laboratory, Wadsworth Center,*
New York State Department of Health, Albany, New York 12201, USA

[b]*Department of Microbiology and Immunology,*
New York Medical College, Valhalla, New York 10595, USA

KEYWORDS: West Nile virus; diluted sera

Investigation of the outbreak of West Nile virus (WNV) infections in New York 1999 has been aided by the use of an IgM capture assay[1] (WN MAC ELISA) and by an IgG ELISA[2] (WN IgG ELISA). These assays have the advantage that the test may be readily modified by the substitution of different antigens and group-specific MAbs to provide a battery of tests for arboviral antibodies. However, recommendations for the assays state that "diluted antibody was stable for only 7 to 10 days" and should be discarded thereafter[1] and that "serum could be diluted appropriately and stored for up to one week at 4°C."[2]

During the course of studies on antibody in relation to WNV, patients' sera from the WNV outbreak, New York 1999 were stored at 4°C in 1:80 or 1:400 dilutions in blocking buffer containing phosphate-buffered saline, 0.2% azide, 0.05% Tween 20, and 2% bovine serum albumin. The sera were retested after six months.

METHODS

The methods were the same as those previously described except that the diluted sera were stored in the above-blocking buffer containing 2% BSA. For the WN IgM capture ELISA,[1] the ELISA plates were coated with goat anti-human IgM, blocked, and then exposed sequentially to test or control sera, WNV antigen (initially infected rat brain and in subsequent tests recombinant E-glycoprotein), and finally MAb 6B6C-1 labeled with horseradish peroxidase. For the WN IgG ELISA,[2] the ELISA plates were coated with MAb DEN2 4G2, blocked, and then exposed sequentially to WNV antigen, test or control sera, and goat anti-human IgG labeled with alkaline

Address for correspondence: Stephen J. Seligman, M.D., Department of Microbiology and Immunology, Room 301, New York Medical College, Valhalla, NY 10595. Voice: 914-594-3130; fax: 914-594-3775.

stephen_seligman@nymc.edu

TABLE 1. Effect of sera storage conditions on IgM West Nile MAC ELISA (P/N)

Specimen No.	Coating Antigen		
	West Nile virus–infected suckling mouse brain[a]	Recombinant West Nile E glycoprotein[b]	Recombinant West Nile E glycoprotein[c]
1	11.2	19.7	qns
2	5.3	18.6	17.9
3	11.6	18.6	19.1
4	12.1	19.3	17.0
5	15.7	17.1	16.9
6	19.6	17.3	15.9
7	15.4	15.3	15.0
8	16.0	16.5	14.5
9	7.8	15.9	13.7
10	12.4	16.4	17.1
11	6.3	19.3	19.9
12	30.2	18.7	18.1
13	16.4	19.4	18.4
14	11.4	14.1	16.2
15	16.9	17.3	15.5
16	33.3	16.9	18.6
17	17.9	13.5	13.8
18	30.1	13.9	13.7
19	6.3	4.9	5.4
20	8.8	17.7	17.5
21	40.0	23.0	23.0

[a]Freshly collected sera, frozen, thawed, and promptly tested.
[b]Sera stored diluted for six months at 4°C.
[c]Sera kept frozen for six months at −70°C.

phosphatase. P/N ratios were calculated as the ratio of optical density in the test serum to the optical density in a known negative serum.

RESULTS AND CONCLUSION

Sera were available from 21 patients in the WNV, New York 1999 outbreak. The P/N ratios for IgM antibodies were similar whether sera were tested at the time of the outbreak, retested after having been stored diluted at 4°C for six months, or retested after having been frozen undiluted at −70°C (TABLE 1) ($P > 0.05$ by ANOVA for three correlated samples). IgG antibodies were only determined after the sera had been stored for six months. At that time, identical interpretations were obtained for

TABLE 2. Effect of sera storage conditions on IgG West Nile ELISA (P/N)

Specimen No.	Coating antigen	
	Recombinant West Nile E glycoprotein	
	Sera stored at 4°C[a]	Sera fragment at −70°C[b]
1	<2	qns
2	9.5	13.1
3	11.1	12.2
4	9.8	11.3
5	10.1	11.2
6	7.9	9.1
7	9.6	11.3
8	3.4	4.2
9	15.4	16.7
10	8.9	9.0
11	5.3	6.6
12	9.3	10.4
13	11.0	12.1
14	5.1	6.4
15	<2	<2
16	2.6	2.5
17	9.1	10.4
18	2.9	2.9
19	11.8	12.6
20	14.4	15.9
21	4.5	4.6

[a]Sera stored diluted for six months at 4°C.
[b]Sera kept frozen for six months at −70°C.

WNV IgG antibodies both with sera stored diluted at 4°C or frozen at −70°C and diluted just prior to testing (TABLE 2). However, P/N ratios ($\times$ avg = 8.5) for the sera stored diluted were slightly lower than the P/N ratios ($\times$ avg = 9.6) for the sera stored frozen ($P<0.001$ by Student's t test for correlated samples) and could indicate an 11% decrease in WNV IgG over the course of six months.

The reasons for the discrepancy in antibody stability found in the present study and that reported by Martin *et al.* have not been determined conclusively. Beaty *et al.* recommend including fetal bovine serum in the antibody diluent.[3] However, Martin *et al.* used phosphate-buffered saline with 0.5% Tween without fetal bovine serum. It is possible that protein in the form of albumin, as in our data, or serum as in the recommendation of Beaty *et al.*, is helpful in antibody preservation during storage at 4°C.

Antibody stability at refrigerator temperatures may be especially relevant when sera are collected in situations in which storage in a deep freeze is not possible, for the acceptance of sera by diagnostic laboratories, and for sharing of specimens for assay development and proficiency testing.

In conclusion, human WNV IgM antibodies were stable, and IgG antibodies declined only slightly for a period of at least six months when stored diluted in phosphate-buffered saline, 0.2% azide, 0.05% Tween 20, and 2% bovine serum albumin at 4°C.

ACKNOWLEDGMENTS

We thank Carol Franchell, Valerie Demarest, Karen Kulas, Lance Kingsley and Reginald Taylor for technical assistance.

REFERENCES

1. MARTIN, D.A., D.A. MUTH, T. BROWN, et al. 2000. Standardization of immunoglobulin M capture enzyme-linked immunosorbent assays for routine diagnosis of arboviral infections. J. Clin. Microbiol. 38: 1823–1826.
2. JOHNSON, A.J., D.A. MARTIN, N. KARABATSOS & J.T. ROEHRIG. 2000. Detection of anti-arboviral immunoglobulin G by using a monoclonal antibody-based capture enzyme-linked immunosorbent assay. J. Clin. Microbiol. 38: 1827–1831.
3. BEATY, B.J., C.H. CALISHER & R.E. SHOPE. 1995. Arboviruses. In Diagnostic Procedures for Viral, Rickettsial and Chlamydial infections. E.H. Lennette, D.A. Lennette & E.T. Lennette, Eds.: 189–212. 7th edit. American Public Health Association. Washington, D.C.

Index of Contributors

(Italic page numbers refer to comments made in discussion.)